www.harcourt-international.com

Bringing you products from all Harcourt Health Sciences companies including Baillière Tindall, Churchill Livingstone, Mosby and W.B. Saunders

W9-AUI-343

▶ **Browse** for latest information on new books, journals and electronic products

▶ **Search** for information on over 20 000 published titles with full product information including tables of contents and sample chapters

▶ **Keep up to date** with our extensive publishing programme in your field by registering with eAlert or requesting postal updates

▶ **Secure online ordering** with prompt delivery, as well as full contact details to order by phone, fax or post

▶ **News** of special features and promotions

If you are based in the following countries, please visit the country-specific site to receive full details of product availability and local ordering information

USA: www.harcourthealth.com

Canada: www.harcourtcanada.com

Australia: www.harcourt.com.au

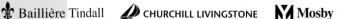 Baillière Tindall   CHURCHILL LIVINGSTONE   Mosby   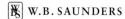 W.B. SAUNDERS

The Desktop Guide to Complementary and Alternative Medicine

For Churchill Livingstone:

Publishing Manager, Health Professions: Inta Ozols
Project Development Manager: Mairi McCubbin
Project Manager: Derek Robertson
Designer: George Ajayi

The Desktop Guide to Complementary and Alternative Medicine

an evidence-based approach

Editor

Edzard Ernst MD PhD FRCP(Edin)

Professor of Complementary Medicine; Director, Department of Complementary Medicine,
School of Postgraduate Medicine and Health Sciences, University of Exeter, Exeter, UK

Associate Editors

Max H. Pittler MD

Research Fellow, Department of Complementary Medicine, University of Exeter, Exeter, UK

Clare Stevinson MSc

Research Fellow, Department of Complementary Medicine, University of Exeter, Exeter, UK

Adrian White MA BM BCh

Senior Lecturer, Department of Complementary Medicine, University of Exeter, Exeter, UK

Contributing Editor

David Eisenberg MD

Director, Division for Research and Education in Complementary and Integrative Medical Therapies,
Harvard Medical School; Associate Professor of Medicine, Harvard Medical School, Beth Israel Deaconess
Medical Center, Boston, Massachusetts, USA

Foreword by

Brian M. Berman MD

Professor of Family Medicine, Director, Complementary Medicine Program,
University of Maryland School of Medicine, Baltimore, Maryland, USA

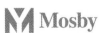 Mosby

EDINBURGH   LONDON   NEW YORK   PHILADELPHIA   ST LOUIS   SYDNEY   TORONTO 2001

MOSBY
An imprint of Harcourt Publishers Limited

© Harcourt Publishers Limited 2001

M is a registered trademark of Harcourt Publishers Limited

The right of Edzard Ernst to be identified as editor of this work has been asserted by him in accordance with the Copyright, Designs and Patents Act 1988.

First published 2001

ISBN 0 7234 3207 4

British Library Cataloguing in Publication Data
A catalogue record for this book is available from the British Library

Library of Congress Cataloging in Publication Data
A catalog record for this book is available from the Library of Congress

Note
The Publisher, the Editors, and the Contributors do not assume any responsibility for any injury and/or damage to persons or property arising out of or related to any use of the material contained in this work. The reader is advised to check the appropriate literature and the product information currently provided by the manufacturer of each therapeutic substance to verify dosages, the method and duration of administration, and contraindications. It is the responsibility of the treating physician, relying on independent experience and knowledge of the patient to determine dosages and the best treatment for the patient.

The
Publisher's
policy is to use
**paper manufactured
from sustainable forests**

Printed in China

II

Contents

Contributors

Michael H Cohen JD MBA MFA
Director of Legal Programs, Center for Alternative Medicine,
Research and Education, Beth Israel Deaconess Medical Center,
Harvard Medical School, USA

Heather Boon BSc Phm PhD
Assistant Professor, Department of Health Administration,
University of Toronto, Toronto, Canada

Marja Verhoef PhD
Associate Professor, Department of Community Health Sciences,
University of Calgary, Canada

Foreword

It is a rare physician these days who has not had a patient ask about an unconventional treatment for their medical condition. In fact, many physicians are themselves wondering if there might be some value to an alternative treatment, particularly when grappling with treating a chronically ill patient who is not responding well to conventional care. The surge of interest in complementary and alternative medicine is well documented in many Western countries but, despite the fact that many of these therapies have been around for hundreds if not thousands of years and are the primary source of health care for over 70% of the world's population, we have had very little access to good information about whether they work or are safe. Physician and consumer are caught in the same bind. With an abundance of claims being made about the curative powers of any number of complementary therapies and a similar number of disclaimers being made about 'quackery', how is either to know where the truth lies?

The authors of this book have been a formidable force in turning these tables and bringing the light of scientific understanding to complementary medicine. Since taking on the first chair position to be created in complementary medicine, Professor Edzard Ernst, more than any other single person, has tackled the impressive task of systematically reviewing the world's research literature on complementary medicine. Dr David Eisenberg, with the publication of his surveys on complementary medicine use in the USA, has helped to identify what therapies people are using and for what problems.

In this book they draw together this information to give us an understanding of the main complementary therapies – their origins, underlying concepts, scientific rationale and method of clinical practice – as well as looking at the main conditions for which the therapies are used. Most important of all, they give us access to the most up-to-date, evidence-based information on safety and effectiveness.

Throughout health care there has been an increasing emphasis on the practice of evidence-based medicine. The premise of the movement is that clinical practice should integrate the expertise of the practitioner with the wishes of the patient and the best available evidence. The evidence-based movement saw a similar growth to that of complementary medicine over the last couple of decades of the old millennium. However, a common criticism of complementary medicine is that it cannot be part of evidence-based medicine because little or no research exists in the field. I would dispute this as an outright claim and am indebted to the authors of this book for their exhaustive work in bringing together and evaluating the evidence that does exist. Although sparse in many areas and often of poor quality, a body of scientific research does exist in complementary medicine that merits examination. As responsible and, above all, caring practitioners, it behooves us to familiarize ourselves with this information so we better comprehend the potential role complementary therapies may play in helping our patients to heal and to maintain health. Complementary medicine is a strong consumer-driven movement. Patients are telling us that this is something that they want. Armed with an understanding of what the therapies are, how they are practiced, and the current best evidence, patients can better define their own wishes and practitioners can better use their own expertise, allowing both to work together and make informed clinical decisions.

Brian M Berman
Baltimore, 2001

Preface

An epitaph to opinion-based medicine

The use of complementary and alternative medicine (CAM) by the general public is increasing and CAM is becoming more relevant to mainstream health-care professionals so the option of CAM will increasingly need to be considered when making clinical decisions. Although much advice on CAM has in the past been based on opinion, both patients and their advisers recognize the need for information based on evidence.

The whole thrust of this book is to help establish an evidence base for CAM. Evidence for the most important parts of our book means data from controlled (preferably randomized) clinical trials or preferably systematic reviews of such studies. But what about expert opinion? Surely years of experience reflected in such opinions must be of considerable value? In a way, this statement amounts to a testable hypothesis – so we decided to test it.

We selected seven recent, general CAM books from our shelves [1-7] which contained chapters devoted to specific medical conditions. From these books, we extracted the CAM treatments which were recommended for specific medical conditions. For the purpose of this exercise a "recommendation" was defined as a mention in a positive context. CAM treatments were recommended for about 300 different conditions. Thus we derived lists of "opinion-based" recommendations for CAM treatments according to each condition. Where possible, we then compared this collective opinion with the evidence from our systematic reviews as summarized in the condition chapters of this book.

The results are both fascinating and disappointing; most of all, they are somewhat worrying. The first striking finding was that an extremely broad range of CAM treatments was recommended for many conditions (Table 1). The second, perhaps more surprising result was the lack of agreement between the authors of the seven books. Most treatments were recommended for a given condition only by one or two, rarely by more than four and never by all authors.

Obviously opinion and evidence can differ without either being wrong. One therapy could, for instance, be recommended without the back-up of trial evidence simply because trials are not yet available. However, we found several instances where a

Table 1
Some conditions for which numerous (>50) CAM treatments were recommended

Condition	Number of treatments recommended
Acne	61
Addictions	120
AIDS/HIV	69
Allergies	57
Anxiety	54
Arthritis	131
Asthma	119
Back pain	65
Cancer	133
Coronary heart disease	71
Chronic fatigue syndrome	64
Common cold	96
Cystitis	57
Depression	87
Dermatitis	57
Diabetes mellitus	89
Eczema	55
Emphysema	54
Fungal infection	75
Hay fever	65
Headache	78
Hemorrhoids	54
Herpes	69
Hypertension	95
Infections	55
Insomnia	74
Irritable bowel syndrome	69
Menopausal problems	68
Pneumonia: bacterial, mycoplasmal and viral	52
Premenstrual syndrome	59
Prostate disorders	63
Psoriasis	57
Sciatica	55
Sinusitis	64
Varicose veins	56

given therapy was being recommended while conclusive trial evidence (i.e. more than one reliable RCT or a systematic review of RCTs) showed that it was not effective for that particular condition. Examples are:

- chelation therapy for cardiovascular disease
- chiropractic for asthma
- guar gum for body weight reduction.

And there were other most remarkable differences between opinion and evidence. For instance, treatments which were supported by compelling evidence from metaanalyses and systematic reviews were not consistently included by all the authors in their recommendation. Examples are:

- acupuncture for nausea
- biofeedback for constipation
- kava for anxiety
- relaxation for anxiety
- saw palmetto for benign prostatic hyperplasia.

One could argue that the books were written before this evidence became available. We checked this notion and found that it did not apply in the above instances.

Truly worrying discrepancies were noted in relation to recommendations for treating a certain condition with a given therapy where the evidence suggests that this therapy should be contraindicated in this particular situation. Examples are:

- chiropractic for osteoporosis
- ginger for morning sickness.

We find such contradictions deeply disturbing. They may exist in other areas of medicine as well but certainly not in such abundance as found here. We believe that they are a reflection of the relative youth (some might say immaturity) of CAM research and of the fact that an evidence-based approach is still a novel concept in CAM. The discrepancies, inconsistencies and contradictions certainly show that opinions, even when originating from CAM 'experts', are not reliable or valid.

We feel that this point is of considerable importance as it touches the core concept of this book. Opinions in various guises seem to dominate today's CAM. Because they are unreliable, they also have the potential of misleading health-care professionals and (more importantly) harming patients. The issue here is not to point an accusing finger at any one book or any one author (in fact, not all the examples used above apply to all the books cited). The issue is rather that CAM (and its literature) is presently far from being evidence-based and ought to become evidence-based sooner rather than later. The best way forward, as far as we can see, lies in objectively and reproducibly establishing and updating the evidence – and this is precisely what our book aims to achieve.

Our main aim was to provide state-of-the-art information and evidence on CAM as a practical reference resource, in a way that is accessible to busy physicians and other health-care professionals. Despite persistent suggestions that the RCT is not an appropriate or feasible method for testing CAM, we have found large numbers of RCTs that cover almost every form of therapy, demonstrating that CAM can be tested in a rigorous manner. As in all branches of medicine, inevitably some evidence is negative. But the overriding conclusions are that some forms of CAM are frequently supported by evidence and therefore do have a role in modern health care.

Edzard Ernst, Max H Pittler,
Clare Stevinson and Adrian White
Exeter, 2001

REFERENCES

1 Pelletier K R. The best alternative medicine. New York: Simon Schuster, 2000

2 Spencer J W, Jacobs J J. (eds) Complementary/alternative medicine. An evidence-based approach. St Louis: Mosby, 1999

3 Springhouse. Nurse's handbook of alternative and complementary medicine. Springhouse, PA: Springhouse, 1998

4 The Burton Goldberg Group. Alternative medicine: the definitive guide. Payallup, WA: Future Medicine, 1994

5 Jamil T. Complementary medicine: a practical guide. Oxford: Butterworth Heinemann, 1997

6 Time-Life. The medical advisor. Alexandria, VA: Time-Life Books, 1997

7 Pizzorno J E, Murray M T (eds). Textbook of natural medicine. Edinburgh: Churchill Livingstone, 1999

Acknowledgements

We wish to thank the following individuals for revising parts of this book:

H Boon (Toronto, Canada)
D Eisenberg (Boston, USA)
A Huntley (Exeter, UK)
L Long (Exeter, UK)
R März (Neumarkt, Germany)
V Schulz (Berlin, Germany)
W Weiger (Boston, USA).

We are also indebted to B Wider for translations as well as R Clark and N Watson for secretarial work.

All unauthored chapters were jointly written by E Ernst, M H Pittler, C Stevinson and A R White, all from the Department of Complementary Medicine, School of Postgraduate Medicine and Health Sciences, University of Exeter, UK.

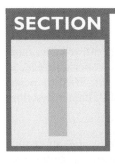

SECTION

1

Using the book

METHODS

The intention of this book is to provide relevant, reliable, thorough and up-to-date information in a clear, concise format. In order to achieve this, a systematic approach was used to locate, select, appraise and present information. This chapter describes the procedures followed.

Definition of complementary and alternative medicine

For the purposes of this book complementary and alternative medicine (CAM) was defined as 'diagnosis, treatment and/or prevention which complements mainstream medicine by contributing to a common whole, satisfying a demand not met by orthodoxy, or diversifying the conceptual framework of medicine'.[1] What constitutes CAM may vary according to national differences and individual viewpoints. The list below indicates many of the treatments that were considered mainstream rather than CAM and were therefore not generally covered in this book. However, some of these treatments are mentioned in Section 5 (Conditions) for particular non-mainstream indications.

- Balneotherapy
- Behavioral therapy
- Cognitive therapy
- Counseling
- Diets and nutritional advice
- Electromagnetic therapy
- Electrotherapy
- Exercise
- Hydrotherapy
- Lifestyle approaches
- Low-dose laser therapy
- Spa therapy
- Specific herbs, e.g. senna (*Cassia* spp), castor oil (*Ricinus communis*), Cayenne pepper (*Capsicum frutescens*)
- Thalassotherapy
- Transcranial magnetic stimulation
- Transcutaneous electrical nerve stimulation (TENS)
- Ultrasound
- Vitamins and minerals

Selection of topics

Sections 2, 3 and 4 cover CAM diagnostic methods and treatments (therapies and medicines) that are popular with patients. Treatments for which evidence relating to effectiveness is available are the subject of individual chapters. Other treatments are covered in tables.

The conditions covered by Section 5 are those which are commonly seen in primary care, frequently treated with CAM and for which the most evidence relating to effectiveness is available. Provisional lists of potential topics for chapters and tables were produced during discussion and amended after inspecting the results of literature searches (see *Literature searches* below) and internal review (see *Review process* below).

Sources and referencing

A number of sources were used to compile information for this book. These included reference books, the department's own files, contact with other experts, a survey of CAM organizations (see *Survey* below) and systematic literature searches (see *Literature searches* below). Rather than provide the reference for each individual piece of information presented, it was decided to keep referencing to a minimum. Since a considerable amount of information is compressed into each chapter, comprehensive referencing would involve lengthy reference lists and much repetition. This would be tedious and distracting for the reader, who needs quick access to clear information. For example, information on risks presented in Sections 3 and 4 is largely based on a vast number of case reports and individual referencing would have been more of a hindrance than a help to the reader. Therefore a bibliography of the main reference sources for the book is provided at the end of this section, which indicates the principal sources of the information. The exception to this is information relating to *Clinical evidence* which provides the major focus of this book. In Sections 2, 3 and 4, key references are provided for the evidence cited. In Section 5 reference details for studies mentioned are provided either directly in boxes or tables or in the reference list at the end of each chapter to allow the interested reader to trace the source.

Survey of CAM professional bodies

In order to obtain up-to-date information about the forms of CAM covered in this book, a survey of professional bodies of CAM was conducted.[2] A list of addresses of 526 CAM organizations was compiled, comprising all 364 addresses of UK CAM organizations (generated by a systematic survey sponsored by the UK Department of Health[3]) and an additional 162 addresses of organizations outside the UK, who have had previous direct contact with our department. Those professional bodies that were dedicated to individual forms of CAM (223 in total) were sent questionnaires asking about indications and contraindications of therapies and training requirements of practitioners. Although the response rate was low (36%), the information obtained was used to supplement material from other sources.

Literature searches for clinical evidence

Systematic searches were carried out in the databases Medline, Embase, Amed and the Cochrane Database of Systematic Reviews. Each database was searched from its respective inception until March 2000. The search strategy used to locate relevant literature was developed and refined at the department (see *Appendix*, p 424). In addition, the department's own files, the bibliographies of relevant papers and the contents pages of all issues of the journals *FACT* (*Focus on Alternative and Complementary Therapies*; London: Pharmaceutical Press) and *Complementary Therapies in Medicine* (Edinburgh: Churchill Livingstone) were searched for further studies. There were no language restrictions imposed. Studies in languages other than English were translated in-house.

Selection of clinical evidence

Each author selected relevant studies on a particular topic by scrutinizing the abstracts. Systematic reviews and metaanalyses of clinical trials were given priority and copies of originals obtained. Where systematic reviews or metaanalyses were not located, the evidence from RCTs and CCTs was considered next. In their absence uncontrolled studies were considered. In most cases, original reports were obtained.

Appraisal of clinical evidence

Formal assessment of methodological quality of the evidence was not performed. However, all authors are familiar with the process of systematic review and consistently evaluated the methodological quality of the studies by assessing important criteria such as randomization, blinding and description of withdrawals and dropouts in an informal review process. For systematic reviews and metaanalyses, the assessment of the methodological quality of included trials by the original authors was accepted. The quality of the review itself was assessed, again informally, and any limitations were noted in the accompanying text. In the *Summary of clinical evidence* tables (Section 5), the methodological quality of the body of evidence of a particular treatment for a particular condition was combined with the level of the evidence and the volume of the evidence to produce a measure of weight. This is intended to indicate the degree of confidence that can be placed on the evidence. Details are given in *How to use this book* (see p 15).

Application of judgement

Clinical judgement was used by the authors in two specific areas: the *Risk–benefit assessment* of each treatment (Sections 3 and 4) and the *Overall recommendation* (Section 5). These judgements are based on personal clinical experience and current medical practice as well as the evidence. In an attempt to minimize bias and achieve standardization, the process was subjected to internal and external review (see *Review process* below). It should be noted that stating that there is a lack of compelling evidence for a treatment does not imply that the treatment is ineffective.

Presentation of information

In most parts of each chapter, the information is presented in a concise narrative form in a predefined format (see *How to use this book*, p 8). However, for *Clinical evidence* in Section 5, tables and boxes are also used for displaying key evidence. The most authoritative systematic review or metaanalysis on a subject has been abstracted into a box. Selected clinical trials are presented in standardized tables; usually these are the most scientifically rigorous or clinically relevant. Data have been extracted into tables according to the predefined criteria of sample size, intervention and main results. The final column provides further relevant information or a critical comment. At the end of Sections 3 and 4, tables are presented containing brief information on other treatments that were not included as full chapters. It is intended that some of these will be presented as full chapters in the next edition of this book. It is also intended to expand the range of condition chapters in Section 5.

Information on safety

Information on safety is central to the assessment of a treatment's value. Hence this material is an important component of the book. Unfortunately, there is often fragmentary knowledge on safety in CAM, making a systematic approach difficult. The treatment chapters (Sections 3 and 4) address risks as fully as is possible from available data. In general, the precautionary principle has been applied, so a treatment is not considered risk free unless evidence suggests otherwise. For herbs, this approach is in contrast with that of the US Food and Drug Administration (and for most herbs, the UK's Medicines Control Agency), which classify herbs as food supplements and therefore essentially safe unless proven otherwise. Pregnancy and lactation are cited as contraindications for all medicines included in this book. Allergic reactions have been mentioned where they have been reported but should be assumed possible for all herbs and many supplements, with the potential to be serious.

For the *Summary of clinical evidence* tables in Section 5, many different ways of summarizing safety data were considered, but it proved impossible to provide sufficient useful detail. It was therefore decided to use a simple Yes/No descriptor to alert the reader in a general way to the existence (however rare) of potentially serious safety concerns, cross-referencing to the sections providing specific details (see *How to use this book*, p 16). Even when a treatment is apparently innocuous, the table entry is 'Yes' if there is insufficient information available to establish safety and serious risks are considered possible. This applies to all herbs and some supplements. Other supplements are marked 'Yes' because overdose is associated with serious consequences. Most products derived from natural sources carry the risk of allergic reactions (see above). In the case of homeopathic remedies, this is unlikely at non-material dilutions, hence homeopathy is marked 'No'. Aromatherapy, on the other hand, is marked 'Yes', due to the allergic reactions possible with essential oils. Therapies marked 'Yes' that cannot be cross-referenced to a specific chapter or table are hydrotherapy (for which cardio-respiratory decompensation and bacterial infections have been reported), exercise (where sudden death has been recorded), electrotherapy (for which psychological disturbance and local injury from electrodes are possible) and fasting and particular diets (where malnutrition can occur). The intention of the book is not to be alarmist, but clearly the priority must be to avoid all possible risks for the patient.

Review process

All information presented in this book was subjected to an internal review by all four authors. Chapters were revised accordingly and additional information was incorporated. Regular consensus conferences were held to ensure a standardized approach. This was performed particularly with a view to minimizing bias in areas where a degree of personal judgement was introduced (see *Application of judgement* above). Any disputes that appeared during the consensus conferences were resolved through discussion.

International experts on CAM were involved in an external review process, in particular the US editor. Information on herbs has been reviewed by three independent experts from Germany and Canada. Specific chapters were reviewed by individuals with relevant expertise (see *Acknowledgements*, p xv).

The ultimate review, however, will be through you, the reader. We welcome constructive criticism on all aspects of this publication and invite readers to contact us via the publisher.

REFERENCES

1 Ernst E, Resch K L, Mills S et al. Complementary medicine – a definition. Br J Gen Pract 1995;309:107–111
2 Long L, Huntley A, Ernst E. Which complementary and alternative therapies benefit which condition? A survey of 223 professional organisations. Comp Ther Med 2001 (in press)
3 Mills S, Peacock W. Professional organisations of complementary and alternative medicine in the United Kingdom 1997: a report to the Department of Health. Centre for Complementary Health Studies, University of Exeter

BIBLIOGRAPHY

Section 2 Diagnostic methods

Ernst E, Hentschel C. Diagnostic methods in complementary medicine. Which craft is witch-craft? Int J Risk Safety Med 1995;7:55–63
Murray M, Pizzorno J. Encyclopedia of natural medicine. Rocklin, CA: Prima, 1998
Novey D W (ed). Clinician's complete reference to complementary and alternative medicine. St. Louis: Mosby, 2000

The Burton Goldberg Group. Alternative medicine: the definitive guide. Payallup, WA: Future Medicine, 1994

Section 3 Therapies

Fugh-Berman A. Alternative medicine: what works. Tucson, AZ: Odonian, 1996
Jonas W B, Levin J S (eds). Essentials of complementary and alternative medicine. Baltimore: Lippincott Williams and Wilkins, 1999
Novey D W (ed). Clinician's complete reference to complementary and alternative medicine. St. Louis: Mosby, 2000
Rowlands B. The Which? guide to complementary medicine. London: Which? 1997
The Burton Goldberg Group. Alternative medicine: the definitive guide. Payallup, WA: Future Medicine, 1994
Schimmel K C (ed). Lehrbuch der Naturheilverfahren. Stuttgart: Hippokrates, 1990
Zollman C, Vickers A. ABC of complementary medicine. London: BMJ Books, 2000

Section 4 Herbal and non-herbal medicines

Blumenthal M (ed). The complete German Commission E monographs. Austin, TX: American Botanical Council, 1998

Blumenthal M, Goldberg A, Brinckmann J (eds). Herbal medicine. Expanded Commission E monographs. Austin, TX: American Botanical Council, 2000

Blumenthal M. Herb market levels after five years of boom. Herbalgram 1999;47:64–65

Boon H, Smith M. The botanical pharmacy. Kingston: Quarry Press, 1999

Brevoort P. The booming US botanical market – a new overview. Herbalgram 1998;44:33–46

Brinker F. Herb contraindications and drug interactions. Sandy, OR: Eclectic Medical Publications, 1998

Cupp M J. Toxicology and clinical pharmacology of herbal products. Totowa, NJ: Humana Press, 2000

Dukes M N G (ed). Meyler's side effects of drugs. Amsterdam: Elsevier, 1996

Ernst E. Possible interactions between synthetic and herbal medicinal products part 1: a systematic review of the indirect evidence. Perfusion 2000;13:4–15

Ernst E. Interactions between synthetic and herbal medicinal products part 2: a systematic review of the direct evidence. Perfusion 2000;13:60–70

Fetrow C W, Avila J R. Professional's handbook of complementary and alternative medicines. Springhouse, PA: Springhouse, 1999

Fugh-Berman A. Herb-drug interactions. Lancet 2000;355:134–138

Hänsel R, Keller K, Rimpler H, Schneider G. Hagers Handbuch der Pharmazeutischen Praxis. Berlin: Springer, 1994

Hildebrandt H (ed). Pschyrembel Wörterbuch Naturheilkunde und alternative Heilverfahren. Berlin: deGruyter, 1996

Lininger S W (ed). A-Z guide to drug-herb-vitamin interactions. Rocklin, CA: Prima, 1999

Meletis C D, Jacobs T. Interactions between drugs and natural medicines. Sandy, OR: Eclectic Medical Publications, 1999

Murray M T. Encyclopedia of nutritional supplements. Rocklin, CA: Prima, 1996

Newall C A, Anderson L A, Phillipson J D. Herbal medicines: a guide for healthcare professionals. London: Pharmaceutical Press, 1996

Reynolds J E F (ed). Martindale: the extra pharmacopoeia. London: Pharmaceutical Press, 1996

Rote Liste. Bundesverband der pharmazeutischen Industrie. Frankfurt: Editio Cantor, 1999

Schulz V, Hänsel R, Tyler V E. Rational phytotherapy: a physician's guide to herbal medicine. Berlin: Springer, 1998

Wagner H, Bauer R, Peigen X, Jianming C, Nenninger A. Chinese drug monographs and analysis. Kötzing: Verlag für Ganzheitliche Medizin Dr. Erich Wühr GmbH, 1996

World Health Organization. Monographs on selected medicinal plants. Geneva: WHO, 1999

Section 5 Conditions

Spraycar M (ed). Stedman's medical dictionary. Baltimore, MD: Williams and Wilkins, 1995

HOW TO USE THIS BOOK

This book is divided into five main sections:

- Diagnostic methods
- Therapies
- Herbal and non-herbal medicines
- Conditions
- General topics.

Standardized structures have been adopted for the chapters within the first four sections. To help the reader understand and make the best use of the information in the individual chapters, there are brief explanations of the material provided under each subheading, with the help of examples taken from the book.

For further details on the methods employed for writing these sections, see p 2.

USING THE BOOK

Section 2 Diagnostic methods

This section includes brief overviews of diagnostic techniques unique to CAM. Methods are presented in alphabetical order. For each one, information is provided relating to its description, the principles on which it is based, evidence of its scientific validity and any direct risks it may pose.

NB: The reader should assume that for all diagnostic methods lacking validity, there is an indirect risk of harming patients through false-positive or false-negative diagnoses.

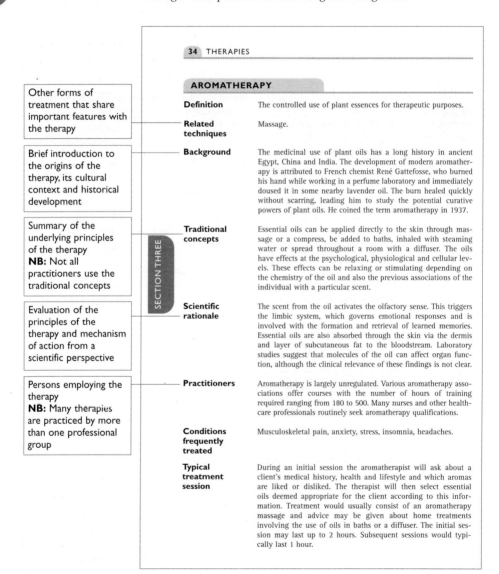

34 THERAPIES

AROMATHERAPY

Other forms of treatment that share important features with the therapy

Definition	The controlled use of plant essences for therapeutic purposes.
Related techniques	Massage.

Brief introduction to the origins of the therapy, its cultural context and historical development

Background — The medicinal use of plant oils has a long history in ancient Egypt, China and India. The development of modern aromatherapy is attributed to French chemist René Gattefosse, who burned his hand while working in a perfume laboratory and immediately doused it in some nearby lavender oil. The burn healed quickly without scarring, leading him to study the potential curative powers of plant oils. He coined the term aromatherapy in 1937.

Summary of the underlying principles of the therapy
NB: Not all practitioners use the traditional concepts

Traditional concepts — Essential oils can be applied directly to the skin through massage or a compress, be added to baths, inhaled with steaming water or spread throughout a room with a diffuser. The oils have effects at the psychological, physiological and cellular levels. These effects can be relaxing or stimulating depending on the chemistry of the oil and also the previous associations of the individual with a particular scent.

SECTION THREE

Evaluation of the principles of the therapy and mechanism of action from a scientific perspective

Scientific rationale — The scent from the oil activates the olfactory sense. This triggers the limbic system, which governs emotional responses and is involved with the formation and retrieval of learned memories. Essential oils are also absorbed through the skin via the dermis and layer of subcutaneous fat to the bloodstream. Laboratory studies suggest that molecules of the oil can affect organ function, although the clinical relevance of these findings is not clear.

Persons employing the therapy
NB: Many therapies are practiced by more than one professional group

Practitioners — Aromatherapy is largely unregulated. Various aromatherapy associations offer courses with the number of hours of training required ranging from 180 to 500. Many nurses and other healthcare professionals routinely seek aromatherapy qualifications.

Conditions frequently treated	Musculoskeletal pain, anxiety, stress, insomnia, headaches.
Typical treatment session	During an initial session the aromatherapist will ask about a client's medical history, health and lifestyle and which aromas are liked or disliked. The therapist will then select essential oils deemed appropriate for the client according to this information. Treatment would usually consist of an aromatherapy massage and advice may be given about home treatments involving the use of oils in baths or a diffuser. The initial session may last up to 2 hours. Subsequent sessions would typically last 1 hour.

**Section 3
Therapies**

This section includes chapters on forms of CAM that are identified as therapeutic modalities and excludes medicines such as herbs or food supplements. Chapters are presented in alphabetical order and are subdivided according to the headings shown in the example below (aromatherapy).

Table

Other therapies without sufficient evidence of effectiveness are presented in a table at the end of this section. Brief information

---

AROMATHERAPY   **35**

Course of treatment

For chronic conditions, one weekly session would be recommended for several weeks, with fortnightly or monthly follow-ups.

Clinical evidence

A systematic review of all RCTs of aromatherapy was conducted.[1] Based on six trials with hospitalized patients, it was concluded that aromatherapy massage has mild, transient anxiolytic effects. Due to lack of independent replication, the results of six other trials were not considered conclusive. These included positive findings for the treatment of alopecia areata[2] and prevention of bronchitis[3] and negative results for postnatal perineal discomfort.[4] Another systematic review included four RCTs of topical applications of tea tree oil.[5] There was some promising but not compelling evidence for acne and fungal infections.

Risks

Contraindications
Pregnancy, contagious disease, epilepsy, local venous thrombosis, varicose veins, broken skin, recent surgery.

Precautions/warnings
Essential oils should not be taken orally or used undiluted on the skin. Some oils cause photosensitive reactions and some have carcinogenic potential. Allergic reactions are possible with all oils.

Adverse effects
Allergic reactions, nausea, headache.

Interactions
Many essential oils are believed to have the potential to either enhance or reduce the effects of prescribed medications including antibiotics, tranquilizers, antihistamines, anticonvulsants, barbiturates, morphine, quinidine.

Quality issues
Products marketed as 'aromatherapy oils' may be synthetic or adulterated rather than the pure essential oil.

Indirect risks
Consulting an aromatherapist for symptoms may delay appropriate treatment for a medical condition. Aromatherapy should generally be considered an adjunctive treatment, not an alternative to conventional care.

Risk–benefit assessment

Aromatherapy appears to have some benefits as a palliative or supportive treatment, particularly in reducing anxiety. In the hands of a responsible therapist there seem to be few risks so it may be worth considering as an adjunctive treatment for chronically ill patients or individuals with psychosomatic illness.

SECTION THREE

Evidence-based summary of the data relating to the effectiveness of the therapy. In cases where a considerable amount of evidence exists, only the most important is presented. Priority is given to systematic reviews/metaanalyses and RCTs

Safety issues specific to the therapy
NB: For a general discussion of CAM safety, see p 412

An evidence-based judgement on whether the therapy does more good than harm
NB: A lack of compelling evidence is not the same as ineffectiveness

USING THE BOOK

is provided for each one, including a description, its main uses and any concerns about its safety.

**Section 4
Herbal and
non-herbal
medicine**

This section includes chapters on forms of CAM that are considered medications such as herbs and non-herbal supplements. Vitamins and minerals are not included. Chapters are presented in alphabetical order and are subdivided according to the headings in the example below (valerian).

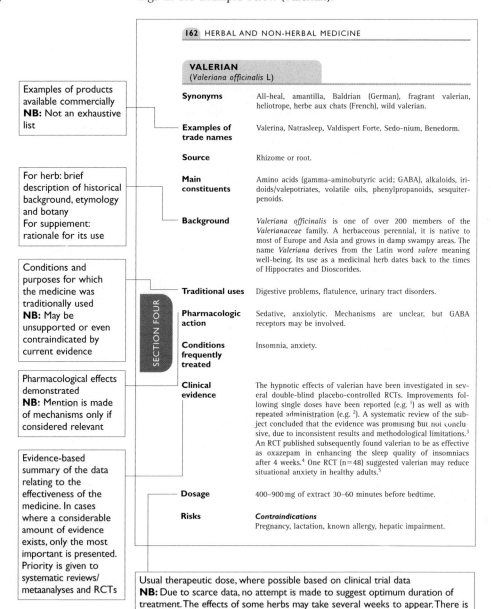

162 HERBAL AND NON-HERBAL MEDICINE

VALERIAN
(*Valeriana officinalis* L)

Synonyms	All-heal, amantilla, Baldrian (German), fragrant valerian, heliotrope, herbe aux chats (French), wild valerian.
Examples of trade names	Valerina, Natrasleep, Valdispert Forte, Sedo-nium, Benedorm.
Source	Rhizome or root.
Main constituents	Amino acids (gamma-aminobutyric acid; GABA), alkaloids, iridoids/valepotriates, volatile oils, phenylpropanoids, sesquiterpenoids.
Background	*Valeriana officinalis* is one of over 200 members of the *Valerianaceae* family. A herbaceous perennial, it is native to most of Europe and Asia and grows in damp swampy areas. The name *Valeriana* derives from the Latin word *valere* meaning well-being. Its use as a medicinal herb dates back to the times of Hippocrates and Dioscorides.
Traditional uses	Digestive problems, flatulence, urinary tract disorders.
Pharmacologic action	Sedative, anxiolytic. Mechanisms are unclear, but GABA receptors may be involved.
Conditions frequently treated	Insomnia, anxiety.
Clinical evidence	The hypnotic effects of valerian have been investigated in several double-blind placebo-controlled RCTs. Improvements following single doses have been reported (e.g. [1]) as well as with repeated administration (e.g. [2]). A systematic review of the subject concluded that the evidence was promising but not conclusive, due to inconsistent results and methodological limitations.[3] An RCT published subsequently found valerian to be as effective as oxazepam in enhancing the sleep quality of insomniacs after 4 weeks.[4] One RCT (n=48) suggested valerian may reduce situational anxiety in healthy adults.[5]
Dosage	400–900 mg of extract 30–60 minutes before bedtime.
Risks	***Contraindications*** Pregnancy, lactation, known allergy, hepatic impairment.

SECTION FOUR

Side annotations (left column):

Examples of products available commercially
NB: Not an exhaustive list

For herb: brief description of historical background, etymology and botany
For supplement: rationale for its use

Conditions and purposes for which the medicine was traditionally used
NB: May be unsupported or even contraindicated by current evidence

Pharmacological effects demonstrated
NB: Mention is made of mechanisms only if considered relevant

Evidence-based summary of the data relating to the effectiveness of the medicine. In cases where a considerable amount of evidence exists, only the most important is presented. Priority is given to systematic reviews/metaanalyses and RCTs

Usual therapeutic dose, where possible based on clinical trial data
NB: Due to scarce data, no attempt is made to suggest optimum duration of treatment. The effects of some herbs may take several weeks to appear. There is generally a lack of adequate data regarding long-term use

Tables

Other herbs and non-herbal supplements without sufficient evidence of effectiveness are presented in tables at the end of this section. Brief information is provided, including a description, main uses and safety concerns. There are also tables relating to the safety of herbs.

VALERIAN **163**

Precautions/warnings
Care should be taken if driving or operating machinery when taking valerian.

Adverse effects
Headache and gastrointestinal symptoms occasionally reported. Morning hangover reported occasionally although RCTs investigating safety factors have found no impairment of reaction time or alertness the morning after intake. Hepatotoxicity has been reported from herbal preparations in which valerian was combined with other herbs, including skullcap.

Overdose
Symptoms of tachycardia, nausea, vomiting, dilated pupils, drowsiness, confusion, visual hallucinations, blurred vision, cardiac disturbance, excitability, headache, hypersensitivity reactions and insomnia have been reported following acute overdoses, with full recoveries made in all cases.

Interactions
Theoretically, potentiation of the effects of sedatives, hypnotics or other central nervous system depressants is possible at high doses. RCTs have shown no potentiation of alcohol.

Quality issues
Composition and purity of extracts vary greatly. Standardized extracts often use valepotriates as the marker substance although valerenic acid is considered more reliable due to its stability. Aqueous extracts are devoid of valepotriates.

> Safety issues specific to the medicine
> **NB:** For a general discussion of CAM safety, see p 412

Risk–benefit assessment
Neither the efficacy nor safety of valerian has been established beyond reasonable doubt. However, the preliminary evidence for both are promising and valerian may be worth considering as a monotherapy for promoting sleep.

> An evidence-based judgement on whether the medicine does more good than harm
> **NB:** A lack of compelling evidence is not the same as ineffectiveness

SECTION FOUR

REFERENCES
1 Leathwood P D, Chauffard F, Heck E, Munoz-Box R. Aqueous extract of valerian root (*Valeriana officinalis* L) improves sleep quality in man. Pharmacol Biochem Behav 1982;17:65–71
2 Vorbach E U, Gortelmeyer R, Bruning J. Therapie von Insomnien: Wirksamkeit und Verträglichkeit eines Baldrianpräparats. Psychopharmakotherapie 1996;3:109–115
3 Stevinson C, Ernst E. Valerian for insomnia: systematic review of randomized placebo-controlled trials. Sleep Med 2000;1:91–99
4 Dorn M. Baldrian versus oxazepam: efficacy and tolerability in non-organic and non-psychiatric insomniacs: a randomized, double-blind, clinical comparative study. Forsch Komplementärmed Klass Naturheilkd 2000;7:79–84
5 Kohnen R, Oswald W D. The effects of valerian, propranolol and their combination on activation, performance and mood of healthy volunteers under social stress conditions. Pharmacopsychiatry 1988;21:447–448

FURTHER READING
Bos R, Woerdenbag H J, De Smet P A G M, Scheffer J J C. Valeriana species. In: De Smet P A G M, Keller K, Hänsel R, Chandler R F (eds) Adverse effects of herbal drugs, volume 3. Berlin: Springer, 1997 *Thorough overview of safety information on valerian.*

USING THE BOOK

Section 5
Conditions

This section includes chapters on conditions commonly seen in primary care for which CAM is popular. Chapters are presented in alphabetical order and are subdivided according to the sub-headings shown in the example below (hay fever).

Information on the use of CAM by patients with the condition

An evidence-based summary of the data relating to the effectiveness of different forms of CAM for the condition. Priority is given to systematic reviews/metaanalyses and RCTs. Treatments are listed in alphabetical order (except *Other therapies*; see below)

Optional standardized tables of RCTs
NB: When several exist, only a few examples appear in the table, selected for their rigor or clinical relevance

Brief overview of the evidence relating to a treatment for the condition

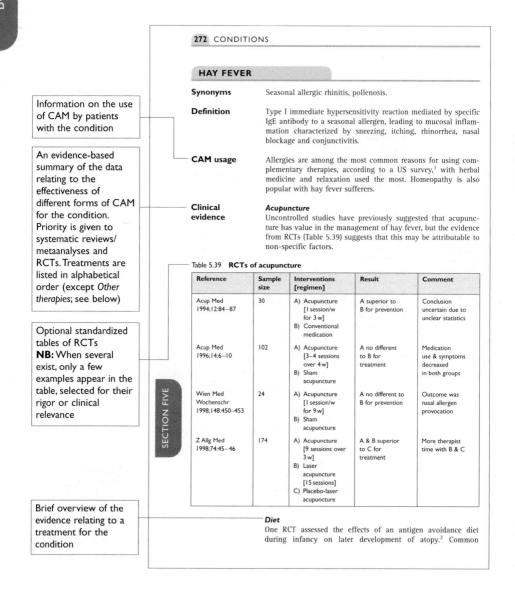

272 CONDITIONS

HAY FEVER

Synonyms	Seasonal allergic rhinitis, pollenosis.
Definition	Type I immediate hypersensitivity reaction mediated by specific IgE antibody to a seasonal allergen, leading to mucosal inflammation characterized by sneezing, itching, rhinorrhea, nasal blockage and conjunctivitis.
CAM usage	Allergies are among the most common reasons for using complementary therapies, according to a US survey,[1] with herbal medicine and relaxation used the most. Homeopathy is also popular with hay fever sufferers.
Clinical evidence	*Acupuncture* Uncontrolled studies have previously suggested that acupuncture has value in the management of hay fever, but the evidence from RCTs (Table 5.39) suggests that this may be attributable to non-specific factors.

Table 5.39   **RCTs of acupuncture**

Reference	Sample size	Interventions [regimen]	Result	Comment
Acup Med 1994;12:84–87	30	A) Acupuncture [1 session/w for 3 w] B) Conventional medication	A superior to B for prevention	Conclusion uncertain due to unclear statistics
Acup Med 1996;14:6–10	102	A) Acupuncture [3–4 sessions over 4 w] B) Sham acupuncture	A no different to B for treatment	Medication use & symptoms decreased in both groups
Wien Med Wochenschr 1998;148:450–453	24	A) Acupuncture [1 session/w for 9 w] B) Sham acupuncture	A no different to B for prevention	Outcome was nasal allergen provocation
Z Allg Med 1998;74:45–46	174	A) Acupuncture [9 sessions over 3 w] B) Laser acupuncture [15 sessions] C) Placebo-laser acupuncture	A & B superior to C for treatment	More therapist time with B & C

SECTION FIVE

Diet
One RCT assessed the effects of an antigen avoidance diet during infancy on later development of atopy.[2] Common

allergens such as cow's milk, egg and peanuts were avoided during gestation and first 3 years of life (n=165). Prevalence of hay fever or other allergies was no different from the control group at age 7 years.

Herbal medicine
A double-blind RCT (n=69) of **stinging nettle** (*Urtica dioica*) taken for one week reported higher global ratings of improvement than for placebo, but no statistical analysis was conducted.[3]

Homeopathy
Seven placebo-controlled RCTs of ***Galphimia glauca*** from one research group were subjected to metaanalysis by the same researchers (Box 5.21). Collectively the results suggested that the remedy is effective for both ocular and nasal symptoms. The success rate of 79% is comparable to conventional treatments, with minimal adverse events reported.

> Summary details of any authoritative systematic review/ metaanalysis on a subject

Box 5.21
Metaanalysis
**Homeopathic
Galphimia glauca
for hay fever**
Forsch
Komplementärmed
1996;3:230–234

- Seven double-blind placebo-controlled RCTs involving 752 patients
- Quality ratings not performed but methods identical for each trial except only two used intent-to-treat analysis
- Superiority over placebo for ocular symptoms (relative risk: 1.25, CI 1.09 to 1.43) and nasal symptoms (relative risk 1.26, CI 1.05 to 1.50)

Promising results were reported from a small pilot RCT (n=36) of homeopathic grass pollens versus placebo.[4] The same research team conducted a larger (n=144) double-blind placebo-controlled RCT testing homeopathic dilutions of specific antigens identified for each hay fever patient by skin tests.[5] Symptom scores and use of antihistamines were reduced significantly more in the homeopathic group.

A double-blind RCT compared a homeopathic nasal spray with a conventional one (cromolyn sodium) over 42 days in 146 hay fever sufferers.[6] Quality of life assessments indicated therapeutic equivalence of the two treatments.

Supplements
Fish oil supplementation was investigated in a double-blind placebo-controlled RCT (n=37) involving pollen-sensitive individuals with hay fever and asthma.[7] Various outcomes measured over a pollen season revealed no differences between the fish oil and placebo groups.

Other therapies
An RCT (n=47) tested the effects of **hypnotic suggestion** on skin reactions to allergen prick tests in individuals with hay

> Treatments for which there is only minimal evidence
> **NB:** Other therapies do not appear in *Summary of clinical evidence* table

SECTION FIVE

USING THE BOOK

fever and asthma.[8] According to the results, undergoing hypnosis was associated with smaller weals, but specific suggestions had no influence. No clinical trials of hypnotherapy for hay fever symptoms were located, making the potential of this therapy difficult to evaluate.

For each treatment, the totality of available evidence is assessed and presented according to 3 criteria:
1) weight of evidence;
2) direction of evidence; 3) serious safety concerns
(see p 15 for explanations)

Table 5.40
Summary of clinical evidence for hay fever

Treatment	Weight of evidence	Direction of evidence	Serious safety concerns
Acupuncture (prevention) (treatment)	O OO	⇨ ⇨	Yes (see p 29)
Diet (prevention)	O	⇩	No
Herbal medicine Nettle	O	⟋	Yes (see p 139)
Homeopathy	OO	⇧	No (see p 55)
Supplements Fish oil	O	⇩	Yes (see p 5)

An evidence-based judgement evaluating the benefits & risks of CAM for the condition in relation to conventional treatments
NB: A lack of compelling evidence is not the same as ineffectiveness

Overall recommendation

There is little clinical trial evidence for the effectiveness of most complementary therapies for the prevention or treatment of hay fever. The one exception is homeopathy for which promising evidence exists, particularly for *Galphimia glauca*. There are suggestions that this may be as effective as conventional medication, but this has not been directly investigated. Adverse effects are rare with homeopathic remedies, so for patients dissatisfied with their orthodox medication, homeopathy may be worth considering.

References to papers that are cited in addition to those already presented in the tables & boxes in *Clinical evidence*

REFERENCES

1 Eisenberg D M, Davis R B, Ettner S L, Appel S, Wilkey S, Rompay M V, Kessler R C. Trends in alternative medicine use in the United States, 1990–1997. JAMA 1998;280:1569–1575

2 Zeiger R S, Heller S. The development and prediction of atopy in high-risk children: follow up at age seven years in a prospective randomized study of combined maternal and infant food allergen avoidance. J Allergy Clin Immunol 1995;95:1179–1190

3 Mittman P. Randomized, double-blind study of freeze-dried *Urtica dioica* in the treatment of allergic rhinitis. Planta Med 1990;56:44–47

4 Reilly D T, Taylor M A. Potent placebo or potency? A proposed study model with initial findings using homoeopathically prepared pollens in hay fever. Br Homoeopath J 1985; 74:65–74

5 Reilly D T, Taylor M A, McSharry C, Aitchison T. Is homoeopathy a placebo response? Controlled trial of homoeopathic potency, with pollen in hay fever as model. Lancet 1986;2:881–886

6 Weiser M, Gegenheimer L H, Klein P. A randomized equivalence trial comparing the efficacy and safety of Luffa comp-Heel nasal spray with cromolyn sodium spray in the treatment of seasonal allergic rhinitis. Forsch Komplementärmed 1999;6: 142–148

7 Thien F C K, Mencia-Huerta J M, Lee T H. Dietary fish oil effects on seasonal hay fever and asthma in pollen-sensitive subjects. Am Rev Respir Dis 1993;147:1138–1143

8 Fry L, Mason A A, Pearson R S. Effect of hypnosis on allergic skin responses in asthma and hay fever. Br Med J 1964;1145–1148

SECTION FIVE

Abbreviations

The following abbreviations are used throughout this book:

CAM	complementary and alternative medicine
RCT	randomized clinical trial
CCT	controlled clinical trial
CI	confidence intervals (95% unless otherwise stated).

The following abbreviations are used in the boxes and tables in Section 5 only:

min	minute(s)	mo	month(s)
h	hour(s)	y	year(s)
d	day(s)	m	meter(s)
w	week(s)	g	gram(s)
wkly	weekly	mg	milligram(s).

**Significance
levels**

When reporting research results, only differences that are statistically significant (p<0.05) are mentioned; p values and the term 'significant' are omitted for conciseness.

**Weight of
evidence**

The weight of the evidence refers to the importance that can be placed on it. There are three discrete categories of weight:

Low	0
Moderate	00
High	000

The judgement of weight is based on a combination of three largely independent factors:

- the **level** of evidence (the highest level being systematic review/metaanalysis, followed by RCT, CCT and uncontrolled study)
- the methodological **quality** of the investigations (the validity and reliability of the studies)
- the **volume** of information (the number of studies and their sample sizes).

Judgements take into account all three of these dimensions of weight. Therefore a treatment where *volume* and *level* are high (e.g. metaanalysis of 50 studies) will not necessarily receive a high weight if the *quality* is low (e.g. methodologically flawed studies). Similarly, even if *quality* and *level* are quite high (e.g. a rigorous RCT), weight can only be considered low if there is a low *volume* of evidence (only a single trial).

**Direction of
evidence**

The direction of the evidence refers to the collective positive or negative outcome of the studies for that treatment. Direction can be reported in one of five ways:

Clearly positive	⇧
Tentatively positive	⤴
Uncertain	⇨
Tentatively negative	⤵
Clearly negative	⇩

Direction is largely judged independently of weight of evidence. The reader must interpret the direction of the evidence in the light of its weight. For example, a *clearly positive* result based on evidence with *low weight* (e.g. a single, small, non-randomized trial) may not be as informative as a *tentatively positive* finding backed by a body of evidence with *high weight* (e.g. a systematic review of RCTs).

Serious safety concerns

Cases where a treatment has been, or may potentially be, associated with life-threatening consequences, hospitalization or sustained harm, even if rare.

No=reports of serious events were not located and are considered unlikely

Yes=serious events have been reported or are considered possible

Whenever possible, page references are provided for the treatment's own chapter or relevant table. In some cases, information is not available about safety. The general principle is to err on the side of caution; so when in doubt, a treatment is marked Yes. This applies to all herbs and some supplements (see Methods, p 5).

NB
- It is imperative that the reader refers to the treatment chapter or table. Even where a treatment is marked No, there may be contraindications and precautions which, if ignored, could have potentially serious consequences.
- Even where a therapy is not associated with serious complications, indirect risks may exist and could have serious consequences. CAM practitioners may not be medically qualified and should not therefore be expected to have competence in orthodox medical management.
- Many of the reported serious adverse events are avoidable by good practice.
- For a general discussion of CAM safety, see p 412.

2

Diagnostic methods

BIORESONANCE

The method was originally called 'Mora-therapy' and was frequently renamed so that a confusing array of terminology persists: biocommunication, biocom, multicom, multiresonance, biophysical information, etc.

Bioresonance is based on a device created by F Morrel MD, a colleague of Reinhold Voll. The apparatus is believed to receive electromagnetic waves directly from a person's body, manipulate the aberrant waveforms and normalize them by increasing or decreasing their amplitude. It then returns the 'treated' normal waves to the patient, thereby effecting first a diagnosis and then a cure. The Mora device is said to be effective for headaches, skin diseases, muscle pain, circulatory defects and many other conditions; it is often used in combination with homeopathic remedies. The method is not associated with specific risks. Its principles lack a scientific rationale. There is no compelling evidence to suggest that it is valid.

In conclusion, it is highly questionable whether bioresonance constitutes a useful diagnostic tool.

CHIROPRACTIC DIAGNOSTIC TECHNIQUES

Chiropractors use a range of diagnostic methods, only some of which are specific to that particular profession. The methods range from manual to radiographic techniques.

The reliability of lumbar spine radiograph readings was tested by four chiropractors evaluating 100 X-rays repeatedly.[1] The reliability was, on average, acceptable.

Various manual diagnostic methods employed by chiropractors have also been tested for reliability. In general the results revealed low values of reliability.[2,3] Manual tests with good reliability were the measurement of passive range of motion[4] and palpation for cervical spine tenderness.[5]

A recent systematic review of the totality of the data suggested that none of the tests for lumbopelvic spine have been sufficiently evaluated in relation to reliability and validity.[6] Other studies examined the diagnostic skills of chiropractors in more general terms. Eighty-three twin pairs were seen by a chiropractor whose aim was to determine the prevalence of positive chiropractic test results in relation to low back pain status. Although no individual test of a battery of 12 tests was accurate, the overall diagnostic discrimination on the basis of these tests was satisfactory.[7]

Finally, the intra- and interexaminer reliability of the following tests was investigated: visual postural analysis, pain description, plain lumbar X-rays, leg length discrepancy, neurologic tests, motion palpation, static palpation and orthopedic tests.[8] The resulting intraexaminer reliability of the decision to manipulate was moderate. The interexaminer agreement pooled across all spinal joints was low. The authors concluded that these commonly used chiropractic diagnostic methods are not reproducible.

The bottom line to this complex situation is that some, but not all, chiropractic diagnostic methods are valid.

REFERENCES

1 Assendelft W J J, Bouter L M, Knipschild P G, Wilmink J T. Reliability of lumbar spine radiography reading by chiropractors. Spine 1997;22:1235–1241

2 Leboeuf C. The reliability of specific sacro-occipital techniques and diagnostic tests. J Manip Physiol Ther 1991;14:512–517

3 Panzer D M. The reliability of lumbar motion palpation. J Manip Physiol Ther 1992;15:518–524

4 Nilsson N, Christensen H W, Hartvigsen J. The inter-examiner reliability of measuring passive cervical range of motion, revisited. J Manip Physiol Ther 1996;19:302–305

5 Hubka M J, Phelen S P. Interexaminer reliability of palpation for cervical spine

tenderness. J Manip Physiol Ther 1994;17:591–596

6 Hestboek L, Leboeuf-Yde C. Are chiropractic tests for the lumbo-pelvic spine reliable and valid? A systematic critical literature review. J Manip Physiol Ther 2000;23:258–275

7 Leboeuf-Yde C, Ohm Kyvik K. Is it possible to differentiate people with or without low back pain on the basis of tests of lumbo-pelvic dysfunction? J Manip Physiol Ther 2000;23:160–167

8 French S D, Green S, Forbes A. Reliability of chiropractic methods commonly used to detect manipulable lesions in patients with chronic low back pain. J Manip Physiol Ther 2000;23:231–237

IRIDOLOGY

Iridology is based on the belief that each body region and organ is represented at one specific location in the iris. Abnormalities in one given region of the iris are assumed to correspond to abnormalities in the respective organ. Iridology was developed more than 100 years ago by a Hungarian physician and became popular in the early part of the 20th century. Iridologists visually assess the irides of their patients by direct examination or study of close-up photographs of the iris.

The method has no scientific basis. Neural connections between the iris and other organs of the body that are required to explain iridology do not exist. A systematic review[1] of all four controlled evaluations available to date concluded that the method is not valid.

REFERENCE

1 Ernst E. Iridology: not useful and potentially harmful. Arch Ophthalmol 2000;118:120–121

KINESIOLOGY

Kinesiology (also 'applied kinesiology') is a system of diagnosis (and treatment) developed by the US chiropractor George Goodheart Jr. It is based on the posit that disease is caused by the accumulation of toxins around major muscle groups which translates into weakness of specific muscle groups. The underlying concept is that the relative strength of a given group of muscles can be used to reveal the status of a patient's health.

The method has no scientific rationale. At least three independent research groups have assessed the validity of this technique under different circumstances in a rigorous manner.[1,2,3] In neither case was validity confirmed. Thus kinesiology cannot be recommended as a useful diagnostic method.

REFERENCES

1 Garrow J S. Kinesiology and food allergy. Br Med J 1988;296:1573–1574

2 Haas M, Peterson D, Hoyer D, Ross G. Muscle testing response to provocative vertebral challenge and spinal manipulation. A randomized controlled trial of construct validity. J Manip Physiol Ther 1994;17:141–148

3 Lüdtke R, Seeber N, Kunz B, Ring J. Health kinesiology is neither reliable nor valid. Focus Alt Compl Ther 2000;5:95

KIRLIAN PHOTOGRAPHY

Kirlian photography is a diagnostic technique in which a high-voltage, high-frequency electric field interacts with the material being photographed (e.g. part of the human body) and is delivered to a photographic plate.

The technique was (re-)discovered by the Russian couple S and V Kirlian. Its concept is that high-frequency currents are applied to the human body and the subsequent electromagnetic discharge is visualized on a photographic plate.[1] The method is used by a minority of CAM providers. The reliability of the method has been found to be better than chance, but less than that of conventional diagnostic tests.[2,3] Specificity and sensitivity have not been defined. Its value as a diagnostic tool therefore seems limited.

REFERENCES

1 Kirlian S D, Kirlian V K. Photography and visual observation by means of high frequency currents. J Sci Appl Photogr 1964;6: 397–403

2 Treugut H, Corner C, Lüdtke R, Mandel P. Kirlian-Fotografie: Reliabilität der energetischen Terminalpunktdiagnose (ETD) nach Mandal bei gesunden Probanden. Forsch Komplementärmed 1997;4:210–217

3 Treugut H, Koppen M, Nickolay B, Fuß R, Schmid P. Kirlian-Fotografie: Zufälliges oder Personen-spezifisches Entladungsmuster? Forsch Komplementärmed Klass Naturheilkd 2000;7:12–16

LABORATORY TESTS

Some CAM providers use a range of laboratory tests for diagnostic purposes. Often, but not always (e.g. hair analysis), blood samples are used for analysis. Proponents of such tests claim that either diseases or (more frequently) predisease stages of medical conditions (e.g. a precancerous state) are being diagnosed with these methods. The conditions tested for are often allergies or malignant diseases. All these diagnostic methods have one thing in common: there is no acceptable evidence to show that they are valid.[1]

REFERENCE

1 Ernst E, Hentschel C H. Diagnostic methods in complementary medicine. Which craft is witchcraft? Int J Risk Safety Med 1995;7:55–63

PULSE DIAGNOSIS

Pulse diagnosis is an integral part of traditional Chinese medicine and is often used in conjunction with tongue diagnosis.

In making a diagnosis, the radial pulse is examined at three adjacent positions on each side in turn and both superficially and deeply. This gives a total of 12 pulses which are believed to yield information on the status of the 12 internal organs or functions. Other systems are also used that are more complex; for example, examining three depths instead of two and checking arteries elsewhere in the body. Yet other systems are simpler and use descriptions of the overall feel of the pulse (such as 'floating', 'deep' or 'choppy'). The pulse may be used to diagnose conditions which have not yet manifested themselves and to gauge the success of acupuncture or herbal treatments. Successful pulse taking is said to require thorough training, long experience and the gift of sensitivity.

One published secondary report of an investigation into pulse diagnosis[1] tested its reliability and validity. Although acupuncturists had some success in distinguishing between ill and healthy people, this was not much more than that of an anesthetist taking the pulse in the conventional way. Interrater reliability was poor between experienced practitioners, and the test-retest reliability was not good. Therefore, the validity of traditional Chinese pulse diagnosis seems questionable.

REFERENCE

1 Vincent C A. Acupuncture research: why do it? Compl Med Res 1992;6:21–24

REFLEXOLOGY CHARTS

Reflexology charts consist of pictures of the soles of the feet on which diagrams of the organs or parts of the body are drawn. While reflexologists formally claim that these relationships are not used for diagnosis, in practice they believe that tenderness or a gritty feeling in the feet represents current or past disease in the corresponding area of the body.

Investigations of reflexology charts have reached inconsistent conclusions. In a multicenter study, three reflexologists selected 76 patients of whom they had no previous knowledge.[1] Each patient and therapist separately graded problems related to 13 areas of the body. Interrater agreement, measured by weighted kappa, ranged between 0.04 and 0.22 and was apparently better than chance for six parts of the body. However, the agreement was too low to be of clinical significance. The examinations were not supervised. Sudmeier and colleagues found an increase in renal blood flow when the corresponding area in the foot was massaged.[2] In a blind study with 18 patients with six chosen conditions, three reflexologists were unable to identify the conditions with any greater reliability than chance.[3]

In conclusion, the validity of reflexology as a diagnostic method is questionable.

REFERENCES

1 Baerheim A, Algory R, Skogedal K R, Stephansen R, Sandvik H. Fottene – et diagnostik hjelpemiddel? Tidsskr Nor Laegeforen 1998;5:753–765
2 Sudmeier I, Bodner G, Egger I, Mur E, Ulmer H, Herold M. Änderung der Nierendurchblutung durch organassoziierte Reflexzonentherapie am Fuss gemessen mit farbkodierter Doppler-Sonographie. Forsch Komplementärmed 1999;6:129–134
3 White A R, Williamson J, Hart A, Ernst E. A blinded investigation into the accuracy of reflexology charts. Compl Ther Med 2000;8:166–172

TONGUE DIAGNOSIS

Tongue diagnosis is part of the evaluation of patients by a traditional acupuncturist in which hues, types of coating, moistness, markings and other changes are assessed. The method is today used by most practitioners of traditional Chinese medicine. Certain medical conditions like iron deficiency or streptococcal infection are, of course, associated with characteristic changes of the tongue and these are used in conventional diagnoses. Beyond that, the method has no scientific rationale.

The validity of tongue diagnosis has rarely been investigated. In one study,[1] 121 patients with circulatory disorders (verified by analysis of nailfold microcirculation) were submitted to tongue diagnosis in parallel; 74% of these individuals had positive tongue signs like dark red color, purple color and presence of petechiae or ecchymoses.

Even though encouraging, such studies give too little information about the validity of tongue diagnosis. Until such data are available, the technique cannot be considered valid.

REFERENCE

1 Fuzhonf M, Weiying Z. Observation on the analysis of nailfold microcirculation and tongue picture in 150 cases of cardio-cerebral angiopathy. Proceedings of the 2nd Asian Congress on Microcirculation, Beijing, August 1995

VEGA-TEST

The Vega-test is a method of diagnosis from abnormalities of the bioelectrical properties of acupuncture points. The method is also claimed to allow selection of appropriate homeopathic and nutritional remedies by including them in the electrical circuit.

The method was developed by Reinhold Voll and is today used by a significant proportion of CAM providers of various disciplines, e.g. homeopaths, acupuncturists. Its proponents claim that it can be employed to detect disease and identify substances of therapeutic use for the individual patient. The method has no scientific rationale. One blinded test apparently showed a good discriminatory power between allergic and non-allergic volunteers.[1] However, this study awaits independent replication. Others have found that the results obtained with this technique are not reproducible.[2] There are no specific risks involved in the technique. At present there is little evidence to indicate that the Vega-test is a valid diagnostic procedure.

REFERENCES

1 Krop J, Lewith G T, Gziut W, Radutescuc A. A double-blind, randomized controlled investigation of electrodermal testing in the diagnosis of allergies. J Alt Compl Med 1997;3:241–248

2 Gloerfeld H. Elektroakupunktur nach Voll. Unpublished MD thesis, University of Marburg, 1987

DIAGNOSTIC METHODS

Therapies

ACUPUNCTURE

Synonyms   Reflexotherapy (in former USSR); sensory stimulation.

Definition   Insertion of a needle into the skin and underlying tissues in special sites, known as points, for therapeutic or preventive purposes.

Related techniques   Point stimulation by: electricity, laser (low-level laser therapy), moxibustion, pressure (acupressure, shiatsu, tui na) or ultrasound; electroacupuncture after Voll, Ryodoraku; neural therapy.

Background   Acupuncture, as practiced in most of the world, originated in China and is one part of oriental medicine. Chinese texts from about the first century BCE describe an already elaborate and systematic therapy. Some authors have suggested that tattoos on human remains may indicate the use of acupuncture in Europe from about 3300 BCE.

Although acupuncture has been used for years within immigrant communities in the West, interest among Westerners has fluctuated. The most recent wave of interest dates from about 1970 and is associated with more open access to China.

Acupuncture is commonly used as a routine treatment in China, Taiwan, Japan, Korea, Singapore and other Eastern countries, although usually separately from Western medicine. In many developed countries it is also available in parallel with orthodox medical care, although in some situations it may be integrated, e.g. for treatment of chronic pain.

Traditional concepts   The fundamental concept is *qi* (pronounced 'chee') which is usually, though inadequately, translated as 'energy'. It is believed that qi is inherited at birth and maintained during life by the intake of food and air. It circulates throughout the body and nourishes and defends every part. One major pathway for its circulation is via 12 meridians which form a continuous pathway through limbs, trunk and head. On these meridians, more than 350 acupuncture points have been defined. Other points lie outside the meridian pathways. Several different approaches to diagnosis have been developed over time, but some concepts are basic to all. For example, health is a balance of two opposites, Yang and Yin. Diseases are associated with disturbances or disharmony (typically 'blockage' or 'deficiency') of energy, often associated with climatic conditions such as cold and damp and revealed as malfunction of tissues or organs.

Acupuncture theory holds that the body can be stimulated to correct its own energy flow and balance by needling or pressing on the points. Practitioners who use traditional, energetic concepts of acupuncture believe that every medical condition reflects a disturbance of energy and therefore may be appropriately addressed by acupuncture. In addition, it is claimed that disturbances may be detected before they develop into conditions and therefore apparently healthy people may benefit from acupuncture.

Scientific rationale

No evidence has been found to confirm the physical existence of qi or the meridians. A possible explanation for the points is that they are sites at which nerves can be stimulated and acupuncture can be understood to some degree as a method of stimulating the nervous and muscular systems. In particular, acupuncture has been found to release various neurotransmitters, including opioid peptides and serotonin.[1,2] Acupuncture may also incorporate a form of trigger point therapy, as there are many similarities between them.[3]

Practitioners

In the US, the National Certification Commission of Acupuncture and Oriental Medicine (NCCAOM) has established standards and its certificates are accepted for licensure in many states. In some states non-medically qualified practitioners are allowed to see patients without medical referral; in other states medical referral is required. In the UK, there are no legal restrictions on the practice of acupuncture and it is used by practitioners trained primarily in acupuncture as well as by primary care practitioners, physiotherapists and manipulative therapists. In many European countries, the practice of acupuncture is officially restricted to medical practitioners but the restrictions may not be applied rigorously. In Germany, it is practiced both by doctors and by *Heilpraktiker* (independent ancillary health workers).

Conditions frequently treated

Pain, especially osteoarthritis and other musculoskeletal disorders, headaches, stress, 'low energy', ear, nose and throat conditions, addictions and allergies, maintaining health and preventing illness.

Typical treatment session

Traditional acupuncturists will take a history of the condition and ask about predisposing factors (such as the weather). They may also explore the personality in order to build up a comprehensive diagnosis in terms of energy disturbance of the body or a particular organ. Traditional examination may include inspection of the tongue, palpation of the pulse and abdomen and a search for tender sites. Doctors or manual therapists who are trained in acupuncture may incorporate it into their usual diagnostic and treatment process.

When the diagnosis has been made, needles will be inserted into selected acupuncture points. Anywhere between one and 12 points may be needled. The needles are typically about 30 mm long, very fine (0.3 mm) and disposable. Insertion is

THERAPIES

often painless. Needles may be placed just under the skin or deeper into muscle and may be stimulated either by repeated manual rotation or by battery-powered electrical apparatus. This may cause an unusual aching sensation called *deqi* (pronounced 'der chee'). The needles may be left in position for a period ranging from a few seconds to 20 minutes, while the patient relaxes. Occasionally, special indwelling needles are inserted which are designed to be left in place for up to 2 weeks before removal. Points in the ear may be used in treatment; this is called auriculoacupuncture.

Points may also be stimulated by pressure, either in the Japanese form, shiatsu, where pressure is applied by fingers, hands, elbows or other parts of the body, or in the Chinese method, tui na, in which a variety of methods of physical stimulation are used such as pulling and rubbing. In moxibustion, points are heated by smoldering a substance called moxa, the powdered leaves of *Artemisia vulgaris*. Points may also be stimulated by laser or ultrasound. Sometimes water, local anesthetic drugs or other substances are injected into points, which may be called neural therapy. Self-treatment versions of acupuncture exist in which pressure pads or electrical apparatus are used. Measurement of electrical characteristics of acupuncture points has been used as a diagnostic and treatment method, two forms of which are electroacupuncture after Voll (EAV) and Ryodoraku.

Course of treatment

Visits usually start at weekly intervals, sometimes more often. The symptoms may typically abate somewhat for a limited period after one or two treatments. When the relief is prolonged the interval between treatments may be increased until a course of six or eight sessions is completed. Chronic conditions may require visits for maintenance treatment at appropriate intervals.

Clinical evidence

The current evidence supports the concept that acupuncture has more than a placebo effect in some conditions (Table 3.1). Systematic reviews have shown acupuncture to be more effective than placebo for treatment of chemotherapy-induced nausea and vomiting,[4] early postoperative nausea and vomiting in adults[5] and for dental pain.[6] The evidence also suggests it has an effect in migraine but the quality of evidence is poor.[7] For musculoskeletal conditions, there is conflicting evidence for the effectiveness of acupuncture for back pain from two independent reviews,[8,9] there is insufficient evidence to draw conclusions for one common indication, osteoarthritis,[10] and there is promising evidence for treatment of fibromyalgia.[11] For nausea and vomiting of pregnancy, an initial review suggested that acupuncture can be effective[4] but a later review concluded that this effect has not definitely been shown to be superior to placebo.[12] Early RCTs of acupuncture for recovery from stroke (e.g. [13,14]) found it

Table 3.1
Evidence of acupuncture's effectiveness from systematic reviews

Conclusively positive	Inconclusive	Conclusively negative
Dental pain Nausea, especially post-operative	Asthma Back pain Drug dependency Fibromyalgia Migraine Neck pain Osteoarthritis Rheumatic disease Stroke Tension headache	Smoking Weight loss

superior to no treatment but a later RCT found no effect compared to placebo.[15] Present evidence suggests it is no better than placebo for nicotine withdrawal[16] or for weight reduction.[17]

Risks

Contraindications
Severe bleeding disorder. Pregnancy (first trimester) is often regarded as a contraindication, except for treatment of nausea. Presence of cardiac pacemaker contraindicates electrical stimulation. Indwelling needles should not be used in patients at risk from bacteremia.

Precautions/warnings
Patients should be treated supine, at least for the first treatment. Acupuncture often causes drowsiness so patients should not drive or operate machinery after acupuncture, particularly after the first treatment. Children should be treated with care, if at all. Special care should be taken when needling points on the thorax. Strict asepsis and close supervision are essential if indwelling needles are used.

Adverse effects
Mild, transient adverse events are quite common. Drowsiness may occur as noted above.[18] Bleeding or bruising, pain on needling and aggravation of symptoms happen occasionally (1–3%). Serious adverse events, such as pneumothorax, appear to occur rather rarely although well-documented cases have occurred, including fatalities.[19] The use of sterile, disposable needles removes all risk of cross-contamination and is mandatory in many states.

Interactions
Electroacupuncture may interfere with cardiac pacemakers (see above).

Indirect risks
Since acupuncture is used by some practitioners as a complete medical system, it may constitute the risk of delaying conventional diagnosis or treatment.

THERAPIES

Risk–benefit assessment

The diagnostic validity of traditional Chinese acupuncture has not been established and may therefore constitute a risk in itself. In cases where conventional medical diagnosis and advice on best management have already been obtained, acupuncture appears to be acceptably safe in trained hands. It appears to be more effective than placebo for some conditions. Although the range of its actions is still not known for certain, it is worth considering for a wide number of indications, particularly pain.

REFERENCES

1 Han J, Terenius L. Neurochemical basis of acupuncture analgesia. Ann Rev Pharmacol Toxicol 1982;22:193–220
2 Andersson S, Lundeberg T. Acupuncture – from empiricism to science: functional background to acupuncture effects in pain and disease. Med Hypotheses 1995;45:271–281
3 Filshie J, Cummings T M. Western medical acupuncture. In: Ernst E, White A (eds). Acupuncture: a scientific appraisal. Oxford: Butterworth Heinemann, 1999, pp 31–59
4 Vickers A. Can acupuncture have specific effects on health? A systematic review of acupuncture antiemesis trials. J Roy Soc Med 1996;89:303–311
5 Lee A, Done M L. The use of nonpharmacologic techniques to prevent postoperative nausea and vomiting: a meta-analysis. Anesthesia and Analgesia 1999;88:1362–1369
6 Ernst E, Pittler M H. The effectiveness of acupuncture in treating acute dental pain: a systematic review. Br Dent J 1998;184:443–447
7 Melchart D, Linde K, Fischer P et al. Acupuncture for recurrent headaches: a systematic review of randomized controlled trials. Cephalalgia 1999;19:779–786
8 Ernst E, White A R. Acupuncture for back pain: a meta-analysis of randomized controlled trials. Arch Intern Med 1998;158:2235–2241
9 Van Tulder M W, Cherkin D C, Berman B, Lao L, Koes B W. The effectiveness of acupuncture in the management of acute and chronic low back pain. Spine 1999; 24:1113–1123
10 Ezzo J, Berman B, Hadhazy V, Jadad A R, Lao L, Singh B B. Is acupuncture effective for the treatment of chronic pain? A systematic review. Pain 2000;86:217–225

11 Berman B M, Ezzo J, Hadhazy V, Swyers J P. Is acupuncture effective in the treatment of fibromyalgia? J Fam Pract 1999; 48:213–218
12 Murphy P A. Alternative therapies for nausea and vomiting of pregnancy. Obstet Gynaecol 1998;91:149–155
13 Johansson B B. Has sensory stimulation a role in stroke rehabilitation? Scand J Rehabil Med 1993;29(suppl):87–96
14 Sallstrom S, Kjendahl A, Osten P E, Stanghelle J K, Borchgrevink C F. Acupuncture in the treatment of stroke patients in the subacute stage: a randomised, controlled study. Compl Ther Med 1996;4:193–197
15 Gosman-Hedstroem G, Claesson L, Klingenstierna U et al. Effects of acupuncture treatment on daily life activities and quality of life. Stroke 1998;29:2100–2108
16 White A, Rampes H, Ernst E. Acupuncture for smoking cessation. Cochrane Library. Oxford: Update Software, 1999
17 Ernst E. Acupuncture/acupressure for weight reduction? A systematic review. Wien Klin Wochenschr 1997;109:60–62
18 Rampes H, James R. Complications of acupuncture. Acupunct Med 1995;8:26–33
19 Ernst E, White A. Life-threatening adverse reactions after acupuncture? A systematic review. Pain 1997;71:123–126

FURTHER READING

Ernst E, White A (eds). Acupuncture: a scientific appraisal. Oxford: Butterworth Heinemann, 1999
A review of the traditional and modern concepts of acupuncture, including likely mechanisms, in addition to the evidence on its safety and effectiveness.

ALEXANDER TECHNIQUE

Definition Process of psychophysical reeducation to improve postural balance and coordination in order to move with minimal strain and maximum ease.

Related techniques Feldenkrais method, Rolfing, Tragerwork, yoga.

Background The Alexander technique was developed around the turn of the last century by Frederick M Alexander, an Australian actor who suffered a recurring loss of voice. By observing himself in a mirror, he concluded that it was due to the tense position in which he habitually held his head. By correcting the relationship between head, neck and spine during activity, he solved the problem over a number of years. This marked the beginning of the Alexander technique.

Traditional concepts The Alexander technique is based on three principles:

- function is affected by use
- an organism functions as a whole
- the relationship of the head, neck and spine is vital to the organism's ability to function optimally.

Human movement is thought to be most fluent when the head leads and the spine follows. This new experience is practiced repeatedly to create new motor pathways, improving proprioception and upright posture and leading to enhanced coordination and balance.

Scientific rationale The notion that learning the Alexander technique allows the conscious changing of habitual and detrimental physiologic reactions receives some support from psychophysiology research, suggesting that the mind can modulate aspects of the autonomic nervous system. Specific investigations of the Alexander technique have demonstrated that it improves the efficiency of moving from the sitting to standing position.

Practitioners There are about 2000 Alexander teachers worldwide. They typically come from a background of performing arts, dance, theater and music or, more recently, physical or occupational therapy and massage. Certified teachers undergo at least three years of training on an approved course involving 1600 hours of training.

Conditions frequently treated Chronic pain, asthma, osteoarthritis, stress, headaches. Also used by performing artists and sportspeople.

THERAPIES

Typical treatment session

Sessions last between 45 and 60 minutes and take place in an Alexander studio with the aid of a bodywork table and mirror. The client or student is encouraged to wear loose, comfortable clothing to facilitate movement. The teacher guides the Alexander process using a gentle hands-on approach to teach movements with the head leading and the spine following. Within 5–10 lessons the student is able to experience and recreate an expansive quality of movement known as poise. The skill can then be refined to specialist activities.

Course of treatment

Thirty lessons are recommended in order to learn the basic concepts. Serious students of the technique may undertake up to 100 lessons.

Clinical evidence

Controlled trials have reported enhanced respiratory function in healthy volunteers,[1] greater functional reach in elderly women[2] and improvements in performance and anxiety in musical students[3] following training in the Alexander technique. An uncontrolled trial of a multidisciplinary program for 67 chronic back pain sufferers incorporating lessons in Alexander technique reported improvements in pain which persisted for 6 months.[4] Another observational study involving seven patients with Parkinson's disease reported improvements in depression and performance of daily activities following instruction in the Alexander technique.[5] Multiple cases of successful application of the Alexander technique to people with learning difficulties[6] and craniomandibular disorders[7] have also been reported.

Risks

Contraindications
None known.

Precautions/warnings
Learning the Alexander technique requires commitment and a great deal of practice by the student.

Adverse effects
None known.

Interactions
None known.

Indirect risks
Learning the Alexander technique cannot replace medical treatment for a condition.

Risk–benefit assessment

Whether learning the Alexander technique has a specific therapeutic effect is not clear, but since it is almost entirely safe and has been associated with positive outcomes in various conditions, it may be worth considering as an adjunctive or palliative therapy for patients who express a strong interest.

REFERENCES

1 Austin J H M, Ausubel P. Enhanced respiratory muscular function in normal adults after lessons in proprioceptive musculoskeletal education without exercises. Chest 1992;102:486–490

2 Dennis R J. Functional reach improvement in normal older women after Alexander technique instruction. J Gerontol – Biol Sci Med Sci 1999;54:8–11

3 Valentine E R, Fitzgerald D F P, Gorton T L, Hudson J A, Symonds E R C. The effect of lessons in the Alexander technique on music performance in high and low stress situations. Psychol Music 1995;23:129–141

4 Elkayam O, Itzhak S B, Avrahami E et al. Multidisciplinary approach to chronic back pain: prognostic elements of the outcome. Clin Exp Rheum 1996:14:281–288

5 Stallibrass C. An evaluation of the Alexander technique for the management of disability in Parkinson's disease – a preliminary study. Clin Rehab 1997;11:8–12

6 Maitland S, Horne R, Burton M. An exploration of the application of the Alexander technique for people with learning disabilities. Br J Learning Disabil 1996;24:70–76

7 Knebelman S. The Alexander technique in diagnosis and treatment of craniomandibular disorders. Basal Facts 1982;5:19–22

FURTHER READING

Alexander F M. The use of the self. London: Gollancz, 1996
Frederick Alexander's account of how he developed his method.

AROMATHERAPY

THERAPIES

Definition	The controlled use of plant essences for therapeutic purposes.
Related techniques	Massage.
Background	The medicinal use of plant oils has a long history in ancient Egypt, China and India. The development of modern aromatherapy is attributed to French chemist René Gattefosse, who burned his hand while working in a perfume laboratory and immediately doused it in some nearby lavender oil. The burn healed quickly without scarring, leading him to study the potential curative powers of plant oils. He coined the term aromatherapy in 1937.
Traditional concepts	Essential oils can be applied directly to the skin through massage or a compress, added to baths, inhaled with steaming water or spread throughout a room with a diffuser. The oils have effects at the psychological, physiological and cellular levels. These effects can be relaxing or stimulating depending on the chemistry of the oil and also the previous associations of the individual with a particular scent.
Scientific rationale	The scent from the oil activates the olfactory sense. This triggers the limbic system, which governs emotional responses and is involved with the formation and retrieval of learned memories. Essential oils are also absorbed through the skin via the dermis and layer of subcutaneous fat to the bloodstream. Laboratory studies suggest that molecules of the oil can affect organ function, although the clinical relevance of these findings is not clear.

Practitioners

Aromatherapy is largely unregulated. Various aromatherapy associations offer courses with the number of hours of training required ranging from 180 to 500. Many nurses and other health-care professionals routinely seek aromatherapy qualifications.

Conditions frequently treated

Musculoskeletal pain, anxiety, stress, insomnia, headaches.

Typical treatment session

During an initial session the aromatherapist will ask about a client's medical history, health and lifestyle and which aromas are liked or disliked. The therapist will then select essential oils deemed appropriate for the client according to this information. Treatment would usually consist of an aromatherapy massage and advice may be given about home treatments involving the use of oils in baths or a diffuser. The initial session may last up to 2 hours. Subsequent sessions would typically last 1 hour.

Course of treatment

For chronic conditions, one weekly session would be recommended for several weeks, with fortnightly or monthly follow-ups.

Clinical evidence

A systematic review of all RCTs of aromatherapy was conducted.[1] Based on six trials with hospitalized patients, it was concluded that aromatherapy massage has mild, transient anxiolytic effects. Due to lack of independent replication, the results of six other trials were not considered conclusive. These included positive findings for the treatment of alopecia areata[2] and prevention of bronchitis[3] and negative results for postnatal perineal discomfort.[4] Another systematic review included four RCTs of topical applications of tea tree oil.[5] There was some promising but not compelling evidence for acne and fungal infections.

Risks

Contraindications
Pregnancy, contagious disease, epilepsy, local venous thrombosis, varicose veins, broken skin, recent surgery.

Precautions/warnings
Essential oils should not be taken orally or used undiluted on the skin. Some oils cause photosensitive reactions and some have carcinogenic potential. Allergic reactions are possible with all oils.

Adverse effects
Allergic reactions, nausea, headache.

Interactions
Many essential oils are believed to have the potential to either enhance or reduce the effects of prescribed medications

including antibiotics, tranquillizers, antihistamines, anticonvulsants, barbiturates, morphine, quinidine.

Quality issues
Products marketed as 'aromatherapy oils' may be synthetic or adulterated rather than the pure essential oil.

Indirect risks
Consulting an aromatherapist for symptoms may delay appropriate treatment for a medical condition. Aromatherapy should generally be considered an adjunctive treatment, not an alternative to conventional care.

Risk–benefit assessment

Aromatherapy appears to have some benefits as a palliative or supportive treatment, particularly in reducing anxiety. In the hands of a responsible therapist there seem to be few risks so it may be worth considering as an adjunctive treatment for chronically ill patients or individuals with psychosomatic illness.

REFERENCES
1 Cooke B, Ernst E. Aromatherapy: a systematic review. Br J Gen Pract 2000;50:493–496
2 Hay I C, Jamieson M, Ormerod A D. Randomised trial of aromatherapy. Successful treatment for alopecia areata. Arch Dermatol 1998;134:1349–1352
3 Ferley J P, Poutignat N, Zmirou D et al. Prophylactic aromatherapy for supervening infections in patients with chronic bronchitis. Statistical evaluation conducted in clinics against a placebo. Phytother Res 1989;3:97–100
4 Dale A, Cornwell S. The role of lavender oil in relieving perineal discomfort following childbirth: a blind randomised clinical trial. J Adv Nurs 1994;19:89–96

5 Ernst E, Huntley A. Tea tree oil: a systematic review of randomized clinical trials. Forsch Komplementärmed Klass Naturheilkd 2000;7:17–20

FURTHER READING
Price S, Price L. Aromatherapy for health professionals, 2nd edn Edinburgh: Churchill Livingstone, 1999
Vickers A. Massage and aromatherapy: a guide for health professionals. Cheltenham: Stanley Thornes, 1998

THERAPIES

AUTOGENIC TRAINING

Synonyms

Autogenic therapy, autogenics.

Definition

Autogenic training (AT) refers to a particular technique of mental exercises involving relaxation and autosuggestion practiced regularly, which aims to teach individuals to recognize the origin of certain mental and physical disorders within themselves and to use that awareness for the self-treatment of those disturbances. In the US, the term 'autogenic' often refers to any method that involves patients using their own resources to help themselves, usually involving relaxation, visualization or autosuggestion.

Related techniques	Relaxation, self-hypnosis.
Background	AT developed out of observations in the last decade of the 19th century that people who had previously undergone hypnotic sessions were able to put themselves readily in a state which appeared to be similar to hypnosis and that the regular use of this state reduced stress and improved efficiency. In the 1930s, Schultz explored these ideas and added autosuggestion, with the aim of developing a practice which avoided the passivity and dependency of hypnosis and gave control to patients themselves. Heaviness and warmth were the two most common sensations during hypnosis, so Schultz taught patients to think about heaviness and warmth of a particular region of the body and then extend these sensations to the whole body. These constitute the first two exercises of AT. Four other instructions, relating to heart rate, breathing, warmth in the stomach and coolness of the forehead, were added to form the six standard exercises.

In the 1940s, a chest physician by the name of Luthe expanded the technique by adding the 'intentional exercises', which are tailored to the individual and involve repetition of therapeutic suggestions, designed, for example, to correct negative patterns of thought. Later, a series of meditative exercises were added for those who have gained considerable experience.

The method has spread via associations of interested practitioners, arriving in the UK in the 1970s. It is now widespread through several European countries, although it is not one of the most common complementary therapies.

Scientific rationale	There is little neurophysiological research on AT. It appears to combine the effects of profound relaxation, which probably involve the limbic system and the hypothalamo-pituitary axis, with psychotherapeutic aspects of autosuggestion.
Practitioners	Practitioners of AT frequently have other health-care training and integrate AT into their practice. German psychiatrists provide an example of this. There is no regulation or restriction on who may practice. In some countries, associations exist which continue to emphasize the classic method of Schultz and Luthe.
Conditions frequently treated	Stress responses, anxiety, phobia, depression, sleep disorders, headache, migraine, premenstrual syndrome, chronic pain, functional disorders of bladder and bowel, dyspepsia, asthma, angina pectoris, hypertension.
Typical treatment session	In a quietened room, patients (training is usually carried out in groups) are first instructed in the three recommended postures. Then they learn to concentrate passively on the heaviness of the

dominant arm and to generalize this sensation to the rest of the body. This is followed by instruction in the other standard exercises. These should be practiced three times daily, for about 10 minutes each time. Students are asked to keep diaries of their experiences in order that the process and reactions can be monitored by the tutor. When the standard exercises have been mastered, intentional exercises will be added, being devised by the instructor after a personal interview with the client. After gaining considerable experience, advanced AT can be learnt, which involves prolonging the autogenic state and performing meditative exercises on increasingly abstract concepts.

Course of treatment

Typically between eight and 10 sessions are required to learn the technique. There is no need for further attendance.

Clinical evidence

A systematic review of all controlled trials reached positive conclusions for some conditions (hypertension, asthma, intestinal diseases, glaucoma and eczema) but made no assessment of the quality of studies.[1] In a systematic review of studies of AT for hypertension, four out of five had positive results;[2] in a review of AT for anxiety (including experimentally induced anxiety) seven out of eight studies were positive.[3] However, in both cases, the quality of studies was too poor to allow firm conclusions to be drawn.

Risks

Contraindications
Severe mental disorders. Latent psychosis and personality disorders, as these may become overt with introspection. Children under 5 years.

Precautions/warnings
For medical conditions, AT should only be used as an adjunct to standard therapy. Some people have difficulty mastering the technique.

Adverse effects
Reactions to AT may occur, such as unusual sensations in the body.

Interactions
Standard therapy (e.g. for hypertension) should be monitored more regularly while learning AT in case alterations of medication are required.

Indirect risks
Use of AT for medical conditions by practitioners without medical training may constitute a risk by delaying conventional diagnosis or treatment.

Risk–benefit assessment

Although there is no firm evidence of its effectiveness compared with appropriate control interventions, patients find AT helpful

THERAPIES

for a number of conditions. It should be safe provided it is learned from someone who recognizes its limitations.

REFERENCES

1 Stetter F, Kupper S. Autogenes Training – qualitative Meta-Analyse kontrollierter klinischer Studien und Beziehungen zur Naturheilkunde. Forsch Komplementärmed 1998;5:211–223
2 Kanji N, White A R, Ernst E. Anti-hypertensive effects of autogenic training: a systematic review. Perfusion 1999;12:279–282
3 Kanji N, Ernst E. Autogenic training for stress and anxiety: a systematic review. Compl Ther Med 2000;8:106–110

FURTHER READING

Luthe W. Autogenic therapy. Vol I, autogenic methods. New York: Grune and Stratton, 1962
Luthe W. Autogenic therapy. Vol II, medical applications. New York: Grune and Stratton, 1969
Luthe W. Autogenic therapy. Vol III, applications in psychotherapy. New York: Grune and Stratton, 1969
A full description of the therapy, written by one of its founders.

BACH FLOWER REMEDIES

Synonyms

Flower remedies; flower essence therapy.

Definition

A therapeutic system that uses specially prepared plant infusions to balance physical and emotional disturbances.

Background

Dr Edward Bach was a microbiologist at the Royal London Homeopathic Hospital in the early part of the 20th century. Inspired by Hahnemann and Jung, he developed his own system of medicine. According to Dr Bach, all human disease and suffering are rooted in emotional imbalances. He identified 38 flower remedies which, he believed, could treat most illnesses.

Traditional concepts

The 38 remedies are divided into seven therapeutic groups according to the following emotions: depression, fear, lack of interest in the present, loneliness, overconcern for the welfare of others, oversensitivity and uncertainty. Bach associated each of these emotions with flowers to be used as remedies.

The remedies are produced by placing freshly picked sun-exposed flowers into spring water, into which brandy is added for preservation. The prescription of these remedies by specialized therapists is highly individualized and intuitive. According to Bach, the remedies work not through their pharmacological actions but through their 'energy'. Thus there are similarities with homeopathy, even though many homeopaths deny this.

Scientific rationale

'Energy' in this context has not been defined in scientific terms. The method is scientifically implausible.

Practitioners

Therapists employing Bach flower remedies are not usually medically qualified and often use these remedies in conjunction with other forms of CAM. Bach flower remedies are also popular for self-treatment and are available in many pharmacies and health food stores.

Conditions frequently treated

According to proponents, Bach flower remedies are not targeted at specific medical conditions but at the underlying emotional imbalances. 'Rescue remedy' (Five-Flower remedy) is promoted as a first aid for emergency situations.

Typical treatment session

Bach flower remedies are sold over the counter for self-medication. Thus many users of these remedies will not see a specialized practitioner. If they do, the therapeutic encounter will entail the taking of a detailed history with little or no physical examination. At the end of the encounter the therapist will prescribe the remedy that is, according to his or her opinion, best suited.

Course of treatment

In many instances, one prescription constitutes a full course of treatment. For persistent complaints several encounters are likely to be deemed necessary. Bach flower remedies are often recommended for long-term use.

Clinical evidence

There are numerous anecdotal reports about therapeutic successes. Very few controlled clinical trials exist and these are inconclusive, not least because of methodological weaknesses. A randomized, placebo-controlled, double-blind trial[1] tested Five-Flower remedy for examination stress in 100 university students. Its results show no significant differences in outcome compared with placebo. A similar RCT found that 61 students responded positively to both Bach flower remedies and placebo.[2] The authors therefore concluded that Bach flower remedies are an 'effective placebo for test-anxiety, which do not have a specific effect'.

Risks

Contraindications
None known.

Precautions/warnings
Contain alcohol.

Adverse effects
Because Bach flower remedies contain only very low concentrations of pharmacologically active ingredients (apart from brandy), there is little risk of adverse effects.

Interactions
None known.

Indirect risks
The possibility of indirect harm exists if treatment with Bach flower remedies hinders access to other vital forms of health care.

THERAPIES

Risk–benefit assessment

According to current evidence, Bach flower remedies are not associated with specific therapeutic effects. They are also devoid of direct risks. Thus their usefulness seems to be limited to that of a placebo therapy.

REFERENCES

1 Armstrong N C, Ernst E. A randomized, double-blind, placebo-controlled trial of Bach Flower Remedy. Perfusion 1999;11:440–446
2 Walach H, Rilling C, Engelke U. Bach flower remedies are ineffective for test anxiety: results of a blinded, placebo-controlled, randomized trial. Forsch Komplementärmed Klass Naturheilkd 2000;7:55

FURTHER READING
Bach E. The twelve healers and other remedies. Saffron Walden: C W Daniel, 1933

BIOFEEDBACK

Definition

The use of apparatus to monitor, amplify and feed back information on physiological responses so that a patient can learn to regulate those responses. It is a form of psychophysiological self-regulation.

Related techniques

Often used as an adjunct to relaxation.

Background

Control of physiological responses (breathing, heart rate, etc.) has long been a part of traditional Eastern practices such as meditation and yoga. In the 1960s, pioneers in the West working in the field of electroencephalograph (EEG) research concentrated on volunteers' attempts to reproduce alpha waves. They found this produced a state of deep relaxation, creative reverie and meditative clarity. Subsequently physiological measures other than EEG were used and the general term biofeedback was coined in 1969.

Traditional concepts

The basic concept is that the process of becoming aware of physiological responses in the body offers the opportunity to learn how to affect them. Simple attention is required, not conscious effort which may hinder the process. Any physiological response that can be monitored is suitable for biofeedback. The most common responses are electrical activity of the brain (EEG biofeedback), skin temperature (thermal), muscle tension or electromyography (EMG), galvanic skin resistance (GSR) or electrodermal resistance (EDR), blood pressure, respiratory rate and blood flow. This information is presented to the patient as a continuous visual or auditory signal. The aim of treatment is to establish the patient's mastery over the response independently of the biofeedback apparatus. Biofeedback is commonly used as an adjunct to other therapies, particularly relaxation with cognitive therapy and stress management.

THERAPIES

Scientific rationale	The ability to alter physiological responses has been repeatedly demonstrated, particularly with EEG phenomena, although the precise mechanism is unknown. This mind–body interaction presumably acts on the limbic system and thereby affects the hypothalamo-pituitary axis and autonomic control.
Practitioners	Biofeedback was originally used by counselors, clinical psychologists and behavioral therapists but its simplicity has meant that it has come to be used much more widely by a variety of health-care professionals, social workers, stress counselors, etc. A certification agency exists in the US which requires a minimum number of education hours and supervised clinical experience with the method.
Conditions frequently treated	Conditions associated with muscle tension, e.g. headaches, chronic pain, muscle spasms. Conditions that are likely to be alleviated by mental calming, e.g. stress, anxiety disorders, asthma, attention deficit disorder, migraine, substance abuse, epilepsy and sleep disorders. Conditions that may be affected directly through the physiological changes achieved, such as hypertension, enuresis, encopresis, irritable bowel syndrome and Raynaud's phenomenon.
Typical treatment session	A standard history will offer the opportunity for patient education about the presenting problem, such as the role of stress in producing symptoms. With the patient seated or lying, monitors for the response being detected (e.g. sphygmomanometer, EMG apparatus) are attached to the body. The response is converted into an audio or visual signal which is played back to the patient, who usually learns quite quickly to influence the signal in the desired direction.
Course of treatment	In many instances, patients return weekly to have their condition monitored and to repeat the biofeedback practice. Courses may vary from four to 10 sessions, depending on the condition and the individual response, and in some cases follow-up sessions will be required over a longer term. Treatment sessions last one hour initially and about 45 minutes thereafter. In many cases, home training with adjunctive techniques is encouraged by the practitioner. Some patients may prefer to purchase the apparatus in order to continue treatments in their own home. Eventually, most patients can exert control on their physiological response without the aid of the apparatus.
Clinical evidence	Systematic reviews of all clinical trials (including observational studies) of the effectiveness of biofeedback in tension headaches[1] and migraine in adults[2] and migraine in children[3] suggest that it is more effective than relaxation alone and that the combination of biofeedback and relaxation is more effective

THERAPIES

than either therapy alone. It has been suggested that the effects are due to improved self-efficacy, rather than any direct effect on the condition.[4] There is also evidence of an effect in attention deficit disorders (e.g. [5]). The physiological changes occurring with biofeedback can be directly used clinically, as shown by the increase in circulation of the lower extremity in diabetics.[6]

Risks

Contraindications
None known.

Precautions/warnings
As with other therapies that induce changes in mental state, biofeedback should be used only under medical supervision in cases of psychosis or severe personality disorder.

Adverse effects
There are occasional reports of biofeedback being associated with acute anxiety, dizziness, disorientation and floating sensations.

Interactions
In patients taking medication involved in homeostasis, such as insulin or antihypertensive therapies, the dose may need to be altered.

Indirect risks
Use of biofeedback for medical conditions without medical supervision of diagnosis and therapy may constitute a risk by delaying conventional management.

Risks–benefit assessment

Although the evidence for biofeedback is still inconclusive, its risks are very small when it is taught by competent personnel, so any perceived benefit must be of value.

REFERENCES

1 Bogaards M C D, ter Kuile M M. Treatment of recurrent tension headache: a meta-analytic review. Clin J Pain 1994,10:174–190
2 Holroyd K A, Penzien D B. Pharmacological versus non-pharmacological prophylaxis of recurrent migraine headache: a meta-analytic review of clinical trials. Pain 1990;42:1–13
3 Hermann C, Kim M, Blanchard E B. Behavioral and prophylactic pharmacological intervention studies of pediatric migraine: an exploratory meta-analysis. Pain 1995;60:239–256
4 Rokicki L A, Holroyd K A, France C R, Lipchik G L, France J L, Kvaal S A. Change mechanisms associated with combined relaxation/EMG biofeedback training for chronic tension headache. Appl Psychophysiol Biofeedback 1997;22:21–41

5 Linden M, Habib T, Radojevic V. A controlled study of the effects of EEG biofeedback on cognition and behavior of children with attention deficit disorder and learning disabilities. Biofeedback Self Regul 1996;21:35–49
6 Rice B I, Schindler J V. Effect of thermal biofeedback-assisted relaxation training on blood circulation in the lower extremities of a population with diabetes. Diabetes Care 1992;15:853–858

FURTHER READING

Basmajian J V. Biofeedback – principles and practice for clinicians. Baltimore: Williams and Wilkins, 1974
The original and classic description of the method and its applications.

CHELATION THERAPY

Synonyms	Chelation, EDTA therapy.
Definition	A method for removing toxins, minerals and metabolic wastes from the bloodstream and vessel walls using intravenous EDTA (ethylene diamine tetraacetic acid) infusions.
Background	The method was introduced in the 1950s. In mainstream medicine it is an established conventional therapy for heavy metal poisoning. Apparently some clinicians noticed that other conditions also improved in patients treated with chelation therapy. Thus it developed as an 'alternative' treatment for a number of conditions unrelated to heavy metal poisoning.
Traditional concepts and scientific rationale	It has been claimed that this therapy, through the chelating mechanism, removes calcium deposits from arteriosclerotic plaques and thus represents a causal treatment for arteriosclerosis. This rationale is based on an outdated understanding of atherogenesis. Newer theories of how chelation therapy might work for arteriosclerosis relate to other mechanisms like antioxidation, free radical scavenging, inhibition of LDL oxidation, reduction of reperfusion injury or hemorheological activity. While these are sound concepts of ischemic injury, it is unclear to what extent chelation therapy does produce such effects in vivo and whether these effects contribute to clinical changes.
Practitioners	Today, chelation therapy is used in the 'alternative' way by more than 1000 US physicians and numerous practitioners in Europe, most but not all of whom are medically qualified.
Conditions frequently treated	In CAM the method is used predominantly with a view to inducing regression of arteriosclerotic lesions, e.g. in ischemic heart disease, intermittent claudication or for stroke prevention or as an alternative to bypass surgery. Other conditions claimed to respond are arthritis, other connective tissue diseases, impaired vision, hearing, sense of smell or memory, cataracts, diabetes, emphysema, gallstones, hypertension, osteoporosis, Parkinson's disease and renal disease.
Typical treatment session	The practitioner would normally take a conventional medical history and establish a conventional diagnosis. For treatment, the patient would receive a slow infusion of EDTA usually in combination with vitamins, trace elements and iron supplements. One session might last for about an hour or longer.
Course of treatment	One single treatment is rarely deemed sufficient. A course of treatments often involves 10–30 sessions over several months.

THERAPIES

The costs for a course of treatments are usually around US $3000.

Clinical evidence

One systematic review of all four randomized, placebo-controlled, double-blind trials of chelation therapy for intermittent claudication found no convincing evidence for efficacy.[1] It concluded, 'Chelation therapy for peripheral arterial occlusive disease is not superior to placebo ... It should now be considered obsolete'.[1]

Another systematic review included all controlled and uncontrolled clinical studies of chelation therapy for ischemic heart disease regardless of trial design.[2] Numerous case reports and case series but only two controlled clinical trials were found. The latter study yielded no convincing evidence for efficacy. It concluded, 'This treatment should now be considered obsolete'.[2]

Risks

Contraindications
Not clearly defined by chelation therapists.

Precautions/warnings
Renal insufficiency, pregnancy, bleeding abnormalities.

Adverse effects
Renal failure, arrhythmias, tetany, hypocalcemia, hypoglycemia, hypotension, bone marrow depression, prolonged bleeding time, convulsions, respiratory arrest and autoimmune diseases have all been described. Several fatalities have been reported with little doubt about the causal role of chelation therapy.

Interactions
Calcium supplementation, renal clearance of drugs.

Indirect risks
Lost time for a potentially life-saving intervention (e.g. bypass surgery).

Risk–benefit assessment

The documented risks of chelation therapy as used in CAM clearly outweigh the benefits. Proponents of chelation therapy might argue that, with more refined treatment regimens, the problems of the 'early days' have been overcome. Yet, in the absence of reliable supporting data, this notion is unconvincing. Thus chelation therapy is not recommended for indications other than heavy metal poisoning.

REFERENCES
1 Ernst E. Chelation therapy for peripheral arterial occlusive disease. Circulation 1997;96:1031–1033
2 Ernst E. Chelation therapy for coronary heart disease. An overview of all clinical investigations. Am Heart J 2000;140:139–141

FURTHER READING
Gier M T, Meyers D G. So much writing, so little science. A review of 37 years of literature on EDTA chelation therapy. Ann Pharmacother 1993;27:1504–1509
A concise review of the postulated mechanisms of action and the clinical evidence.

CHIROPRACTIC

Definition   A system of health care which is based on the belief that the nervous system is the most important determinant of health and that most diseases are caused by spinal subluxations which respond to spinal manipulation.

Related techniques   Osteopathy, manual therapy, spinal manipulation, spinal mobilization.

Background   Some therapeutic elements which chiropractors use, such as spinal manipulation, go back to antiquity and were used by bonesetters throughout the history of (folk) medicine. In 1895 the founder of chiropractic, D D Palmer (1845–1913), a grocery store owner in the US Midwest, manipulated the neck of a janitor, thereby allegedly curing his deafness. Chiropractic was born. The term chiropractic was derived by Palmer from the Greek *cheir* (hand) and *praxis* (action).

During subsequent decades, chiropractic had a colorful history dominated by the bickering between various subsets of the chiropractic profession. The 'straights' adhere to Palmer's teaching as to a dogma, while the 'mixers' have a more liberal attitude. During much of the last century, a fierce debate also raged between mainstream medicine and chiropractic. More recently, chiropractors have become accepted health-care professionals and their treatments are now being evaluated objectively according to the principles of evidence-based medicine.

Traditional concepts   Palmer reasoned that the normal muscular tone produced pressure on nerves. Disease, he argued, is caused by malalignment or subluxation of the vertebral joints, causing excessive or deficient pressure on the spinal nerves. Adjusting vertebrae was deemed to be the only correct way of restoring health. Chiropractors use several manual therapeutic and diagnostic techniques. Their most important therapeutic method is spinal manipulation. It entails high-velocity, low-amplitude manual thrusts to spinal joints to extend them slightly beyond their normal passive range of motion. Spinal mobilization, by contrast, is the application of manual force to such joints without thrust and within the normal passive range of motion.

Scientific rationale   The primary premise that subluxation is the cause of all illness has no scientific rationale. Spinal mobilization has been shown to have a number of physiological effects (such as reduction of muscle spasm, inhibition of nociceptive transmissions) and intuitively one may feel that this and related techniques improve joint function and alleviate pain related to spinal abnormalities.

THERAPIES

Practitioners

By definition, chiropractic is what chiropractors do. However, spinal manipulation and mobilization are also used by osteopaths, naturopaths, physical therapists and doctors. Both in the US and the UK, chiropractors need a license for practice.

Conditions frequently treated

Musculoskeletal problems, more specifically spinal pain syndromes; asthma, cardiovascular problems, migraine, headache, irritable bowel syndrome.

Typical treatment session

A chiropractor takes the patient's medical history and conducts a thorough physical examination. In most cases, this is supplemented by spinal X-rays and possibly other tests. The initial encounter can be purely diagnostic. During subsequent treatment sessions, the patient is required to partly undress. Treatment invariably involves hands-on techniques, usually with the patient sitting or lying. Sessions may last for 20 minutes or longer.

Course of treatment

The number of sessions required is highly variable. One series of treatment might require 5–20 sessions. Often repetitive courses of treatments or continuing prophylactic sessions are recommended.

Clinical evidence

Numerous systematic reviews of (chiropractic) spinal manipulation have been published. A recent and thorough 'best evidence synthesis' conducted by a chiropractor[1] suggested that 'There is moderate evidence of short-term efficacy for spinal manipulation in the treatment of acute low back pain (LBP)' and 'Moderate evidence that it is efficacious when compared with placebo and commonly used therapies such as general practitioners' management for chronic LBP'. For mixed acute and chronic low back pain and for sciatica, the evidence was deemed inconclusive. Other systematic reviews arrive at a considerably more negative judgement (see Back pain, p 223). In the light of various national guidelines which include recommendations to use chiropractic in the treatment of LBP, these results may seem surprising. Yet, two recent trials, which were not included in the above analysis[1] and did not demonstrate a convincing benefit of chiropractic over other forms of routine LBP treatments[2,3] suggest that these judgements might even be overoptimistic. The bottom line of this somewhat confusing situation is that the effectiveness of chiropractic treatment of back pain is uncertain.

A systematic review of spinal manipulation for non-migrainous headaches included six RCTs with a total of 286 patients and suggested encouraging, albeit not fully convincing therapeutic effects.[4] In particular, the authors comment that no high-quality studies exist in this area.

Numerous other conditions have been assessed by CCTs. However, the paucity of data and their low average quality prevent firm conclusions.

Risks

Contraindications

Advanced osteoporosis, bleeding abnormalities, malignant or inflammatory spinal disease, patients on anticoagulants.

Precautions/warnings

Elderly patients, people who feel uncomfortable with close contact.

Adverse effects

Serious adverse effects are probably rare and include arterial dissection and stroke (upper spinal manipulation) and cauda equina syndrome (lower spinal manipulation).[5,6] Mild and transient adverse effects such as local discomfort are reported by about 50% of all patients.[7,8]

Interactions

Patients on anticoagulants are at a higher risk of cerebrovascular accidents.

Indirect risks

Hindering or delaying access to effective conventional treatment for serious conditions, overuse of X-ray diagnostics, advice of some chiropractors against immunization (see p 413), unreliability of diagnostic techniques used by chiropractors (see p 18).

Risk–benefit assessment

Even though the evidence is by no means fully convincing, chiropractic treatment might be helpful for acute and chronic low back pain. In view of the lack of truly effective conventional treatments for LBP, chiropractic might therefore be worth considering for such patients. The risks of chiropractic may be infrequent in relation to life-threatening events but seem to be considerable as far as mild, transient complaints are concerned.

THERAPIES

REFERENCES

1 Bronfort G. Spinal manipulation, current state of research and its indications. Neurol Clin North Am 1999;17:91–111

2 Cherkin D C, Deyo R A, Battie M, Street J, Barlow W. A comparison of physical therapy, chiropractic manipulation and provision of an educational booklet for the treatment of patients with low back pain. New Engl J Med 1998;339:1021–1029

3 Skargren E, Oberg B E. Predictive factors for 1-year outcome of low-back and neck pain in patients treated in primary care: comparison between the treatment strategies chiropractic and physiotherapy. Pain 1998;77:201–207

4 Vernon H, McDermaid C S, Hagino C. Systematic review of randomized clinical trials of complementary/alternative therapies in the treatment of tension-type and cervicogenic headache. Compl Ther Med 1999;7:142–155

5 Assendelft W J, Bouter L M, Knipschild P G. Complications of spinal manipulation. J Fam Pract 1996;42:475–480

6 Fibio R. Manipulation of the cervical spine: risks and benefits. Physical Ther 1999; 79:50–65

7 Senstad O, Leboeuf-Yde C, Borchgrevink C. Frequency and characteristics of side effects of spinal manipulative therapy. Spine 1997; 22:435–441

8 Leboeuf-Yde C, Hennius B, Rudberg E,
Leufvenmark P, Thunman M. Side effects of
chiropractic treatment: a prospective study.
J Manip Physiol Therapeut 1997;20:511–515

FURTHER READING
Grieve G P. Modern manual therapy of the
vertebral column. Churchill Livingstone,
Edinburgh, 1986

CRANIOSACRAL THERAPY

Synonyms/subcategories

Cranial osteopathy, craniooccipital technique.

Definition

A proprietary form of therapeutic manipulation which is 'tissue-, fluid-, membrane-, and energy-oriented and more subtle than any other type of cranial work'.

Related techniques

Osteopathy.

Background

The technique was developed in the 1970s by J E Upledger as a refinement of concepts originally put forward by W G Sutherland (cranial osteopathy) in the 1930s. It became popular first in the US and subsequently also in Europe.

Traditional concepts

Craniosacral therapy is based on the notion that movement restrictions at the sutures of the skull negatively affect rhythmic impulses conveyed through the cerebrospinal fluid from the cranium to the sacrum. Through gentle manipulation on the skull, therapists aim at normalizing these movement restrictions which, in turn, is thought to alleviate a large range of symptoms. According to Upledger, an osteopathic physician and the originator of craniosacral therapy, the circulation of the cerebrospinal fluid can be sensed in a similar way to a peripheral pulse. Therapy consists of light touch over various points of pulsation which is claimed to normalize the cerebrospinal circulation and thus improve function of the nervous system.[1]

Scientific rationale

Even though small movements between cranial bones are possible,[2] there is no good evidence to suggest that restrictions of these movements have any health-related relevance.

Practitioners

Craniosacral therapy is practiced by chiropractors, osteopaths, naturopaths, physiotherapists, dentists, physicians and other regulated or unregulated health-care professionals.

Conditions frequently treated

According to Upledger the following conditions respond to craniosacral therapy: birth trauma, chronic pain, cerebral dysfunction, cerebral palsy, colic, depression, dyslexia, ear infections, headaches, learning disabilities, Ménière's disease, musculoskeletal problems, migraine, sinusitis, strabismus, stroke, trigeminal neuralgia. Young children are believed to respond particularly well.

Typical treatment session

The initial diagnostic session is conducted by a craniosacral therapist in order to evaluate the nature of the problem. The patient may be lying down or sitting. The procedure mainly involves touching the skull and/or sacrum of the patient and applying mild pressure. The first session may take about half an hour. Subsequent therapeutic sessions are usually shorter.

Course of treatment

The number of sessions required is extremely variable and depends on the nature and severity of the condition(s) treated. Upledger states that if no effect is seen after about six sessions, craniosacral therapy may not be effective.

Clinical evidence

Upledger claims that his method 'is helpful in at least 90% of the patients'.[1] However, a thorough review of the evidence by the Canadian Office of Health Technology Assessment concluded that there is 'insufficient evidence to support craniosacral therapy'.[2] No controlled trials seem to exist and none are cited by Upledger himself.[1]

Risks

Contraindications
Intracranial aneurysm, cerebral hemorrhage, subdural or subarachnoid bleeding, increased intracranial pressure.

Precautions/warnings
None known.

Adverse effects
Some undesired effects were reported in patients with traumatic brain syndrome;[3] temporary worsening of symptoms and mild discomfort may occur.[1]

Interactions
According to proponents of the technique, the possibility exists of enhancement of antidiabetic, antiepileptic or psychoactive medications.[1]

Indirect risks
Access to conventional treatments might be hindered.

Risk–benefit assessment

There are no well-documented benefits beyond non-specific (e.g. placebo) effects but several indirect and direct risks have been associated with craniosacral therapy. On balance, therefore, craniosacral therapy cannot be recommended for any condition.

THERAPIES

REFERENCES

1 Upledger J E. Craniosacral therapy. In: Novey D W (ed) The complete reference to complementary and alternative medicine. St Louis: Mosby, 2000

2 Green C, Martin C W, Bassett K, Kazanjian A. A systematic review of craniosacral therapy: biological plausibility, assessment reliability

and clinical effectiveness. Compl Ther Med
1999;7:201–207

3 Greenman P E, McPartland J M. Cranial
findings and iatrogenesis from craniosacral
manipulation in patients with traumatic brain
syndrome. J Am Osteopath Assoc
1995;95:182–188

FURTHER READING

Hollenberg S, Dennis M. An introduction to
craniosacral therapy. Physiotherapy 1994;
80:528–532
A concise introduction to the subject.

HERBALISM

Synonyms/ subcategories

Ayurveda, botanical medicine, Chinese herbalism, European herbalism, herbal medicine, kampo, medical herbalism, phyto-medicine, phytotherapy.

Definition

The medical use of preparations that contain exclusively plant material.

Background

Plants have been used since the dawn of humanity for medicinal purposes and form the origin of much of modern medicine (e.g. digoxin from *Digitalis purpurea* or artemether from *Artemisia annua* for severe malaria). Modern Western herbalism or phytomedicine as practiced in many European countries (e.g. Germany) is integrated into conventional medicine with compulsory education and training for physicians and pharmacists. Other more traditional systems include Chinese herbal medicine, which is based on the concepts of Yin and Yang and qi energy. Ill health is viewed as a pattern of disharmony or imbalance and Chinese herbal medicines are believed to harmonize these energies and ultimately restore health. In Japan this system of traditional herbal medicine has evolved into kampo. Ayurveda, the traditional medical system of India, also frequently uses herbal mixtures.

Characteristic of these systems is a high degree of individualization of treatment, e.g. two patients with the same disease according to Western criteria could receive two different herbal preparations. Contrary to modern phytotherapy, all traditional herbal medicine systems predominantly employ complex mixtures of different herbs.

Traditional concepts

Whole plants, parts of plants or extracts are used. The different constituents of a single plant or of herbal mixtures are claimed to work synergistically to produce a greater effect than the sum of the effects of the single constituents. It is also claimed that the combined actions of the various constituents reduce the toxicity of the extract as compared with the single isolated constituent. These concepts of synergy and buffering extend to the use of different plant extracts in combination preparations. In traditional herbal medicine the diagnostic principles used differ considerably from those in mainstream medicine, with less emphasis on conventional disease categories and modern diagnostic techniques. Modern herbalism as practiced in most European countries follows the diagnostic principles of conventional medicine.

Scientific rationale

Herbal extracts contain plant material with pharmacologically active constituents. The active principle(s) of the extract, which is in many cases unknown, may exert its effects on the molecular level and may have, for instance, enzyme-inhibiting effects (e.g. escin). A single main constituent may be active or, more often, a complex mixture of structurally related compounds produces a combined effect. Known active constituents or marker substances may be used to standardize preparations.

Practitioners

Most traditional herbalists in the UK and the US are not medically qualified. In contrast to the situation in continental Europe, there is little integration into the conventional healthcare systems. In countries such as Germany and France much of herbalism, particularly modern Western herbalism, is practiced by conventionally trained physicians and integrated into routine medical care.

Conditions frequently treated

A wide range of conditions are treated; for instance, anxiety, depression, benign prostatic hyperplasia, intermittent claudication and many more.

Typical treatment session

During an initial treatment session the practitioner will usually take the patient's medical history to get an overall impression of the medical status and to screen for contraindications. Herbalists of the Chinese, Japanese and Ayurvedic traditions will also seek information on the patient's personality and background, which may influence the selection of herbs. Individualized combinations of herbs are prescribed and may be taken as extracts, tinctures, infusions or decoctions. Follow-up appointments are arranged as necessary and herbal preparations and regimen reviewed and changed if appropriate. Practitioners may advise on lifestyle factors such as diet and exercise. Consultations and treatment as practiced on the European continent generally follow the principles of a conventional medical appointment.

Course of treatment

Depending largely on the nature and severity of the condition but generally 1–2 appointments per week for a treatment period of one to several weeks.

Clinical evidence

The clinical evidence has to be evaluated according to each individual herbal preparation (see Section 4) or traditional approach. There is good clinical evidence for the effectiveness of

THERAPIES

a number of herbal monopreparations for the treatment of, for instance, anxiety,[1] benign prostatic hyperplasia,[2] depression[3-5] and intermittent claudication.[6] Traditional Chinese herbal mixtures have been assessed in a number of studies, although many are of poor methodological quality.[7] Little evidence exists, for instance, for the treatment of eczema,[8] while some positive findings relate to irritable bowel syndrome.[9] The latter study is one of the few which compared individualized prescriptions with a non-individualized approach. No superiority of the former over the latter was reported.[9] There is also limited evidence for the effectiveness of Ayurvedic herbal treatments.[10] Generally, there is a lack of comparative trials of any type of medical herbalism against conventional medications.

Risks

Contraindications

Contraindications and precautions vary for each individual herbal preparation (see Section 4) but usually include pregnancy and lactation.

Precautions/warnings

Precautions vary for each individual herbal preparation (see Section 4).

Adverse effects

Plant extracts may have powerful pharmacological effects and therefore the risk of adverse effects is probably greater than with most other complementary therapies. The reader is referred to the information on the individual herbs in Section 4.

Interactions

Possible interactions between different herbal preparations or with conventional drugs should generally be assumed and relevant patients should be closely monitored. Patients should be asked about self-prescription drug use.

Quality issues

The amount of active constituent may vary and depends on a variety of different factors such as time of harvest, type of soil or amount of sunlight and rain. Products may be contaminated with other plant material or adulterated or plants may be misidentified.

Indirect risks

In cases where the therapist is not medically qualified, appropriate treatment of a medical condition may be delayed.

Risk–benefit assessment

The most convincing evidence that exists in the area of complementary medicine probably relates to a number of herbal extracts (monopreparations), suggesting effectiveness for various conditions. The possibility of adverse effects has to be considered and the risk–benefit ratio has to be assessed for each herbal preparation individually. A number of conditions exist for which conventional medical treatment is not satisfactory and herbalism may provide a possible option.

REFERENCES

1 Pittler M H, Ernst E. Efficacy of kava for treating anxiety: systematic review and meta-analysis. J Clin Psychopharmacol 2000; 20:84–89

2 Wilt T J, Ishani A, Stark G, MacDonald R, Lau J, Mulrow C. Saw palmetto extracts for treatment of benign prostatic hyperplasia. JAMA 1998;280:1604–1609

3 Linde K, Ramirez G, Mulrow C D, Pauls A, Weidenhammer W, Melchart D. St John's wort for depression – an overview and meta-analysis of randomised clinical trials. Br Med J 1996;313:253–258

4 Stevinson C, Ernst E. Hypericum for depression. An update of the clinical evidence. Eur Neuropsychopharmacol 1999;9:501–505

5 Gaster B, Holroyd J. St John's wort for depression. Arch Intern Med 2000; 160:152–156

6 Pittler M H, Ernst E. The efficacy of Ginkgo biloba extract for the treatment of intermittent claudication. A meta-analysis of randomized clinical trials. Am J Med 2000; 108: 276–281

7 Kaptchuk T J. The state of clinical research in traditional Chinese medicine in China. Focus Compl Alt Ther 2000;5:26–27

8 Armstrong N C, Ernst E. The treatment of eczema with Chinese herbs: a systematic review of randomized clinical trials. Br J Clin Pharmacol 1999;48:262–264

9 Bensousson A, Talley N J, Hing M, Menzies R, Guo A, Ngu M. Treatment of irritable bowel syndrome with Chinese herbal medicine. A randomized controlled trial. JAMA 1998; 280:1585–1589

10 Lodha R, Bagga A. Traditional Indian systems of medicine. Ann Acad Med Singapore 2000; 29:37–41

FURTHER READING

Ernst E (ed). Herbal medicine. Oxford: Butterworth Heinemann, 2000
A concise overview for professionals.
Boon H, Smith M. The botanical pharmacy. Canada: Quarry Press, 1999
An evidence-based approach to the pharmacology and therapeutic use of 47 common herbs.

THERAPIES

HOMEOPATHY

Definition	A therapeutic method using preparations of substances whose effects when administered to healthy subjects correspond to the manifestations of the disorder (symptoms, clinical signs and pathological states) in the unwell patient.
Related techniques	Autoisopathy, bioemic medicine, homotoxic therapy, isopathy, tautopathy.
Background	Homeopathy became popular first in Europe and later in the US during the second half of the 19th century. With the advent of effective drug treatments in the early part of the 20th century, its popularity significantly decreased in most countries. Today, it is again becoming more widely available due to a general trend towards CAM. Many schools of homeopathy exist.

Traditional concepts

Homeopathy is built on two independent assumptions. The law of similars or 'like cures like' principle states that a remedy which causes a certain symptom (e.g. a headache) in healthy volunteers can be used to treat a headache in individuals who suffer from it. According to the second assumption, homeopathic remedies become stronger rather than weaker when submitted to 'potentization', which describes stepwise dilution combined with 'sucussion', i.e. vigorous shaking of the mixture. Thus remedies are believed to be clinically effective even if they are so dilute that they are likely not to contain a single molecule of the substance.

Scientific rationale

Even though examples can be found where the 'like cures like' principle does apply (e.g. digitalis), it is not a universal principle or natural law. There is no scientific rationale for assuming that remedies devoid of pharmacologically active molecules can produce clinical effects. Moreover, homeopathic 'provings', which form the basis for therapeutic selection, often lack scientific rigor and are therefore unconvincing.

Practitioners

Homeopathy is practiced by both medically qualified and non-medically qualified practitioners.

Conditions frequently treated

Homeopaths do not usually use conventional disease categories. Their aim is to match a patient's individual symptoms with a 'drug picture' (i.e. a set of symptoms caused by a remedy in healthy volunteers). Homeopaths often see patients with benign chronic conditions.

Typical treatment session

A first consultation might take 1 1/2 hours or longer. Homeopaths take a most detailed history and explore the patient's problems in much detail, with a view to finding the optimally matching homeopathic drug ('simile'). They put considerably less emphasis on physical examination than conventional physicians.

Course of treatment

Homeopaths believe that the treatment of a long-standing problem is necessarily prolonged. Thus they would typically insist on numerous consultations during which the prescriptions can be altered according to the changes in symptomatology.

Clinical evidence

Homeopathy (and other forms of CAM) was strongly promoted by Nazi officials in Germany. During this time a thorough scientific evaluation of homeopathy was initiated. Its results have never been published, but a thorough eyewitness report suggests that no evidence in favor of homeopathy emerged.[1] A more recent metaanalysis[2] of all homeopathic, placebo-controlled RCTs showed that the risk ratio for clinical improvement with homeopathy was 2.45 times that with placebo. This positive overall result for homeopathy has attracted much criticism. Similar analyses of the efficacy of a specific remedy[3] or condition[4,5] yielded no convincing evidence of clinical effectiveness.

Risks

Contraindications
Life-threatening conditions.

Precautions/warnings
Do not expose remedies to bright light or other radiation.

Adverse effects
In about 20% of cases homeopaths observe an aggravation of symptoms (which they believe is a positive sign indicating that the correct remedy has been given); in low dilutions homeopathic remedies can have adverse effects such as allergic reactions.

Interactions
Several medicines (e.g. corticosteroids, antibiotics) are believed to block the actions of homeopathic drugs; convincing evidence is not available.

Indirect risks
Access to conventional treatments might be hindered; for instance, many non-medically trained homeopaths advise their clients against immunization of children.[6]

Risk–benefit assessment

Based on the available trial evidence to date, the effectiveness of homeopathic remedies can be neither confirmed nor ruled out. There are few risks associated with homeopathy. Thus the evidence is insufficient for firm recommendations. The adjunctive use of homeopathic remedies for chronic, stable conditions might be tolerated in cases where patients feel a desire to be treated homeopathically.

THERAPIES

REFERENCES

1 Donner F. Bemerkungen zu der Überprüfung der Homöopathie durch das Reichsgesundheitsamt 1936–1939. Perfusion 1995;8:3–7 (Part 1), 35–40 (Part 2), 84–88 (Part 3), 124–129 (Part 4), 164–166 (Part 5)

2 Linde K, Clausius N, Ramirez G, Melchart D, Eitel F, Hedges L V, Jonas W. Are the clinical effects of homeopathy placebo effects? A meta-analysis of placebo-controlled trials. Lancet 1997;350:834–843

3 Ernst E, Pittler M H. Efficacy of homeopathic arnica. A systematic review of placebo-controlled clinical trials. Arch Surg 1998;133:1187–1190

4 Ernst E, Barnes J. Are homeopathic remedies effective for delayed-onset muscle soreness? A systematic review of placebo-controlled trials. Perfusion 1998;11:4–8

5 Ernst E. Homeopathic prophylaxis of headaches and migraine? A systematic review. J Pain Sympt Manage 1999;18:353–357

FURTHER READING

Bellavite P, Signorini A. Homeopathy, a frontier in medical science. Berkeley, CA: North Atlantic Books, 1995
A thorough justification of homeopathic concepts from a homeopathic perspective.

Ernst E, Hahn E G (eds). Homeopathy. A critical appraisal. Oxford: Butterworth Heinemann, 1998
An introduction to several aspects of homeopathy written for health-care professionals.

Swayne J. International dictionary of homeopathy. Edinburgh: Churchill Livingstone, 2000
A definitive clarification of terms and concepts.

HYPNOTHERAPY

Definition

The induction of a trance-like state to facilitate the relaxation of the conscious mind and make use of enhanced suggestibility to treat psychological and medical conditions and effect behavioral changes.

Related techniques

Self-hypnosis, imagery, autogenic training, meditation, relaxation.

Background

Hypnotic practices have been traced at least as far back as ancient Egypt, but the first therapeutic use has been attributed to charismatic Austrian physician Franz Anton Mesmer in 1778 from whom the word mesmerism came. He devised a treatment based on magnetism that was hugely successful until a Royal Commission investigated the method and concluded that the effects were due entirely to imagination. Mesmerism saw a revival in the 1800s when British surgeon James Esdaile used it as the sole anesthetic when performing major operations in India. Another British doctor, James Braid, is credited with making hypnosis respectable to the medical community and in the 1950s the British and American Medical Associations recognized hypnosis as a legitimate medical procedure.

Traditional concepts

The goal of hypnotherapy is to gain self-control over behavior, emotions or physiological processes. This is achieved by the induction of the hypnotic trance (often called an altered state of consciousness) where the conscious mind is subdued, thereby allowing easier access to the non-critical unconscious mind which is more receptive to suggestion. A good rapport between the therapist and patient or client is vital, but a fundamental principle of hypnotic phenomena is that the hypnotized individual is under his own control and not that of the hypnotist or anyone else. It is argued consequently that all hypnosis is really self-hypnosis and the therapist should actually be called a facilitator.

Scientific rationale

Hypnosis is associated with a deep state of relaxation. Whether this represents a specific altered state of consciousness has been the subject of fierce scientific debate. It has repeatedly been shown that analgesia and many other hypnotic phenomena can be achieved by means of suggestion alone without hypnotizing individuals. However, in defense of the genuineness and importance of the hypnotic trance it has been argued that highly suggestible (or hypnotizable) individuals are easily able to enter a hypnotic state without requiring formal induction. The means by which hypnotic suggestion enables involuntary processes such as skin temperature, heart rate and gut secretions to be deliberately controlled is not fully understood. It may be that hypnosis is essentially just a specific type of relaxation technique.

Practitioners

The credentials and duration of training of hypnotherapists vary widely. The number of hours of training may range from 300 to 1600. Most therapists are not medically qualified. However, many doctors, dentists and psychologists are trained as clinical hypnotherapists and make use of hypnosis during their practice.

Conditions frequently treated

Psychosomatic conditions, anxiety, stress, pain, addictions, phobia.

Typical treatment session

Sessions typically last between 30 and 90 minutes. The initial visit involves the gathering of history and discussion about hypnosis, suggestion and the client's expectations of the therapy. Tests for hypnotic suggestibility may also be conducted. Hypnotic induction may or may not be part of the first session. The hypnotic state is achieved by first relaxing the body, then shifting attention away from the external environment towards a narrow range of objects or ideas suggested by the therapist. Sometimes hypnotherapy is carried out in group settings, e.g. antenatal classes as preparation for labor.

Course of treatment

Varies according to the individual, but an average course is 6–12 weekly sessions.

Clinical evidence

A metaanalysis of 18 controlled trials suggested that hypnotherapy enhances the effects of cognitive-behavioral psychotherapy for various conditions, including anxiety, insomnia, pain, hypertension and obesity.[1] A subsequent review reiterated the positive results but concluded that due to methodological limitation, efficacy was unresolved.[2] A systematic review of nine RCTs of smoking cessation concluded that hypnotherapy was no more effective than no treatment or other interventions.[3] Another review of 59 studies of various designs also suggested that hypnosis was not effective for this indication.[4] A metaanalysis of 18 studies of the analgesic effects of hypnosis found a moderate to large positive effect in pain management.[5] A review of a wide range of medical conditions suggested that there is reasonable evidence from clinical trials for the use of hypnosis in preparation for surgery, treatment of asthma, dermatological conditions, irritable bowel syndrome, hemophilia and nausea and emesis in oncology.[6] A systematic review of studies of hypnotherapy for posttraumatic conditions[7] located only one RCT,[8] preventing a firm conclusion regarding effectiveness. A review of 15 controlled trials of hypnosis in children found promising findings for

THERAPIES

pain, enuresis and chemotherapy-related distress, but no compelling evidence.[9]

Risks

Contraindications
Psychosis, personality disorders, epilepsy, children under 5 years.

Precautions/warnings
Information elicited under hypnosis is subject to confabulation.

Adverse effects
Recovering repressed memories can be painful and psychological problems may be exacerbated. False memory syndrome has been reported. Studies investigating negative consequences of hypnosis have concluded that when practiced by a clinically trained professional, it is safe.

Indirect risks
Visiting a hypnotherapist rather than consulting a doctor for a medical condition may delay appropriate treatment.

Risk–benefit assessment

Although the evidence in favor of hypnotherapy is not compelling and risks do exist, it appears on balance to be a valuable tool for pain management and various other conditions with a psychosomatic component, when performed by a qualified and responsible practitioner. It may be particularly effective with children.

REFERENCES

1 Kirsch I, Montgomery G, Sapirstein G. Hypnosis as an adjunct to cognitive-behavioural psychotherapy: a meta-analysis. J Consult Clin Psychol 1995;63:214–220

2 Schoenberger N E. Research on hypnosis as an adjunct to cognitive-behavioural psychotherapy. Int J Clin Exp Hypn 2000;48:154–169

3 Abbot N C, Stead L F, White A R, Barnes J, Ernst E. Hypnotherapy for smoking cessation (Cochrane Review). In: Cochrane Library. Oxford: Update Software,1998

4 Green J P, Lynn S J. Hypnosis and suggestion-based approaches to smoking cessation: an examination of the evidence. Int J Clin Exp Hypn 2000;48:195–224

5 Montgomery G H, Du Hamel K N, Redd W H. A meta-analysis of hypnotically induced analgesia: how effective is hypnosis? Int J Clin Exp Hypn 2000;48:138–153

6 Pinnell C M, Covino N A. Empirical findings on the use of hypnosis in medicine: a critical review. Int J Clin Exp Hypn 2000;48:170–194

7 Cardeña E. Hypnosis in the treatment of trauma: a promising, but not fully supported, efficacious intervention. Int J Clin Exp Hypn 2000;48:125–138

8 Brom D, Kleber R J, Defares P B. Brief psychotherapy for posttraumatic stress disorders. J Consult Clin Psychol 1989;57:607–612

9 Milling L S, Costantino C A. Clinical hypnosis with children: first steps toward empirical support. Int J Clin Exp Hypn 2000; 48:113–137

FURTHER READING

Lynn S J, Kirsch I, Barabasz A, Cardeña E, Patterson D. Hypnosis as an empirically supported clinical intervention: the state of the evidence and a look to the future. Int J Clin Exp Hypn 2000;48:239–259
Summary of the state of the evidence according to recent systematic reviews and metaanalyses.

MASSAGE

Definition	A method of manipulating the soft tissue of whole body areas using pressure and traction. (This discussion predominantly focuses on 'Swedish massage'.)
Related techniques	Aromatherapy, reflexology.
Background	Massage is one of the oldest forms of treatment. The development of modern massage is attributed to the Swede Per Henrik Ling, who developed an integrated system consisting of massage and exercises, which was later termed 'Swedish massage'. In the middle of the 19th century it was introduced in the US and was practiced predominantly by physicians until the early 20th century. The interest in massage therapy gradually declined but increased again in the 1970s. Today massage is considered a complementary therapy in many countries and more gentle techniques than the vigorous treatment recommended by Ling are frequently used. In some European countries (e.g. Germany), however, massage continues to be part of conventional medicine.
Traditional concepts	Massage is applied using various manual techniques, applying pressure and traction to manipulate the soft tissues of the body. Touch is fundamental to massage therapy and allows the therapist to locate areas of muscle tension. These areas can be treated, conveying a sense of caring using touch with the optimal amount of pressure for each person.
Scientific rationale	The friction of the hands and the mechanical pressure exerted on cutaneous and subcutaneous structures affect the body. The circulation of blood and lymph is generally enhanced, resulting in increased oxygen supply and allegedly in the removal of waste products. Direct mechanical pressure and effects mediated by the nervous system beneficially affect areas of increased muscular tension.
Practitioners	In the US massage is often practiced by nurses and a variety of training courses are available aimed specifically at nurses and other health-care professionals. The number of hours of training required varies greatly and examinations by the International Therapy Examinations Council are the most widely accepted. The number of professional massage therapists employed in hospitals and general practices is increasing. In other countries such as Germany, massage is fully registered and a recognized profession.

THERAPIES

THERAPIES

Conditions frequently treated

Back pain and other musculoskeletal disorders, constipation, anxiety, depression, stress and many other conditions.

Typical treatment session

During an initial treatment session the therapist will usually take the patient's medical history to get an overall impression of the medical status and screen for contraindications. The duration of individual treatment sessions varies depending on the condition, but will usually be about 30 minutes. Patients are normally treated unclothed with a sheet or towel provided.

Usually the massage is performed on a specially designed massage couch. Therapists often use oil to facilitate movement of their hands over the patient's body. The five fundamental techniques used in massage are effleurage, pétrissage, friction, tapotement and vibration. Sometimes sessions are followed by other treatments such as external heat applications. Most patients are advised to rest for about 20 minutes after a treatment session.

Course of treatment

Usually, 1–2 sessions per week for a treatment period of 4–8 weeks would be initially recommended.

Clinical evidence

A systematic review assessed the evidence on abdominal massage for constipation.[1] Based on four CCTs, it was cautiously concluded that abdominal massage could be a promising treatment option for this condition. Another systematic review[2] of four CCTs for the treatment of low back pain concluded that it seems to have some potential. A Cochrane Review reported that the evidence to support massage as a treatment to promote development in preterm and/or low birth-weight infants is weak.[3] Some evidence from RCTs suggested positive effects of massage for anxiety, for instance in depressed adolescent mothers,[4] women with premenstrual syndrome[5] and in elderly institutionalized patients.[6] In patients with fibromyalgia it has been suggested to relieve pain and depression and improve quality of life.[7]

Risks

Contraindications
Phlebitis, deep vein thrombosis, burns, skin infections, eczema, open wounds, bone fractures, advanced osteoporosis.

Precautions/warnings
Cancer, myocardial infarction, osteoporosis, pregnancy, individuals who feel uncomfortable with close contact.

Adverse effects
Adverse effects are extremely rare. However, bone fractures and liver rupture have been reported.

Interactions

Interactions and adverse effects attributable to oils, which may be used, are not considered in the assessment of risks involved in massage. The medical history should, however, include questions relating to any allergic predisposition.

Indirect risks

Massage should generally be considered as an adjunctive treatment, not as an alternative to conventional care.

Risk–benefit assessment

Massage appears to have some beneficial effects in a number of conditions such as constipation, back pain, anxiety, depression and stress. Given the few risks involved when performed by a responsible, well-trained practitioner, it may be worth considering. Its comparative effectiveness against other complementary therapies or against conventional treatment approaches is unclear. Given its relaxing effects, massage may have some, albeit non-specific, beneficial influence on the well-being of most patients.

REFERENCES

1 Ernst E. Abdominal massage therapy for chronic constipation: a systematic review of controlled clinical trials. Forsch Komplementärmed 1999;6:149–151
2 Ernst E. Massage therapy for low back pain: a systematic review. J Pain Symptom Manage 1999;17:65–69
3 Vickers A, Ohlsson A, Lacey J B, Horsley A. Massage therapy for premature and/or low birth weight infants to improve weight gain and/or decrease hospital length of stay. Cochrane Library. Oxford: Update Software, 1998
4 Field T. Grizzle N, Scafidi F, Schanberg S. Massage relaxation therapies' effects on depressed adolescent mothers. Adolescence 1996;31:903–911
5 Hernandez-Reif M, Martinez A, Field T, Quintero O, Hart S, Burman I. Premenstrual symptoms are relieved by massage therapy. J Psychosom Obstet Gynecol 2000;21:9–15
6 Fraser J, Kerr J R. Psychophysiological effects of back massage on elderly institutionalised patients. Nursing 1993;18:238–245
7 Brattberg G. Connective tissue massage in the treatment of fibromyalgia. Eur J Pain 1999;3:235–245

FURTHER READING

Vickers A. Massage and aromatherapy: a guide for health professionals. Cheltenham: Stanley Thornes, 1998
A thorough review of the background and clinical literature, which however ignores much of the evidence published in languages other than English.

NATUROPATHY

Synonym	Naturheilkunde (German).
Definition	An eclectic system of health care, which integrates elements of complementary and conventional medicine to support and enhance self-healing processes.
Related techniques	Hydrotherapy, Kneippkur (German), physical medicine, physiotherapy, Naturheilverfahren (German).

THERAPIES

Background

The philosophy of naturopathy can be traced back as far as Hippocrates (about 460–377 BCE). The power of natural means to cure ill health gained interest during the 18th and 19th centuries when the Germans Vinzenz Prießnietz (1799–1851) and particularly Sebastian Kneipp (1821–1897) established complex hydrotherapeutic interventions as a cure for many ailments. A disciple of Kneipp, Benedict Lust (1870–1945), introduced hydrotherapy to the US and later used the term naturopathy to describe the concept that he developed. In the UK one of the early nature cure resorts was established at Champneys near Tring in Hertfordshire in the 1930s.

Traditional concepts

Naturopathy is based on the belief that health is influenced by nature's own healing power (*vis medicatrix naturae*), which is understood as an inherent property of the living organism. Ill health is viewed as a direct result of ignoring or violating general principles of a healthy lifestyle. These principles are thought to be determined by an internal and external environment that optimizes the health of an individual. Naturopathy aims to correct and stabilize the condition of the internal and external environment.

Scientific rationale

The general principles of a healthy lifestyle, including a diet that is rich in fresh fruit and vegetables and a sufficient amount of physical exercise, are now well recognized in mainstream medicine. The different therapeutic interventions and techniques that are used include herbal medicine, hydrotherapy and iridology as well as physical treatments (e.g. spinal manipulation) and the scientific rationale varies according to each individual treatment. For some interventions a plausible scientific rationale is lacking, while for others the rationale is supported by the results of scientific investigation.

Practitioners

In the US, licensed naturopathic physicians have completed a relatively extensive training including basic medical sciences and conventional diagnostic techniques. A number of accredited colleges of naturopathic medicine offer 4-year training programs, which may lead to licensure. Naturopaths are currently licensed as primary care providers in a limited number of US states.

Conditions frequently treated

Naturopaths treat any condition but are trained to refer patients with serious medical conditions for conventional treatment.

Typical treatment session

During an initial consultation the naturopath will usually take a detailed medical history of the patient to get an overall impression of the medical status and screen for any serious conditions. This will also include questions relating to lifestyle and diet and may be followed by a more conventional diagnostic evaluation, including laboratory analyses. According to the diagnosed condition, the treatment plan will vary but often includes a change in lifestyle. The treatment of a particular condition may vary between practitioners. Follow-up appointments are arranged as necessary and medicines and regimen reviewed and changed if appropriate.

Course of treatment

Depending largely on the nature and severity of the condition but generally 1–2 appointments per week for a treatment period of one to several weeks. Lifestyle changes should be permanent.

Clinical evidence

The clinical evidence has to be evaluated according to each individual therapy (see respective chapters). There is clinical evidence from RCTs and systematic reviews for some complementary therapies, such as certain herbal extracts[1,2] and hydrotherapy.[3] For other elements there is little evidence to support their use (e.g. [4]). Spa therapy, which also integrates a number of different interventions, has been investigated in RCTs and was found to have some beneficial effects.[5] The effectiveness of the totality of the naturopathic approach, however, has not been evaluated in RCTs.

Risks

Contraindications
Contraindications and precautions vary for each individual therapy (see respective chapters) and often include pregnancy and lactation.

Precautions/warnings
Precautions may vary for each individual therapy (see respective chapters).

Adverse effects
The risk of adverse effects exists. The reader is referred to the respective chapters in this book and the conventional medical literature.

Interactions
Possible interactions, for instance between different herbal preparations or with conventional drugs or other intervention, should be considered (see respective chapters) and relevant patients should be closely monitored. Patients should be asked about self-prescription drug use.

Indirect risks
In cases where the practitioner is not aware of the limitations of certain treatments, appropriate therapy may be delayed.

Risk–benefit assessment

The possibility of adverse effects exists and the risk–benefit ratio has to be assessed for each treatment individually (see respective chapters). However, given the nature and relative lack of risks associated with many interventions, naturopathy may be worth considering when performed by a responsible, well-trained and licensed therapist.

REFERENCES

1 Pittler M H, Vogler B K, Ernst E. Efficacy of feverfew for the prevention of migraine. Cochrane Library. Oxford: Update Software, 2000

2 Stevinson C, Pittler M H, Ernst E. Garlic for treating hypercholesterolemia. A meta-analysis of randomized clinical trials. Ann Intern Med 2000;133:420–429

3 Hartmann B R, Bassenge E, Hartmann M. Effects of serial percutaneous application of carbon dioxide in intermittent claudication: results of a controlled trial. Angiology 1997;48:957–963

4 Ernst E. Iridology. Arch Ophthalmol 2000;118:120–121

5 Ernst E, Pittler M H. How efficacious is spa treatment? A systematic review of randomized studies. Dtsch Med Wochenschr 1998;123:273–277

FURTHER READING

Pizzorno J E, Murray M T (eds). Textbook of natural medicine. Edinburgh: Churchill Livingstone, 1999
A comprehensive but frequently misleading standard text.

OSTEOPATHY

Synonyms   Osteopathic medicine.

Definition   Form of manual therapy involving massage, mobilization and spinal manipulation.

Related techniques   Craniosacral therapy, chiropractic, manual therapy, spinal manipulation and mobilization.

Background   Osteopathy was founded in the US by Dr Andrew Taylor Still in 1874, since when it has had a turbulent history. It is now an accepted conventional form of health care in the US and a well-established form of CAM in the UK and many other countries.

Traditional concepts   Osteopaths believe that the primary role of the physician is to facilitate the body's inherent ability to heal itself, that the structure and function of the body are closely related and that problems of one organ affect other parts of the body.[1] For osteopaths, a perfect alignment of the musculoskeletal system eliminates obstructions in blood and lymph flow which, in turn, maximize health. To ensure perfect alignment, osteopaths have developed a range of manipulative techniques. These can be grouped into six major categories:

- high-velocity, low-amplitude thrusts
- muscle energy techniques
- counterstrain
- myofascial release
- craniosacral techniques (see Craniosacral therapy)
- lymphatic pump techniques.[1]

Scientific rationale	Some of the traditional osteopathic concepts ring intuitively true, yet their scientific rationale is not fully convincing. In particular, the theory of the overriding importance of perfect alignment lacks a scientific rationale.
Practitioners	In the US, osteopaths today constitute the smaller of the two major schools of medicine. US osteopaths (doctors of osteopathy, DOs) use most allopathic therapeutic options alongside osteopathic manipulative techniques and are regarded as mainstream health-care professionals. Outside the US, osteopaths mainly use spinal manipulation and mobilization and are usually considered as complementary therapists.
Conditions frequently treated	Typically, osteopaths treat musculoskeletal problems, particularly back and neck pain. US osteopaths would treat many other conditions as well, combining allopathic treatments with manual osteopathic techniques. The majority of US osteopaths, however, do not routinely use manipulative techniques.
Typical treatment session	A visit to a DO would normally be very similar to a consultation with a conventional physician. Outside the US, an osteopath would take a medical history and perform a careful physical examination of the musculoskeletal system, particularly the spine. In most cases this would be followed by treatment consisting of spinal manipulation and mobilization.
Course of treatment	One such treatment would rarely be considered to be sufficient. Depending on the condition and on clinical progress, 6–12 (or more) treatments would constitute a full course.
Clinical evidence	There is some evidence to suggest that osteopathy is helpful for low back pain, particularly acute and subacute stages.[1,2] A recent large RCT compared US-style osteopathy with standard care for patients with low back pain and concluded that the clinical outcomes were similar.[3] For other indications the clinical trial evidence is sparse and not compelling.[1,2]
Risks	***Contraindications*** Osteoporosis, neoplasms, infections, bleeding disorders. ***Precautions/warnings*** None known. ***Adverse effects*** Spinal trauma after high-velocity thrusts, vertebral artery dissection, stroke. ***Interactions*** None known.

THERAPIES

Indirect risks
Access to conventional treatments might be hindered.

Risk–benefit assessment

Osteopathic spinal manipulation and mobilization may be helpful in cases of low back pain. In as far as the techniques are often gentler than those used by chiropractors. the risk of spinal injury should be smaller. On balance, therefore, such techniques may be worth trying for patients with low back pain. For all other conditions data are insufficient for issuing strong recommendations.

REFERENCES

1 Lesho E P. An overview of osteopathic medicine. Arch Fam Med 1999;8: 477–483
2 Schwerla F, Hass-Degg K, Schwerla B. Evaluierung und kritische Bewertung von in der europäischen Literatur veröffentlichten, osteopathischen Studien im klinischen Bereich und im Bereich der Grundlagenforschung. Forsch Komplementärmed 1999;6:302–310
3 Andersson G B J, Lucente T, Davis A M, Kappler R E, Lipton J A, Leurgans S. A comparison of osteopathic spinal manipulation with standard care for patients with low back pain. New Engl J Med 1999;341:1426–1431

REFLEXOLOGY

Synonyms

Zone therapy, reflex zone therapy. (Note that the term 'reflexology' is sometimes used to describe treatment of segmental nerve reflexes with needles. 'Reflexotherapy' was used historically to describe acupuncture in the former USSR.)

Definition

A therapeutic method that uses manual pressure applied to specific areas, or zones, of the feet (and sometimes the hands or ears) that are believed to correspond to areas of the body, in order to relieve stress and prevent and treat physical disorders.

Related techniques

Reflexology may be used together with other techniques by manual therapists of various disciplines. Other therapies that use the concept of correspondence to parts of the body include acupuncture techniques such as auriculotherapy and Korean hand acupuncture.

Background

Egyptian papyri from about 2500 BCE show manual treatment of the feet and there is evidence that similar treatment was part of Chinese culture. Zone therapy is recorded in various ancient European medical systems and those of the North American Indians. It was from this latter group that Dr William Fitzgerald learnt the technique in the early 20th century. He investigated the effects of pressure in inducing analgesia elsewhere in the body and concluded that the body was divided into 10 vertical zones, each represented by a part of the foot including one toe.

From this idea, the charts of bodily correspondences evolved, initially drawn up by Eunice Ingham and published from the 1930s onwards.

Traditional concepts

The organs, glands and other components of each half of the body are believed to be represented at the foot on that side, mainly on the sole but also on the dorsum, heel and toes. The health of the body can be assessed by examining the feet to detect imbalances or obstructions to the flow of energy, which are expressed as tenderness or feelings of grittiness or crystal formation at the site. Bodily function can then be influenced by stimulating these areas with pressure or massage, thus activating a reflex mechanism involving nerves or meridians. Reflexology is claimed to reduce stress, improve circulation, eliminate toxins and promote metabolic homeostasis.

Scientific rationale

There is no known neurophysiological basis for connections between organs or glands and specific areas of the feet. Three investigations into the claimed correspondences are known: reflexologists' diagnoses were no better than chance in identifying medical conditions in one blinded study[1] whereas in another[2] their diagnostic success was better than chance but not clinically relevant. Pressure on the kidney area was claimed to produce changes in renal blood flow.[3]

Reflexology foot massage may have general health benefits independently of whether the reflex correspondences with particular organs are valid.

Practitioners

Practitioners range from those who teach themselves from books to those who follow training courses and join professional associations. No regulatory systems exist, as there are currently no state licensure or training requirements. Reflexology is commonly used by other health professionals including conventionally trained nurses.

Conditions frequently treated

Functional disorders including asthma, back and neck pain, migraine and headaches, chronic fatigue, sinusitis, arthritis, insomnia, digestive problems such as irritable bowel syndrome and constipation, stress-related disorders and postmenopausal symptoms.

Typical treatment session

The reflexologist usually takes a full history before examining the bare feet systematically, with the patient lying on a couch or reclining in a chair. Tender or gritty areas will be massaged as soon as they are found. The strength of pressure used varies greatly between practitioners. For lubrication, therapists may use oils which may contain specific aromatherapy products. Often the reflexologist and patient will converse throughout,

THERAPIES

though some patients prefer to be treated in silence. The whole session usually lasts 45–60 minutes. Some practitioners will use sticks or other instruments to treat the feet.

Course of treatment

This varies considerably between practitioners and on the condition. In the West, treatment is often offered weekly for a course of 6–8 sessions. For chronic conditions follow-up treatments may be offered.

Clinical evidence

One RCT found reflexology to be superior to placebo reflexology for the treatment of premenstrual symptoms, but the protocol included foot, hand and ear treatment so no conclusions can be drawn about any one independently.[4] One RCT showed beneficial effects on blood glucose in diabetics but the details are too sparse to be regarded as convincing.[5] Another RCT in patients with multiple sclerosis showed symptomatic improvements but the drop-out rate was high.[6] A large observational study found that 81% of patients with headache reported themselves helped or cured at 3 months follow-up[7] and an RCT found a non-significant trend in the same condition but important details are missing from the report.[8] Other RCTs have shown no effect on asthma[9] or on concentrations of serum cortisol during surgery.[10]

Risks

Contraindications
Relevant conditions of the feet such as gout, ulceration or vascular disease.

Precautions/warnings
Individuals with bone or joint conditions of the feet or lower leg should be treated cautiously.

Adverse effects
Fatigue, foot tenderness, changes in micturition or bowel function. Allergy to aromatherapy oils, if used.

Interactions
Possible interference with the effects of some drugs, e.g. insulin.

Indirect risks
Although professional associations insist that reflexologists should not make diagnostic claims, there have been incidents where reflexologists have made false-positive or -negative diagnoses and thus interfered with medical management to the patient's detriment.

Risk–benefit assessment

In the hands of responsible practitioners, reflexology seems to do little harm and possibly some good in the management of many functional disorders. Reflexology should never be used to make, or suggest, a diagnosis.

REFERENCES

1 White A R, Williamson J, Hart A, Ernst E. A blinded investigation into the accuracy of reflexology charts. Compl Ther Med 2000;8:166–172

2 Baerheim A, Algroy R, Skogedal K R, Stephansen R, Sandvik H. Fottene – et diagnostisk hjelpemiddel? Tidsskr Nor Laegeforen 1998;5:753–755

3 Sudmeier I, Bodner G, Egger I, Mur E, Ulmer H, Herold M. Änderung der Nierendurchblutung durch organassoziierte Reflexzonentherapie am Fuss gemessen mit farbkodierter Doppler-Sonographie. Forsch Komplementärmed 1999;6:129–134

4 Oleson T, Flocco W. Randomised controlled study of premenstrual symptoms treated with ear, hand and foot reflexology. Obstet Gynaecol 1993;82:906–911

5 Wang X M. Treating type II diabetes mellitus with foot reflexotherapy [Chinese]. Chung-Kuo Chung Hsi i Chieh Ho Tsa Chih 1993;13:536–538

6 Siev-Ner I, Gamus D, Lerner-Geva L et al. Reflexology treatment relieves symptoms of multiple sclerosis: a randomized controlled study. Focus Alt Compl Ther 1997;2:196

7 Launso L, Brendstrup E, Arnberg S. An exploratory study of reflexological treatment for headache. Alt Ther Health Med 1999;5:57–65

8 Lafuente A, Noguera M, Puy C, Molins A, Titus F, Sanz F. Effekt der Reflexzonenbehandlung am Fuss bezüglich der prophylaktischen Behandlung mit Funarizin bei an Cephalea-Kopfschmerzen leidenden Patienten. Erfahrungsheilkunde 1990;39:713–715

9 Peterson L N, Faurschou P, Olsen O T, Svendsen U G. Reflexology and bronchial asthma. Ugeskr Laeger 1992;154:2065–2068

10 Engquist A, Vibe-Hansen H. Zone therapy and plasma cortisol during surgical stress. Ugeskr Laeger 1977;139:460–462

FURTHER READING

Ernst E, Koeder K. An overview of reflexology. Eur J Gen Pract 1997;3:52–57
A systematic review of clinical trials together with some background information.

THERAPIES

RELAXATION THERAPY

Definition

Techniques for eliciting the 'relaxation response' of the autonomic nervous system.

Related techniques

Autogenic training, biofeedback, hypnotherapy, meditation. Many CAM interventions include an element of relaxation.

Background

One of the most common relaxation techniques is progressive muscle relaxation, pioneered in 1930 by Dr Edmund Jacobson, an American physician. It has been modified over time by others, but is still based on the original principles. Other relaxation techniques involve passive muscle relaxation, refocusing, breathing control or imagery.

Traditional concepts

Progressive muscle relaxation is based on the notion that it is impossible to be tense in any part of the body where the muscles are completely relaxed. Furthermore, tension in involuntary muscles and organs can be reduced if the associated skeletal muscles are relaxed. The method is learnt by first tensing a muscle before relaxing it, to help recognize the difference between tension and relaxation. Subsequently, it is possible to relax a limb without tensing it first. Systematic relaxation involves a more passive release of tension while focusing on muscle groups. Benson's relaxation response contains an attention control element where the focus is on slow rhythmical breathing combined with repetition of a single word. With imagery-based relaxation, the idea is to imagine oneself in a place or situation associated with relaxation and comfort using visualization and involving all the other senses in creating a vivid image.

Scientific rationale

Progressive muscle relaxation has been shown to be effective in eliciting the relaxation response, resulting in the normalizing of blood supply to the muscles, decreases in oxygen consumption, heart rate, respiration and skeletal muscle activity and increases in skin resistance and alpha brain waves. Other relaxation techniques have also been shown to be effective in diffusing muscle tension.

Practitioners

Relaxation techniques are taught by various complementary practitioners, physicians, psychotherapists, hypnotherapists, nurses, clinical psychologists and sports therapists. There is no formal credentialling for relaxation therapies.

Conditions frequently treated

Anxiety, headaches, stress disorders, musculoskeletal pain.

Typical treatment session

With progressive muscle relaxation, subjects usually lie on their back with arms to the side in a quiet environment without bright light. Occasionally a sitting posture in a comfortable chair is adopted instead. Muscle groups are systematically contracted then relaxed in a predetermined order. In the early stages, an entire session will be devoted to a single muscle group. With practice it becomes possible to combine muscle groups and then eventually relax the entire body all at once.

Course of treatment

With progressive muscle relaxation, several months of practice at least three times a week are needed after learning the technique in order to be able to evoke the relaxation response within seconds.

Clinical evidence

A large body of evidence suggests that relaxation therapies are useful in anxiety. Positive results from RCTs exist for relaxation in association with desensitization for agoraphobia and panic disorder (e.g. [1,2]) and anxiety associated with serious conditions such as cancer[3] or with undergoing medical interventions such as radiation therapy.[4] A systematic review including 22 studies of progressive muscle relaxation reported a moderate effect on trait anxiety in non-psychiatric patients.[5] Systematic reviews of RCTs in both acute[6] and chronic[7] pain have found only weak and contradictory evidence that relaxation is an effective form of treatment on its own. Other conditions for which there is promising evidence from RCTs include depression,[8-10] insomnia[11-13] and menopausal symptoms[14-16] although effects appear to be generally short-lived. Various other conditions have been investigated, but no compelling evidence exists.

Risks

Contraindications
Schizophrenic or actively psychotic patients.

Precautions/warnings
Techniques requiring inward focusing may intensify depressed mood.

Adverse effects
None known.

Interactions
Adjunctive relaxation therapy may reduce the required dosage of certain medications, i.e. antihypertensive or anxiolytic drugs.

Indirect risks
Attempting to use relaxation therapy rather than consulting a doctor for a medical condition may delay appropriate treatment.

Risk–benefit assesment

Relaxation techniques may be useful for treating anxiety disorders or states, although they do not appear to be as effective as psychotherapy. For conditions with a strong psychosomatic element, relaxation appears to have some potential benefits although these may not be long term. However, since relaxation therapies are almost risk free, they can be recommended as an adjunctive therapy for most conditions.

THERAPIES

REFERENCES

1 Ost L G, Westling B E, Hellstrom K. Applied relaxation, exposure *in vivo* and cognitive methods in the treatment of panic disorder with agoraphobia. Behav Res Ther 1993;31:383–394

2 Beck J G, Stanley M A, Baldwin L E, Deagle E A 3rd, Averill P M. Comparison of cognitive therapy and relaxation training for panic disorder. J Consult Clin Psychol 1994;62:818–826

3 Bindemann S, Soukop M, Kaye S B. Randomized controlled study of relaxation training. Eur J Cancer 1991;27:170–174

4 Kolcaba K, Fox C. The effects of guided imagery on comfort of women with early stage breast cancer undergoing radiation therapy. Oncol Nurs Forum 1999;26:67–72

5 Eppley K R, Abrams A I, Shear J. Differential effects of relaxation techniques on trait anxiety. J Clin Psychol 1989;45:957–974

6 Seers K, Carroll D. Relaxation techniques for acute pain management: a systematic review. J Adv Nurs 1998;27:466–475

7 Carroll D, Seers K. Relaxation for the relief of chronic pain: a systematic review. J Adv Nurs 1998;27:476–487

8 Reynolds W M, Coats K I. A comparison of cognitive-behavioural therapy and relaxation training for the treatment of depression in adolescents. J Consult Clin Psychol 1986;54:653–660

9 Broota A, Dhir R. Efficacy of two relaxation techniques in depression. J Pers Clin Stud 1990;6:83–90

10 Murphy G E, Carney R M, Knesevich M A, Wetzel R D, Whitworth P. Cognitive behaviour therapy, relaxation training and tricyclic antidepressant medication in the treatment of depression. Psychol Rep 1995;77:403–420

11 Greeff A P, Conradie W S. Use of progressive relaxation training for chronic alcoholics with insomnia. Psychol Rep 1998;82:407–412

12 Engle Friedman M, Bootzin R R, Hazlewood L, Tsao C. An evaluation of behavioural treatments for insomnia in the older adult. J Clin Psychol 1992;48:77–90

13 Hauri P J. Can we mix behavioural therapy with hypnotics when treating insomniacs? Sleep 1997;20:1111–1118

14 Irvin J H, Domar A D, Clark C, Zuttermeister P C, Friedman R. The effects of relaxation response training on menopausal symptoms. J Psychosom Obstet Gynecol 1996;17: 202–207

15 Freedman R R, Woodward S. Behavioural treatment of menopausal hot flushes: evaluation by ambulatory monitoring. Am J Obstet Gynecol 1992;167:436–439

16 Germaine L M, Freedman R R. Behavioural treatment of menopausal hot flashes: evaluation by objective methods. J Consult Clin Psychol 1984;52:1072–1079

SPIRITUAL HEALING

Synonyms/ subcategories

Distant healing, faith healing, intercessory prayer, paranormal healing, psychic healing, Reiki, therapeutic touch.

Definition

The direct interaction between one individual (the healer) and a second (sick) individual with the intention of bringing about an improvement or cure of the illness.[1]

Related techniques

All types of energy healing systems.

Background

Spiritual healing can be traced back to the Bible (New Testament, *1 Corinthians* 12:9) where it was listed amongst the gifts bestowed on the faithful. It has always had its adherents and in recent years has gained widespread popularity.

Traditional concepts

Spiritual healers believe that the therapeutic effect results from the channeling of 'energy' from an assumed source via the healer to the patient. The central claim of healers is that they promote or facilitate self-healing in the patient.

Scientific rationale

There is no scientific evidence to support the existence of this 'energy', nor is there a scientific rationale for any other concept underlying spiritual healing.

Practitioners

In the UK almost 13 000 members are today registered in nine separate healing organizations. In the US its sister therapies, therapeutic touch (TT) and Reiki, boast many thousands of healer therapists. TT was developed in the early 1970s by Dora Kunz and Dolores Krieger. The technique is taught at 75 US institutions and universities. Krieger claims she has personally taught TT to more than 48 000 health-care professionals in 75 countries. Most healers are not medically qualified and there is no mandatory training. Members of the UK Confederation of Healing Organizations have, however, a minimum of 2 years' training. Most US practitioners of TT are trained nurses.

Conditions frequently treated

Healers do not usually relate to the disease entities of conventional medicine. Their aim is to help the patient in more general terms, for instance by increasing well-being. Many healers treat patients with emotional problems or chronic pain.

Typical treatment session

The healer discusses the problem with the patient in order to gain some understanding of it. Subsequently the patient may be asked to lie or sit down and the therapist may scan the patient's body with his or her hands at a distance and channel healing 'energy' through his or her body towards the patient. Treatments are often given without charge.

Course of treatment

One treatment is rarely deemed to suffice. A typical course may consist of eight or more single sessions. Often several courses of treatment are given within a year.

Clinical evidence

A systematic review[2] included 23 placebo-controlled RCTs involving almost 3000 patients. About half of these studies yielded a positive result, suggesting that spiritual healing is efficacious. However, due to numerous methodological limitations of these trials, no firm conclusions could be drawn. A similar review with slightly different inclusion criteria included 22 RCTs, of which 10 were positive.[3] For the same reasons as above, the author abstained from firm conclusions regarding efficacy.

Risks

Contraindications
Psychiatric illness.

Precautions/warnings
None known.

Adverse effects
Sensations like heat or tingling are often reported in areas under the hands of the healer.

Interactions
None known.

Indirect risks
Access to conventional treatments might be hindered.

Risk–benefit assessment

Whether spiritual healing is associated with specific therapeutic effects is unclear. Healing has few risks. There is insufficient evidence for strong recommendation for or against this form of therapy.

THERAPIES

REFERENCES

1 Hodges R D, Scofield A M. Is spiritual healing a valid and effective therapy? J Roy Soc Med 1995;88:203–207

2 Astin J, Harkness E, Ernst E. The efficacy of spiritual healing: a systematic review of randomised trials. Ann Intern Med 2000;132:903–910

3 Abbot N C. Healing as a therapy for human disease: a systematic review. J Alt Compl Med 2000;6:159–169

FURTHER READING

Benor D J. Healing research: holistic energy medicine and spirituality. Volume 1 Research in healing. Helix Editions, Deddington, Oxford, 1992

An introduction to healing written by an outspoken advocate.

TAI CHI

Definition	A system of movements and postures rooted in ancient Chinese philosophy and martial arts used to enhance mental and physical health.
Related techniques	Qi gong.
Background	Tai chi has a long history in China and is today widely practiced there. It has also become increasingly popular in many Western countries. A number of different styles and forms were developed from the original 13 postures, believed to have been created in the early 12th century. The various forms of tai chi comprise a series of postures linked by gentle and graceful movements.
Traditional concepts	Influenced by Confucian and Buddhist philosophy, tai chi is based on the principles of the two opposing life forces, Yin and Yang. Ill health is viewed as an imbalance between Yin, the female, receptive principle, and Yang, the male, creative principle. The alternating movements and postures are thought to stabilize these flowing energies, create inner and outer harmony and emotional balance.
Scientific rationale	The slow movement between different postures that are normally held for a short period of time are physical stimuli with effects on the cardiovascular and muscular system. These stimuli, much like other physical exercise, result in muscular adaptation, which ultimately leads to increased muscle strength, if performed regularly. In addition to adaptation processes at the level of the nervous system, these effects may produce better cardiovascular function, coordination and balance.
Practitioners	Teachers should have a basic understanding of human anatomy and physiology and should have some knowledge of the philosophy and historical background of tai chi. Ideally, teachers have had at least 5 years of experience and study with a master before independent teaching. There is, however, no generally acknowledged minimum requirement.
Conditions frequently treated	Stress-related conditions, depression, osteoporosis, high or low blood pressure.

Typical treatment session

Tai chi is usually taught in classes of 5–10 or more people. The atmosphere during practice is usually quiet, relaxed but intense. The student should maintain a level of concentration and should not be distracted by external influences. The movements are performed simultaneously by the group responding to advice and corrections by the teacher. Tai chi is a lifelong endeavor and regular practice is essential in achieving beneficial effects.

Course of treatment

The various forms take between 5 and 30 minutes to complete. Daily practice is ideal but at least twice-weekly exercises are recommended. The best time for practice is said to be early in the morning.

Clinical evidence

Evidence from RCTs suggested beneficial effects of tai chi as an intervention to maintain balance and strength[1] and to reduce the risk of falls[2] in elderly individuals. The results of another RCT suggested beneficial effects on depression, anger and fatigue.[3] CCTs suggested beneficial effects on cardiorespiratory function in elderly individuals.[4,5]

Risks

Contraindications
Contraindications and precautions are largely based on common sense (e.g. severe osteoporosis, acute back pain, knee problems, sprains and fractures). Usually it can be safely practiced during pregnancy and lactation.

Precautions/warnings
Before starting tai chi older individuals should be carefully examined for any of the above or other contraindications. Teachers should have certified knowledge of first aid in medical emergencies.

Adverse effects
Adverse effects are rare, but may include delayed-onset muscle soreness, pulled ligaments or ankle sprains.

Interactions
None known.

Indirect risk
Tai chi should be viewed as an adjunctive treatment, not as an alternative to conventional medical care.

Risk–benefit assessment

There is only limited evidence from rigorous clinical trials but it appears that tai chi increases cardiovascular function, muscle strength and balance. This may decrease the risk of falls, which is of particular relevance in the elderly. Tai chi may also have other health benefits, for instance for depression and anxiety, as has been suggested for physical exercise. Given the nature and frequency of the risks involved when instructed by a responsible

THERAPIES

teacher, it is worth considering as a general measure for promoting a healthy lifestyle and may thus benefit most individuals.

REFERENCES

1 Wolfson L, Whipple R, Derby C et al. Balance and strength in older adults: intervention gains and tai chi maintenance. J Am Geriatr Soc 1996;44:498–506

2 Wolf S L, Barnhart H X, Kutner N G et al. Reducing frailty and falls in older persons: an investigation of tai chi and computerized balance training, Atlanta FISCSIT Group. J Am Geriatr Soc 1996;44:489–497

3 Putai Jin. Changes in heart rate, noradrenaline, cortisol and mood during tai chi. J Psychosom Res 1989;33:197–206

4 Lai J-S, Wong M-K, Lan C, Chong C-K, Lien I-N. Cardiorespiratory responses of tai chi chuan practitioners and sedentary subjects during cycle ergometry. J Formos Med Assoc 1993;92:894–899

5 Lai J-S, Lan C, Wong M-K, Teng S-H. Two-year trends in cardiorespiratory function among older tai chi chuan practitioners and sedentary subjects. J Am Geriatr Soc 1995;43:1222–1227

YOGA

Definition

A practice of gentle stretching, exercises for breath control and meditation as a mind–body intervention.

Related techniques

Tai chi, qi gong.

Background

The word yoga is derived from the Sanskrit word *yuj*, which means 'to yoke', reflecting its purpose in joining mind and body in harmonious relaxation. Indian symbols dating from 3000 BCE are believed to indicate that yoga was in existence at that time. Records of the Yoga Sutras, the eight aspects of spiritual enlightenment, date from about 2300 years ago and include ethical principles of behavior. The three yoga practices mostly used in the West, called hatha yoga, are the poses (*asanas*), breath control (*pranayama*) and meditation, which are aimed at achieving heightened awareness of the body and stillness of the mind. Yoga devotees practice regularly and increase their skills and techniques throughout their lifetime. Yoga is widely practiced in both Eastern and Western countries, but yoga masters from India are still held in great reverence.

Although yoga developed within Indian culture and religion, the practice of yoga does not require spiritual beliefs or religious observances.

Traditional concepts

Yoga is believed to increase the body's stores of *prana*, or vital energy, and to facilitate its flow by improved posture. The body becomes a 'fit vehicle for the spirit'. Poor diet, stress and other factors can block the natural flow of prana, leaving the body vulnerable.

THERAPIES

Scientific rationale

The regular practice of yoga induces a deep sense of relaxation which is beneficial in itself, at least temporarily. Physical benefits of regular practice that have been described include bodily suppleness and muscular strength. Mental benefits include feelings of well-being and, possibly, reduction of sympathetic drive. Yoga breathing exercises counter the rapid breathing that accompanies the stress response and may in addition reduce muscular spasm and expand the available lung capacity.

Practitioners

Although yoga can be self-taught through various media, it is preferable to learn with supervision in classes. Practitioners (usually called yoga teachers) should have the knowledge and experience to ensure that benefit is obtained without over-stretching joints and muscles. No uniform credentialling exists and no licensure is currently required to teach yoga.

Conditions frequently treated

Stress, insomnia, headaches, anxiety, premenstrual syndrome, arthritis, back pain, gastrointestinal, respiratory and cardiovascular problems. Also used in pregnancy as preparation for childbirth. Yoga can also be used by healthy people to gain self-mastery.

Typical treatment session

Classes last about one hour and involve some theoretical introduction, supervised postures and breathing exercises usually leading to a period of deep relaxation or sometimes meditation. Precise content and form vary considerably.

Course of treatment

Yoga is used daily by enthusiastic adherents and is probably best practiced more than once a week for maximum benefit. It should be regarded as a long-term commitment.

Clinical evidence

Many uncontrolled observational studies have found that yoga practice by healthy people has beneficial effects on mood, emotional well-being and quality of life indicators, as well as some physiological measures such as autonomic arousal.[1] There is a small number of controlled trials that suggest that yoga may have a useful long-term effect in the treatment of hypertension (e.g. [2]) and, more questionably, of asthma.[3] It may have a role in reducing joint stiffness in osteoarthritis.[4]

Risks

Contraindications
No absolute contraindications exist, but certain postures are contraindicated in pregnancy. Meditation may precipitate feelings of unreality and depersonalization and should therefore not be used by people with a history of psychotic or personality disorder.

Precautions/warnings
Physical damage can occur from overstretching either healthy or, more particularly, diseased joints and ligaments. Those learning

yoga for treatment of medical conditions are advised to seek supervision by an experienced and knowledgeable teacher who will adapt the postures in appropriate ways.

Adverse effects
Drowsiness may occur.

Interactions
None known. It is possible that the dose of antihypertensive medication, etc. may need to be altered.

Indirect risks
Yoga teachers are generally not medically qualified and formal medical advice should be sought in the usual way for management of clinical conditions.

Risk–benefit assessment

Regular practice of yoga is a largely safe method of improving general health and well-being, but its role as an adjunct to the management of any medical conditions has not been firmly established.

REFERENCES

1 Collins C. Yoga: intuition, preventive medicine, and treatment. J Obstet Gynecol Neonatal Nurs 1998;September/October:563–568

2 Patel C. Twelve month follow-up of yoga and bio-feedback in the management of hypertension. Lancet 1975;1:62–64

3 Vedanthan P K, Kesavalu L N, Murthy K C et al. Clinical study of yoga techniques in university students with asthma: a controlled study. Allergy Asthma Proc 1998;19:3–9

4 Garfinkel M S, Schumacher H R, Husain A, Levy M, Reshetar R A. Evaluation of a yoga based regimen for treatment of osteoarthritis of the hands. J Rheumatol 1994;21:2341–2343

TABLE 3.2 OTHER THERAPIES **79**

Table 3.2 Other therapies without sufficient evidence of effectiveness

Therapy	Description	Conditions frequently treated	Safety concerns
Anthroposophical medicine	An approach that integrates conventional medicine with an exploration of inner feelings and the meaning of illness. Treatment may involve both conventional and CAM interventions	Any condition	None other than those of the individual therapies
Art therapy	Use of creative art as a means of expression for rehabilitation and personal development	Adjunct to psychotherapy for many psychological and psychiatric conditions	Use of potentially harmful chemicals, e.g. solvents; problems with disturbed behavior
Autologous blood therapy	Taking of small amounts of blood, usually from an antecubital vein, and intramuscular reinjection	Asthma, eczema, psoriasis, pemphigus, urticaria and many other chronic conditions	Pain around the injection sites, bruising, infection
Bowen technique	Gentle soft tissue mobilization procedures using pressure from thumb and fingers	Musculoskeletal conditions; stress-related disorders; symptoms of chronic conditions	None known
Colonic irrigation, colon therapy, hydrotherapy	Use of standard enemas for rectosigmoid area or apparatus for prolonged irrigation of higher colon. Uses water, sometimes with enzymes, herbs or coffee added	Constipation, diarrhea, gastrointestinal disorders; removal of 'toxins' in wide range of conditions inc. addictions, allergies	Infections, perforations, electrolyte imbalance and deaths have been reported
Color (light, photo-) therapy	Single or mixed colors (inc. laser) shone on whole body or particular areas, e.g. chakras	Psychological problems including seasonal affective disorder, attention deficit disorder; visually related disorders; conventional use in skin disease and hyperbilirubinemia	Direct eye injury; strobic light may produce seizures; photosensitivity
Crystal therapy, crystal healing, gem therapy	Use of crystals, individually selected for their wavelength, to influence the body's 'energy field'	Wide range of mental and physical conditions	None known

table continues

THERAPIES

Therapy	Description	Conditions frequently treated	Safety concerns
Dance (movement) therapy	Use of dance to express emotions for therapeutic purposes	Communication disorders; physical and learning disabilities; stress and other psychological problems	None known
Enzyme therapy	Plant-derived and pancreatic enzymes given orally with the aim of improving the digestive and immune system	A wide variety of conditions including chronic digestive disorders, inflammatory and viral diseases, multiple sclerosis and cancer	Increased risk of bleeding
Feldenkrais method	A method of relearning dysfunctional movement habits; based on classes of 'awareness through movement' and 'functional integration'	Disabilities from injury, disease or degeneration; anxiety, other psychological and stress-related disorders	Possible exacerbation of symptoms
Flotation therapy	Form of sensory deprivation from lying in a tank filled with saline to counteract gravitational stress, with low or absent light and sound	Stressful states, for relaxation, arthritis and low back pain, drug abuse and smoking cessation	Hygiene problems from reuse of water; frightening for those with claustrophobia
Hellerwork, structural integration	Deep tissue bodywork, movement education and dialogue to improve posture (see Rolfing)	Postural and musculoskeletal conditions; headaches; stress	Possible exacerbation of symptoms
Imagery, guided imagery, visualization	Controlled use of mental images for therapeutic purposes	Psychological symptoms, especially anxiety, stress-related disorders, depression; physical symptoms, especially pain; cancer	None known (but excessive inward focusing may reveal latent psychoses or personality disorders)
Magnetic field therapy	Permanent or pulsed magnetic fields applied to head or other part of body; often used with acupuncture	Non-union of fracture (FDA approved); wide variety of indications (self-use)	Contraindicated in pregnancy, pacemakers; myasthenia gravis, bleeding disorders, pacemakers
Meditation, transcendental meditation	Self-regulation of attention; may be used outside its original religious and cultural context	Stress and stress-related disorders; functional disorders of body	Risks with latent psychoses or personality disorders; excessive meditation may lead to mental disturbance

TABLE 3.2 OTHER THERAPIES **81**

Therapy	Description	Uses	Cautions
Music therapy	Listening to or making music for therapeutic purposes	Communication disorders; stress and other psychological problems; pain; neurological disability	Music should not exceed 90 dB as this may lead to hearing impairment
Neural therapy	Injection of 'trigger' areas, usually with local anesthetic	Chronic conditions, especially pain	Allergy to anesthetic agent
Neurolinguistic programming	Use of mental strategies and changes to thought patterns in problem solving	Anxiety, stress, other psychological problems; personal development	Abreaction has been reported
Oxygen therapy	Use of oxygen injections; use of hyperbaric oxygen for unconventional indications (sometimes used for ozone therapy)	Stroke and other brain injury; many conditions, especially chronic; physical fitness enhancement	Excess free radicals, peroxidation; risk of embolism or infection with IV injection
Ozone therapy	Injection of ozone (or hydrogen peroxide) or reinjection of own blood enriched with ozone	Degenerative diseases; HIV/AIDS; cancer	Serious complications reported including infections and embolism
Polarity therapy	Use of hands in order to influence flow of body energy; may also involve exercise and lifestyle changes	Anxiety, stress, other psychological and functional physical conditions	None known
Qi gong	Branch of Chinese medicine using meditation to strengthen own qi (see p 26); also exercises, self-massage; many individual styles; Qi gong masters use 'emitted qi' for healing	Health promotion; wide range of functional disorders; symptom control	Psychosis reported, probably in those with latent condition
Reiki	A form of spiritual healing (see p 72)	Chronic pain, emotional problems	None known
Rolfing, structural integration	Improves posture of body by soft tissue techniques, including strong massage, often in an ordered sequence, designed to free fascia	Postural problems, musculoskeletal conditions; headaches; stress	Possible exacerbation of symptoms, risk of fracturing osteoporotic bones
Shiatsu	Japanese form of massage on acupressure points (see p 26)	Numerous, especially chronic conditions and general ill health	Tissue trauma from excessive force
Tragerwork	Use of therapist's hands and mind to communicate lightness and encourage 'playfulness'	Many chronic physical and psychological conditions	None known
Water injection	Subcutaneous injection of sterile water over trigger points	Painful conditions, particularly due to myofascial trigger points	Local pain, bruising, infection

THERAPIES

Herbal and non-herbal medicine

ALOE VERA
(*Aloe barbadensis* Miller)

Synonyms	Barbados aloe, burn plant, Curaçao aloe, elephant's gall, first-aid plant, Hsiang-Dan, lily of the desert, Lu-Hui, medicine plant, miracle plant, plant of immortality.
Examples of trade names	Avistol, Rhemogen.
Source	Aloe vera gel is made of mucilaginous tissue from the center of the leaf. Aloe vera juice (also sap or aloes) is produced from the peripheral bundle sheath cells.
Main constituents	Aloe vera gel contains several polysaccharides. Aloe vera juice contains aloin, anthraquinones and barbaloine.
Background	A cactus-like plant which grows in hot, dry climates, Aloe vera has been used in most ancient medical cultures. At present it is heavily promoted for numerous purposes ranging from diabetes to wound healing.
Traditional uses	Wound healing, various skin problems, laxative.
Pharmacologic action	*Gel*: antimicrobial, antiinflammatory, moisturizing, antipruritic. *Juice*: laxative, hypoglycemic, hypolipo-proteinemic. The best-documented mechanism of action is irritation of the large intestines by a metabolite of aloin, responsible for the laxative properties of aloe vera juice.
Conditions frequently treated	Various skin conditions, constipation and many other indications.
Clinical evidence	A systematic review included 10 CCTs, seven with topical and three with oral administration.[1] Taken orally, aloe vera juice might lower blood glucose and blood lipids levels, according to these trials. Applied topically, aloe vera gel might be effective for genital herpes and psoriasis. Its effects on wound healing are contradictory and two trials did not show a protective effect of aloe vera gel on radiation-induced skin injury. For none of these indications is the available evidence compelling.
Dosage	*Gel*: apply liberally to the skin as needed. *Juice* (orally): 50–100 mg daily.
Risks	***Contraindications*** Pregnancy, lactation, known allergy to plants from the *Liliaceae* family (e.g. garlic, onions, tulips), intestinal obstruction.

Precautions/warnings

Reflex stimulation of uterus could theoretically cause abortion in pregnant women. Aloe vera products should not be injected; this has been associated with serious complications and death.

Adverse effects

Allergic reactions, damage to intestinal mucosa, delayed healing of deep wounds (topical use), red discoloration of urine, intestinal pain, fluid or electrolyte loss (frequent oral use).

Overdose

Life-threatening hemorrhagic diarrhea and kidney damage with oral use.

Interactions

Increased effects of antiarrhythmics, cardiac glycosides, diuretics and steroids.

Quality issues

Stability of preparations is not established.

Risk–benefit assessment

Topical use has few risks but also few well-documented benefits. The oral administration of aloe vera juice is associated with considerable risks and has no benefit over conventional treatments. Its use should therefore be discouraged until compelling evidence to the contrary is available.

REFERENCE

1 Vogler B K, Ernst E. Aloe vera: a systematic review of its clinical effectiveness. Br J Gen Pract 1999;49:823–828

FURTHER READING

Atherton P. Aloe vera revisited. Br J Phytother 1998;4:176–183

Shelton R M. Aloe vera: its chemical and therapeutic properties. Int J Dermatol 1991;30:679–683

ARTICHOKE
(Cynara scolymus L)

Synonyms

Artischocke (German), bur artichoke, garden artichoke, globe artichoke.

Examples of trade names

Cynafol, Hepagallin N, Hepar SL Forte, Hewechol Artischocken-dragees.

Source

Leaf.

Main constituents

Phenolic acids, sesquiterpene lactones, flavonoids, phytosterols, sugars and inulin.

Background

Artichoke is a herbaceous perennial, which can grow to a height of up to 2 meters. The plant is native to southern Europe, northern Africa and the Canary Islands. Its cultivation dates back to ancient Roman and Greek times. Galen (129–199 AD) knew of its pleasant taste and Plinius called it the 'food of the rich'. For pharmaceutical use the first-year rosette of leaves is preferred and harvested from plants especially produced for medicinal purposes.

Traditional uses

As a choleretic and diuretic.

Pharmacologic action

Hepatoprotective, hepatostimulating, diuretic, lipid lowering, carminative, antiemetic, choleretic. Indirect inhibitory effects at the level of HMG-CoA reductase have been suggested as a possible mechanism of action.[1] Cynarine (1.5-di-caffeoyl-D-quinic acid) may be one of the principal active components of artichoke extract. Other findings indicate that the flavonoid luteolin may be responsible for its effects.

Conditions frequently treated

Dyspepsia, hyperlipidemia.

Clinical evidence

Artichoke extract has been the subject of a small number of clinical trials investigating its potential cholesterol-lowering effects. A systematic review[1] identified one double-blind RCT, which assessed 44 healthy volunteers who received 640 mg artichoke extract or placebo three times daily for 12 weeks. No significant effects on serum cholesterol levels were reported. Subgroup analyses suggested positive effects in individuals with total cholesterol levels of 210 mg/dl or above. A double-blind RCT (n=143), which became available after the systematic review, corroborated this finding and suggested a significant reduction of the total cholesterol level of 18.5% in the artichoke group compared with 8.6% in the placebo group.[2] Other evidence reported by a small (n=20) double-blind RCT suggests an increase in bile secretion after a single dose of 1.92 g artichoke extract.[3]

Dosage

0.5–1.92 g of dry extract daily in divided doses.

Risks

Contraindications
Known allergies to artichoke and related species (*Asteraceae* or *Compositae*), obstruction of bile duct.

Precautions/warnings
Gallstones.

Adverse effects
Flatulence, allergic reactions.

Interactions
None known.

Quality issues

Standardized extracts contain a 3.8–5.5:1 artichoke extract ratio, which is equivalent to about 1500 mg dried artichoke leaves for a 320 mg capsule.

Risk–benefit assessment

The clinical evidence for the medicinal use of artichoke extract is not compelling for any indication. In the light of the nature and frequency of adverse effects, however, its potential beneficial effects for total cholesterol reduction and dyspeptic complaints might outweigh possible adverse effects.

REFERENCES

1 Pittler M H, Ernst E. Artichoke leaf extract for serum cholesterol reduction. Perfusion 1998;11:338–340

2 Englisch W, Beckers C, Unkauf M, Ruepp M, Zinserling V. Efficacy of artichoke dry extract in patients with hyperlipoproteinemia. Arzneim-Forsch/Drug Res 2000;50:260–265

3 Kirchhoff R, Beckers C H, Kirchhoff G M, Trinczek-Gärtner H, Petrowicz O, Reimann H J. Increase in choleresis by means of artichoke extract. Phytomedicine 1994;1:107–115

ASIAN GINSENG
(Panax ginseng C A Meyer)

Synonyms

Allheilkraut (German), Chinese ginseng, Korean ginseng, ninjin (Japanese), true ginseng.

Examples of trade names

Cimexon, Gincosan, Ginsana, Ginseng Curarina, Gintec Ginseng, Red Kooga.

Source

Roots.

Main constituents

Triterpene saponins known as ginsenosides or panaxosides.

Background

Asian ginseng is a perennial herb reaching a height of about 60–80 cm. It is native to the mountain forests of China and Korea and grows at altitudes of about 1000 meters. Today, however, it is rarely found in the wild. The common name ginseng is derived from the Chinese *gin* (man) and *seng* (essence) and stands for the ideogram 'crystallization of the essence of the earth in the form of a man'. The genus name *Panax* is derived from the Greek *pan* (all) and *akos* (cure), which refers to the cure-all or *panacea* quality often attributed to the herb.

Ginseng comprises a number of different species, which all belong to the same family, the *Aaraliaceae*. However, Korean, Japanese and American ginseng belong to the genus *Panax*, while Siberian ginseng belongs to the genus *Eleutherococcus*. Ginseng is included in the pharmacopoeias of several countries, such as China, Germany and the UK. The German Commission E recommends its use as a tonic. It is widely available as an over-the-counter food supplement.

Traditional uses

To reduce susceptibility to illness, promote health and longevity and as an aid during convalescence.

Pharmacologic action

Immunomodulatory, antiinflammatory, antitumor, smooth muscle relaxant, stimulant and hypoglycemic.

Conditions frequently treated

Modern therapeutic claims refer to vitality, immune function, cancer, cardiovascular diseases, sexual function and diabetes.

Clinical evidence

A systematic review assessed the clinical evidence from all double-blind RCTs of Asian ginseng for any indication.[1] Relevant literature was translated from various languages including Chinese, Japanese, Korean and Russian. The limited number of rigorous clinical trials which could be identified relate to physical performance, psychomotor performance and cognitive function, immunomodulation, type II diabetes mellitus and herpes simplex type II infections. The review concluded that the effectiveness of Asian ginseng root extract is not established beyond reasonable doubt for any indication. With regard to improving physical performance this finding is largely corroborated by a non-systematic but reasonably comprehensive review.[2] One placebo-controlled RCT that was not reported as double blind assessed 90 patients with erectile dysfunction who were treated with either ginseng or Trazodone.[3] It is reported that ginseng was superior for penile rigidity, girth, libido and patient satisfaction but no intergroup differences were found, for instance, for frequency of intercourse. Another small (n=15) double-blind RCT reports positive effects for psychomotor performance in young athletes.[4]

Dosage

100 mg of standardized extract (4% total ginsenosides) two to three times daily.
0.5–2.0 g of dry root daily in divided doses.

Risks

Contraindications
Pregnancy, lactation.

Precautions/warnings
Hypertension, cardiovascular disease, hypotension, diabetes, patients receiving steroid therapy.

Adverse effects
Insomnia, diarrhea, vaginal bleeding, mastalgia, swollen tender breasts, increased libido, manic episodes, a possible cause of Stevens–Johnson syndrome.

Overdose
'Ginseng abuse syndrome' (dose approximately 3 g daily) with symptoms including hypertension, sleeplessness, skin eruptions,

morning diarrhea, agitation. Doses of 15 g daily and over were associated with depersonalization, confusion and depression.

Interactions

MAO inhibitors such as phenelzine, increased effects of hypoglycemics.

Quality issues

Evidence in the scientific literature mostly relates to G115® standardized ginseng extract (containing 100 mg of a 4% ginsenoside concentration from Korean *Panax ginseng*) and G115S® standardized ginseng extract (containing 100 mg of a 7% ginsenoside concentration from Korean *Panax ginseng*). Considerable inconsistencies in terms of active ingredients in commercial preparations exist.

Risk–benefit assessment

The data from rigorous clinical trials suggest that the effectiveness of ginseng root extract from *Panax ginseng* is not established beyond reasonable doubt for any indication. The possibility of serious adverse effects exists and thus may outweigh any potentially beneficial effects. Therefore (and contrary to the opinion of the German Commission E), the use of Asian ginseng as a therapeutic intervention cannot, at present, be recommended.

REFERENCES

1 Vogler B K, Pittler M H, Ernst E. The efficacy of ginseng. A systematic review of randomised clinical trials. Eur J Clin Pharmacol 1999; 55:567–575

2 Bahrke M S, Morgan W P. Evaluation of the ergogenic properties of ginseng. Sports Med 2000;29:113–133

3 Choi H K, Seong D H, Rha K H. Clinical efficacy of Korean red ginseng for erectile dysfunction. Int J Impot Res 1995; 7:181–186

4 Ziemba A W, Chmura J, Kaciuba-Uscilko H, Nazar K, Wisnik P, Gawronski W. Ginseng treatment improves psychomotor performance in young athletes. Int J Sports Nutr 1999; 9:371–377

HERBAL AND NON-HERBAL MEDICINE

BLACK COHOSH
(*Cimicifuga racemosa* L)

Synonyms

Actaea racemosa L, black snakeroot, bugbane, rattleroot, rattletop, rattleweed, Traubensilberkerze (German), Wanzenkraut (German).

Examples of trade names

Biophylin, Cimisan, Estroven, Femilla N, Femtrol, GNC Menopause, Klimadynon, Ligvites, Remifemin, Vegetex.

Source

Rhizome.

Main constituents

Steroidal terpenes. cimifugoside, actein, 27-deoxyactein, salicylic acid, tannin.

Background

Black cohosh is a perennial plant and a member of the buttercup family native to the eastern parts of North America. It grows up to a height of 2 meters and is found particularly in shady forests. Its Latin genus name *cimicifuga* derives from the Latin *cimex*, which is the genus name of the bedbug (*Cimex lectularius* L) and the Latin verb *fugare* ('to repel'), indicating that the unpleasant smell of the plant was used as an insect repellent, hence its synonyms 'bugbane' and 'Wanzenkraut'. Black cohosh was frequently used by the early settlers in North America as a remedy for rheumatism and rheumatic pain. Today, it is one of the best selling herbal remedies for reducing menopausal symptoms in the US.

Traditional uses

Inflammation, diarrhea, rheumatism. Promotion of lactation and menses.

Pharmacologic action

Vascular and estrogenic activity, hypotensive.

Conditions frequently treated

Premenstrual syndrome, dysmenorrhea, climacteric symptoms.

Clinical evidence

Several RCTs have been conducted on black cohosh extract and relate to symptoms associated with menopause.[1-3] One double-blind RCT (n=80) reported significant beneficial effects for menopausal symptoms as assessed by the Kupperman Index after 12 weeks of treatment compared with placebo.[1] Two RCTs reported a significant reduction of the Kupperman Index compared with baseline and no difference compared with reference medication.[2,3] Evidence from another double-blind RCT (n=179) suggested that a fixed combination of St John's wort and black cohosh administered over a treatment period of 6 weeks significantly reduces psychovegetative complaints compared with placebo.[4] There is no evidence from rigorous clinical trials for other indications.

Dosage

8 mg of standardized extract (1% 27-deoxyactein) daily in divided doses.
40 mg of dried rhizome and root daily in divided doses.

Risks

Contraindications
Pregnancy, lactation, estrogen-dependent tumors.

Precautions/warnings
Patients receiving antihypertensive medication.

Adverse effects
Gastrointestinal complaints, hypotension, headache, dizziness, nausea, allergic reactions.

Overdose

A review found no evidence for toxic or mutagenic effects in animal experiments after administering the extract for 6 months at about 90 times the human dose.[5]

Interactions

May interact with antihypertensive agents.

Quality issues

Quality and purity may vary between preparations. The majority of clinical trials were conducted using the same brand (Remifemin).

Risk–benefit assessment

Positive results from a few rigorous clinical studies indicate the potential of black cohosh for the treatment of symptoms associated with menopause. Its adverse effects profile is encouraging and it seems worth considering for symptoms associated with menopause. Conflicting evidence exists on its alleged estrogen-like activity and its effects in estrogen-dependent tumors. Thus it seems wise to view the latter condition as a contraindication for black cohosh extract.

REFERENCES

1 Stoll W. Phytopharmacon influences atrophic vaginal epithelium: double-blind study – Cimicifuga vs estrogenic substances. Therapeuticum 1987;1:23–31
2 Lehmann-Willenbrock E, Riedel H H. Clinical and endocrinological examinations concerning therapy of climacteric symptoms following hysterectomy with remaining ovaries. Zentralblatt für Gynäkologie 1988; 110:611–618
3 Warnecke G. Influence of a phytopharmaceutical on climacteric complaints. Med Welt 1985; 36:871–874
4 Boblitz N, Schrader E, Hennicke-von Zeppelin H-H, Wüstenberg P. Benefit of a drug containing St John's wort and black cohosh for climacteric patients – results of a randomised clinical trial. Focus Alt Compl Ther 2000;5:85–86
5 Beuscher N. Cimicifuga racemosa L. – Die Traubensilberkerze. Zeitschr für Phytotherapie 1995;16:301–310

CHASTE TREE
(Vitex agnus castus L)

Synonyms

Agneau chaste (French), agnus castus, chasteberry, gatillier (French), hemp tree, Keuschlamm (German), monk's pepper, vitex.

Examples of trade names

Agnolyt, Agnucaston, Femicur, Mastodynon.

Source

Root bark and fruit.

Main constituents

Flavonoids, iridoids, volatile oil, linoleic acid.

Background

A member of the *Verbenaceae* family, chaste tree is a deciduous shrub originating in Mediterranean Europe and western Asia. In Greek and Roman times the plant was used for promoting chastity in women and celibacy in monks. A wide range of medicinal uses was described by Hippocrates, Dioscorides and Pliny. The main uses that have persisted to modern times are in women's health care.

Traditional uses

Injuries, inflammation, snake bite, diarrhea, epilepsy, women's health, i.e. insufficient lactation, dysmenorrhea, amenorrhea, infertility, premenstrual and menopausal symptoms.

Pharmacologic action

Hypoprolactinemic, dopaminergic, antiinflammatory, antiandrogenic, antimicrobial.

Conditions frequently treated

Premenstrual syndrome, menopausal complaints, female infertility.

Clinical evidence

Double-blind placebo-controlled RCTs have suggested that chaste tree extracts are effective for cyclical mastalgia,[1–3] luteal phase deficiency[4] and female infertility due to secondary amenorrhea or luteal insufficiency.[5] For premenstrual syndrome, uncontrolled trials have produced positive results[6] but a placebo-controlled RCT was negative,[7] while an RCT comparing chaste tree and vitamin B_6 had an ambiguous result.[8]

Dosage

40 mg of standardized extract daily in divided doses.

Risks

Contraindications
Pregnancy, lactation.

Precautions/warnings
Increases in menstrual flow and changes in cycle are possible.

Adverse effects
Adverse effects have been reported only rarely and include allergic reaction, dry mouth, headache, and nausea.

Overdose
Studies with male volunteers have found no adverse effects with doses 12 times higher than the recommended dose. Routine animal toxicology studies have revealed no specific risks of large doses.

Interactions
Theoretically, interactions are possible with oral contraceptives, hormone replacement therapy and dopamine agonists and antagonists.

Quality issues
The whole plant extract is considered necessary for a therapeutic action. Authenticity is usually measured by agnuside content.

Risk–benefit assessment

Although the body of evidence from clinical trials for chaste tree is small, there are some promising results and the safety profile is encouraging. As a monotherapy, therefore, the potential benefits of this herb probably outweigh the risks.

REFERENCES

1 Wuttke W, Splitt G, Gorkow C. Sieder C. Behandlung zyklusabhängiger Brustschmerzen mit einem Agnus castus-haltigen Arzneimittel. Ergebnisse einer randomisierten, plazebokontrollierten Doppelblindstudie. Geb Fra 1997;57:569–574
2 Kubista E, Müller G, Spona J. Behandlung der Mastopathie mit zyklischer Mastodynie. Klinische Ergebnisse und Hormonprofile. Gynak Rdsch 1986;26:65–79
3 Halaska M, Beles P, Gorkow C, Sieder C. Treatment of cyclical mastalgia with a solution containing an extract of Vitex agnus castus: recent results of a placebo-controlled double-blind study. Breast 1999;8:175–181
4 Milewicz A, Gejdel E, Sworen H, Sienkiewicz K, Jedrzejak J, Teucher T, Schmitz H. Vitex agnus castus extract in the treatment of luteal phase defects due to latent hyperprolactinemia: results of a randomised, placebo-controlled, double-blind study. Arzneim-Forsch/Drug Res 1993;43:752–756
5 Gerhard I, Patek A, Monga B, Blank A, Gorkow C. Mastodynon bei weiblicher Sterilität. Randomisierte, plazebokontrollierte klinische Doppelblindstudie. Forsch Komplementärmed 1998;20:272–278
6 Loch E G, Selle H, Boblitz N. Treatment of premenstrual syndrome with a phytopharmaceutical formulation containing Vitex agnus castus. J Wom Health Gender-Based Med 2000;9:315–320
7 Turner S, Mills S. A double blind clinical trial on a herbal remedy for premenstrual syndrome: a case study. Compl Ther Med 1993; 1:73–77
8 Lauritzen C H, Reuter H D, Repges R, Bohnert K J, Schmidt U. Treatment of premenstrual tension syndrome with Vitex agnus castus. Controlled, double-blind study versus pyrodoxine. Phytomedicine 1997;4:183–189

FURTHER READING

Christie S, Walker A F. Vitex agnus castus L. (1) A review of its traditional and modern therapeutic use; (2) current use from a survey of practitioners. Eur J Herbal Med 1997–98; 3(3):29–45
An overview of some of the clinical trials of chaste tree and an insight into its use by herbalists.

CHITOSAN

Examples of trade names

Chitorich, Fat breaker, Fatmagnets.

Source

Shells of crustacea and various fungi.

Main constituent

Chitosan is a hydrophilic, positively charged polysaccharide.

Background

Chitosan, a co-polymer of glucosamine and N-acetylglucosamine, is generally obtained from the crustacean industry. The shells are collected and immediately processed for the isolation of chitin. It is used, for instance, in the cosmetic and textile industries but also as an ingredient in over-the-counter remedies in the US, UK and other countries.

Traditional uses

Chitosan has only relatively recently been used for medical purposes.

HERBAL AND NON-HERBAL MEDICINE

Pharmacologic action	Hypocholesterolemic, hypolipidemic, fat binding (in vitro and, according to manufacturers' claims, in human intestines).
Conditions frequently treated	Hypercholesterolemia, overweight, obesity.
Clinical evidence	A metaanalysis assessed five double-blind RCTs of chitosan for body weight reduction including 386 patients.[1] Although some positive evidence is reported, it was concluded that due to methodological limitations, the effectiveness of chitosan for lowering body weight is not established beyond reasonable doubt. Two double-blind RCTs conducted after the metaanalysis suggested that chitosan does not lower body weight.[2,3] Overall, there is no convincing evidence that chitosan is beneficial for body weight reduction.[4]
	Several clinical RCTs which administered calorie-restricted diets (1000–1200 kcal/day) corroborated findings from animal experiments and suggested cholesterol-lowering effects in hyper-cholesterolemic patients.[5,6] However, two double-blind RCTs which administered chitosan without dietary alterations found no relevant effects on total cholesterol.[2,3] There were, however, some positive effects on LDL cholesterol levels in a subgroup of obese patients.[3] No significant effects on fat-soluble vitamins are reported.
Dosage	2 g of deacetylated chitin biopolymer daily in divided doses.
Risks	*Contraindications* Pregnancy, lactation.
	Precautions/warnings There is a lack of relevant safety data relating to effects in women taking oral contraception.
	Adverse effects Constipation.
	Interactions May slow the absorption of oral contraceptives.
	Quality issues Products may vary in their content of deacetylated chitin.
Risk–benefit assessment	The few clinical studies available report mixed findings on the effects of chitosan for cholesterol reduction. The effectiveness of chitosan for hypercholesterolemia is therefore not established beyond reasonable doubt. Similarly, there is no convincing evidence that chitosan lowers body weight and more conventional behavioral approaches to change diet and physical activity should be encouraged. Chitosan seems to be relatively safe but it is costly.

REFERENCES

1 Ernst E, Pittler M H. Chitosan as a treatment for body weight reduction? A meta-analysis. Perfusion 1998;11:461–465

2 Pittler M H, Abbot N C, Harkness E F, Ernst E. Randomised, double blind trial of chitosan for body weight reduction. Eur J Clin Nutr 1999;53:379–381

3 Wuolijoki E, Hirvela T, Ylitalo P. Decrease in serum LDL cholesterol with microcrystalline chitosan. Methods Find Exp Clin Pharmacol 1999;21:357–361

4 Egger G, Cameron-Smith D, Stanton R. The effectiveness of popular, non-prescription weight loss supplements. Med J Aust 1999;171:604–608

5 Veneroni G, Veneroni F, Contos S, Tripodi S, de Bernardi M, Guarino C, Marleti A M. Effect of a new chitosan dietary integrator and hypocaloric diet on hyperlipidemia and overweight in obese patients. Acta Toxicol Ther 1996;17:53–70

6 Sciutto A M, Colombo P. Lipid-lowering effect of chitosan dietary integrator and hypocaloric diet in obese patients. Acta Toxicol Ther 1995;16: 215–230

CHONDROITIN

Synonyms

Chondroitin sulfate.

Examples of trade names

Arteparon.

Source

Bovine tracheal cartilage.

Main constituents

Glycosaminoglycans (GAGS), principally chondroitin-4-sulfate (CSA) and chondroitin-6-sulfate (CSC), and disaccharide polymers composed of equimolar amounts of D-glucuronic acid. N-acetyl-galactosamine and sulfates in 30 to 100 disaccharide units.

Background

Chondroitin is thought to rebuild cartilage and is promoted as a treatment for conditions associated with cartilage degeneration. There is some debate over the extent to which large molecules like glycosaminoglycans are absorbed after oral administration.

Traditional uses

Osteoarthritis, joint pain.

Pharmacologic action

Chondroitin has antiinflammatory activity, controls the formation of new cartilage matrix, inhibits leukocyte elastase and hyaluronidase. It also stimulates production of highly polymerized hyaluronic acid in synovial cells, thus increasing synovial viscosity and therefore possibly contributing to a 'lubrication effect'. Furthermore, it reduces inflammatory activity by inhibiting the recognition process of complement. These actions are believed to work in concert and constitute chondroitin's complex mechanisms of action.

Conditions frequently treated

Osteoarthritis.

HERBAL AND NON-HERBAL MEDICINE

**Clinical
evidence**

Several good-quality trials suggest symptomatic improvement in patients suffering from osteoarthritis (e.g. [1]). A metaanalysis of seven RCTs, including 372 patients in total, also came to a cautiously positive conclusion.[2] Yet it also pointed to the lack of long-term data. A further metaanalysis combined 15 RCTs of chondroitin and glucosamine for treatment of osteoarthritis.[3] It disclosed several methodological weaknesses of the primary studies and raised the suspicion of publication bias. Nevertheless, it came to a positive overall conclusion and stated that 'moderate to large effects' can be expected from these supplements.

Dosage

800–1200 mg of chondroitin sulfate daily in divided doses.

Risks

Contraindications
Pregnancy, lactation.

Precautions/warnings
Bleeding disorders.

Adverse effects
Dyspepsia, headache, euphoria, nausea.

Interactions
Potentiation of anticoagulants theoretically possible.

Quality issues
Many commercially available products do not contain the stated dosage.

**Risk–benefit
assessment**

Effectiveness seems likely and risks seem to be minor. The size of the effect is usually such that chondroitin is best used as an adjuvant to other interventions for osteoarthritis.

REFERENCES

1 Morreale P, Manopulo R, Galati M. Boccanera L, Saponati G, Bocchi L. Comparison of the anti-inflammatory efficacy of chondroitin sulfate and diclofenac sodium in patients with knee osteoarthritis. J Rheumatol 1996;23:1385–1391

2 Leeb B F, Scweitzer H, Montag K, Smolen J S. A metaanalysis of chondroitin sulfate in the treatment of osteoarthritis. J Rheumatol 2000;27:1

3 McAlindon T E, LaValley M P, Gulin J P, Felson D T. Glucosamine and chondroitin for treatment of osteoarthritis. A systematic quality assessment and meta-analysis. JAMA 2000;283:1469–1475

CO-ENZYME Q10

Synonyms

Ubiquinone; 2,3 dimethoxy-5 methyl-6-decaprenyl benzoquinone.

**Examples of
trade names**

Adelir, Heartcin, Neuquinone, Q10, Taidecanone, Udekinon.

Source Co-enzyme Q10 is present in most cells and the highest concentrations are found in heart, liver, kidneys and pancreas. Today it is synthesized in large quantities for the food supplement market.

Main constituent Ubiquinones.

Background The compound is thought to enhance cell function. Patients with congestive heart failure have low levels of co-enzyme Q10. It is commercially produced according to a Japanese patent and marketed for a wide range of conditions.

Traditional uses Oral supplementation with co-enzyme Q10 has been promoted for a wide variety of indications ranging from heart failure to general tonic.

Pharmacologic action On the cellular level co-enzyme Q10 participates in the electron transfer within the oxidative respiration chain in the mitochondria, thus preventing ATP depletion as well as oxidant and ischemic cellular damage. It also acts as a membrane stabilizer and free radical scavenger.

Conditions frequently treated Congestive heart failure (CHF) and, increasingly, neurological disorders.

Clinical evidence Several RCTs have been published but their results are highly contradictory. Some trials included patients with CHF NYHA stage III–IV and showed superiority over placebo (e.g. [1]). A rigorous crossover trial included 30 patients suffering from ischemic or idiopathic dilated cardiomyopathy and chronic left ventricular dysfunction. Its results showed no subjective or objective improvements during 3 months of co-enzyme Q10 therapy.[2] In a larger (n=55) RCT patients with CHF NYHA stage III–IV received either 200 mg/day of co-enzyme Q10 or placebo for 6 months.[3] The results show no advantage over placebo in terms of ejection fraction, peak oxygen consumption or exercise duration. Moreover, there were no intergroup differences related to subjective improvement. There is no compelling evidence to demonstrate that co-enzyme Q10 is effective for any other indication.

Dosage 50–300 mg of co-enzyme Q_{10} daily.

Risks ***Contraindications***
Pregnancy, lactation, known allergy (probably rare).

HERBAL AND NON-HERBAL MEDICINE

Precautions/warnings
Excessive exercise should be avoided while taking co-enzyme Q10 supplements.

Adverse effects
Anorexia, diarrhea, other gastrointestinal symptoms, nausea.

Interactions
Theoretically it could decrease the effects of warfarin; HMG-CoA reductase inhibitors might decrease co-enzyme Q10 levels.

Quality issues
Products should state concentration and purity.

Risk–benefit assessment
The effectiveness of co-enzyme Q10 for CHF is uncertain but risks are few. Several effective conventional treatments exist for this condition so co-enzyme Q10 cannot be recommended as therapy for CHF. No conclusive evidence exists for any other indications.

REFERENCES
1 Morisco C, Trimarco B, Condorelli M. Effect of coenzyme Q10 therapy in patients with congestive heart failure. A long-term multicenter, randomized study. Clin Invest 1993; 71:134–136
2 Watson P S, Scalia G M, Galbraith A, Burstow D J, Bett N. Lack of effect of Coenzyme Q on left ventricular function in patients with congestive heart failure. J Am Coll Cardiol 1999;33:1549–1552
3 Khatta M, Alexander B S, Krichten C M, Frendenberger R, Robinson S W. Gottlieb S S. The effect of Coenzyme Q10 in patients with congestive heart failure. Ann Intern Med 2000; 132:636–640

FURTHER READING
Sinatra S T. Co-enzyme Q10: a vital therapeutic nutrient for the heart with special application in congestive heart failure. Conn Med 1997;65:707–711

CRANBERRY
(*Vaccinium marcocarpon*)

Synonyms
Kronsbeere (German), marsh apple, Moosbeere, Preisselbeere (German), *Vaccinium oxycoccos*.

Examples of trade names
Cran Fastic, Cran Relief.

Source
Berries.

Main constituents
Catechin, flavone glycosides, fructose, organic acids, proanthocyanidins, vitamin C.

Background
Cranberries are evergreen shrubs which grow in most temperate climates. In the US, cranberries are native to the area from Tennessee to Alaska. In 1840, German scientists postulated that cranberry juice had antibacterial activity. Ever since, it has been

advocated as a remedy for urinary tract infections. Several clinical trials have confirmed its efficacy but a degree of controversy and uncertainty remains. In particular, it is now clear that cranberry has no antibacterial activity.

Traditional uses   Urinary tract infection.

Pharmacologic action   The mechanism(s) by which cranberry prevents urinary tract infections is (are) still controversial. A current theory suggests that its mode of action is the inhibition of the adhesion of bacteria to the uroepithelial surface.

Conditions frequently treated   Prevention of recurrent urinary tract infections.

Clinical evidence   The most rigorous RCTs show that cranberry juice (300 ml/day) taken regularly for 6 months reduces the incidence of urinary tract infections when compared with placebo.[1] A recent Cochrane Review[2] included four RCTs, three of which yielded positive results. However, due to the poor quality of these studies, the authors question the reliability of these findings. Cranberry juice is not an effective therapy for manifest infections.[3] Cranberry has also been suggested as an anticancer remedy, but no good evidence exists in support of this claim.

Dosage   300–400 mg of standardized extract twice daily.
150–600 ml of cranberry juice daily.

Risks
Contraindications
Pregnancy, lactation.

Precautions/warnings
Cranberry should not be taken as a substitute for antibiotic treatment; diabetics must consider the sugar content of the juice.

Adverse effects
None known.

Overdose
Diarrhea.

Interactions
Theoretically cranberry juice could enhance the elimination of drugs excreted in urine or increase effects of some antibiotics in the urinary tract.

Quality issues
Standardized extracts or juice should be used for medicinal purposes; diabetics should use sugar-free preparations.

HERBAL AND NON-HERBAL MEDICINE

Risk–benefit assessment	On balance, the evidence is only marginally in favor of cranberry's efficacy in the prevention of urinary tract infections. However, its safety profile is excellent so it might be considered as a preventive in patients prone to such infections, particularly as long-term antibiotic prophylaxis has significant adverse effects.

REFERENCES

1 Avorn J, Manone M, Gurwitz J H, Glynn R J, Choodnovskiy I, Lipsitz L A. Reduction of bacteriuria and pyuria after ingestion of cranberry juice. JAMA 1994;272:590

2 Jepson R G, Mihaljevic L, Craig J. Cranberries for preventing urinary tract infections. Cochrane Library. Oxford: Update Software, 2000

3 Jepson R G, Mihaljevic L, Craig J. Cranberries for treating urinary tract infections. Cochrane Library. Oxford: Update Software, 2000

DEVIL'S CLAW
(Harpagophytum procumbens Burchell)

Synonyms	Grapple plant, Teufelskralle (German), wood spider.
Examples of trade names	Artrosan, Devil's Claw Vegicaps, Harpagon.
Source	Root and tubers.
Main constituents	The major active ingredient is harpagoside. Other compounds are harpagide, procumbide, stigmasterol, beta-sitosterol, triterpenes and flavonoids.
Background	The name devil's claw is derived from the plant's unique fruits which are covered with claw-like hooks. It grows wild in South Africa and the recent popularity of devil's claw has nearly resulted in it becoming an endangered species.
Traditional uses	Digestive problems, rheumatic conditions, climacteric problems, dysmenorrhea, gastrointestinal complaints, headaches, liver and kidney diseases, malaria, nicotine poisoning and skin cancer.
Pharmacologic action	Antiinflammatory, negative chronotropic, positive inotropic, antiarrhythmic.
Conditions frequently treated	Musculoskeletal and arthritic pain.
Clinical evidence	Several RCTs have so far been carried out. The most rigorous studies[1] suggest that devil's claw is superior to placebo in

alleviating musculoskeletal pain. Another RCT[2] demonstrated a dose-dependent analgesic effect in 183 patients with back pain. The effect size. however, is moderate. A recent RCT[3] included 122 patients with osteoarthritis and compared the effects of 6×435 mg powdered devil's claw with 100 mg oral diacerhein given daily for 4 months. Both treatments were associated with similar reductions in pain and there were fewer adverse effects in the devil's claw group.

Dosage

400–500 mg of dried extract three times daily.

Risks

Contraindications
Pregnancy, lactation, gastric or duodenal ulcer.

Precautions/warnings
See above.

Adverse effects
Gastrointestinal symptoms.

Overdose
Cardiac effects.

Interactions
May increase anticoagulation effects of warfarin; theoretically it could interact with cardiac drugs.

Quality issues
The harpagoside content and pharmacokinetic profile have been shown to vary considerably between commercial preparations.

Risk–benefit assessment

Effectiveness for musculoskeletal pain is reasonably well documented and only mild adverse effects are on record. The effectiveness of devil's claw compared to conventional treatment options (e.g. NSAIDS) cannot be judged on the basis of only one comparative trial.[3] Thus devil's claw can be tried in selected cases but the risks of herb/drug interactions must be considered.

HERBAL AND NON-HERBAL MEDICINE

REFERENCES

1 Ernst E, Chrubasik S. Phyto-antiinflammatories. A systematic review of randomized, placebo-controlled, double-blind trials. Rheum Dis Clin North Am 2000;1:13–27

2 Chrubasik S, Junck H, Breitschwerdt H, Conradt C H, Zappe H. Effectiveness of *Harpagophytum* extract WS 1531 in the treatment of exacerbation of low back pain: a randomized, placebo-controlled, double-blind study. Eur J Anaesthesiol 1999;16:118–129

3 Chantre P, Cappelaere A, Leblan D, Guedon D, Vandermander J, Fournie B. Efficacy and tolerance of *Harpagophytum procumbens* versus diacerhein in treatment of osteoarthritis. Phytomedicine 2000;7:177–183

ECHINACEA
(*Echinacea* spp.)

Synonyms	American cone flower, black Sampson hedgehog, Indian head, snakeroot, red sunflower, scurvy root.
Examples of trade names	Glycerite, Herbal Comfort, Echinacin.
Source	Roots of *E. angustifolia* and *E. pallida*, roots and other parts of *E. purpurea*.
Main constituents	Polysaccharides, glycoproteins, alkamides, flavonoids.
Background	Echinacea was used for medicinal purposes by the American Indians. It started to be scientifically investigated in the late 19th century, mainly in Germany, and has now become one of the most popular herbal remedies on the US and European markets. Three different species are used for medicinal purposes.
Traditional uses	Externally for wound healing, mouth sores, toothache, burns, eczema. Internally for varicose ulcers and prevention of infections, snake bites, fever, urinary tract infections.
Pharmacologic action	Stimulant of cellular and hormonal immune defense, local anesthetic, antiinflammatory, activation of adrenal cortex, antiviral, free radical scavenger. The main mechanism of action is believed to lie in stimulating macrophages to produce interleukins and tumor necrosis factor.
Conditions frequently treated	Prevention and treatment of common infections such as respiratory tract infections.
Clinical evidence	A Cochrane Review[1] summarized 16 CCTs of echinacea for the common cold. Five placebo-controlled prevention trials tested five different echinacea preparations. Overall, the results were not conclusive. Three prevention trials with no-intervention control groups suggested a beneficial effect. Of the eight treatment trials (all placebo-controlled) only two showed no significant effect in favor of echinacea. The authors conclude that, to date, there is insufficient evidence to recommend a specific echinacea product.
Dosage	1 g of dried herb or equivalent three times daily. 0.5–1.0 ml of liquid extract (1:1 45% ethanol) three times daily.
Risks	***Contraindications*** Pregnancy, lactation.

Precautions/warnings

Patients suffering from progressive systemic diseases such as AIDS, MS, collagen or autoimmune diseases and leukoses should not use echinacea for prolonged periods of time (theoretical concerns).

Adverse effects

Allergic reactions (uncommon).

Interactions

Could theoretically decrease effects of immunosuppressants.

Quality issues

Cold-pressed juice of *E. purpurea* seems to be the most active preparation for prevention of upper respiratory tract infections. Controversy continues as to which parts of the plants are best suited for medicinal use.

Risk–benefit assessment

There is some encouraging evidence relating to the treatment and prevention of the common cold. Treatment seems most promising in the very early stages of the condition. No serious risks have been reported. Thus echinacea preparations may be worth considering for such patients.

REFERENCE

1 Melchart D, Linde K, Fischer P, Kaesmayr J. Echinacea for the prevention and treatment of the common cold. Cochrane Library. Oxford: Update Software, 1999

FURTHER READING

Hobbs C. The chemistry and pharmacology of Echinacea species. Herbalgram l994;30(suppl):1–7
Bauer R. Wagner H. Echinacea species as potential immunostimulatory drugs. Economic Med Plant Res 1991;5:253–321

HERBAL AND NON-HERBAL MEDICINE

EVENING PRIMROSE
(Oenothera biennis L)

Synonyms

Fever plant, king's cureall, Nachtkerze (German), night willow-herb, scabish, sundrop, tree primrose.

Examples of trade names

Efamast, Efamol, Epogam, Evoprim.

Source

Oil from seeds.

Main constituents

The seeds contain 14% fixed oil comprising approximately 70% cis-linoleic acid (LA), 9% cis-gamma-linolenic acid (GLA), 2–16% oleic acid, 7% palmitic acid, 3% stearic acid.

Background

Evening primrose is not actually a primrose but belongs to the fuchsia (*Onagraceae*) family. It is native to North America and naturalized in western Europe and parts of Asia and blooms in early summer, producing large yellow flowers which open in the evenings – hence its name. Originally the root was used as a vegetable for culinary purposes and the whole plant was used for its medicinal properties to treat a wide range of conditions. Today it is mainly the oil that is used for therapeutic purposes.

Traditional uses

Gastrointestinal disorders, neuralgia, asthma, whooping cough.

Pharmacologic action

For individuals in whom the conversion of LA to GLA by the enzyme delta-6 desaturase is impaired, the rich GLA content of evening primrose oil allows this conversion to be bypassed.

Conditions frequently treated

Dermatological conditions (atopic eczema, psoriasis), inflammatory/autoimmune conditions (rheumatoid arthritis, multiple sclerosis), cardiovascular conditions, psychiatric conditions (schizophrenia, hyperactivity, dementia), female conditions (premenstrual syndrome, menopausal complaints, mastalgia).

Clinical evidence

Positive results from a metaanalysis of nine controlled trials of atopic eczema in 1989[1] have been contradicted by subsequent RCTs.[2–4] A systematic review of premenstrual syndrome trials suggested that evening primrose oil had little value for treating this condition.[5] A large range of other conditions have been investigated, including asthma,[6,7] psoriasis,[8,9] hyperactivity,[10,11] multiple sclerosis,[12,13] menopausal flushing,[14] schizophrenia,[15] obesity,[16,17] chronic fatigue syndrome,[18,19] rheumatoid arthritis,[20–22] and mastalgia.[23–25] Results have been largely negative or ambiguous. Diabetic neuropathy is one condition where results appear promising.[26,27]

Dosage

Mastalgia: 3–4 g (8% GLA) daily in divided doses.

Atopic eczema: 6–8 g (adults), 2–4 g (children) daily in divided doses.

Risks

Contraindications
Pregnancy, lactation, mania, epilepsy.

Precautions/warnings
There is a risk of undiagnosed temporal lope epilepsy being manifested in schizophrenics or other patients taking epileptogenic agents.

Adverse effects
Gastrointestinal symptoms, headache.

Overdose
Gastrointestinal symptoms have been observed with large doses.

Interactions
Theoretically, interactions with antiinflammatory drugs, corticosteroids, beta-blockers, antipsychotics and anticoagulants are

possible. Concomitant use with epileptogenic agents such as phenothiazines may increase the risk of seizures.

Quality issues

Standardized preparations usually contain 8% GLA. Some products contain a combination of evening primrose oil and fish oil (omega-3).

Risk–benefit assessment

Despite having been subjected to a reasonably large number of clinical trials, evening primrose oil has not been established as an efficacious treatment for any condition. It appears to be generally safe, however, so for conditions where preliminary evidence offers some promise (e.g. diabetic neuropathy), it may merit consideration.

REFERENCES

1 Morse P F, Horrobin D F, Manku M S et al. Meta-analysis of placebo-controlled studies of the efficacy of Epogam in the treatment of atopic eczema. Relationship between plasma essential fatty acid changes and clinical response. Br J Dermatol 1989;121:75–90

2 Whitaker D K, Cilliers J, De Beer C. Evening primrose oil (Epogam) in the treatment of chronic hand dermatitis: disappointing therapeutic results. Dermatology 1996;193:115–120

3 Berth-Jones J, Brown G. Placebo-controlled trial of essential fatty acid supplementation in atopic dermatitis. Lancet 1993;341:1557–1560

4 Hederos C A, Berg A. Epogam evening primrose oil treatment in atopic dermatitis and asthma. Arch Dis Child 1996;75:494–497

5 Budeiri D, Li Won Po D, Dornan J C. Is evening primrose oil of value in the treatment of premenstrual syndrome? Controlled Clin Trials 1996;17:60–68

6 Ebden P, Bevan C, Banks J, Fennerty A, Walters E H. A study of evening primrose seed oil in atopic asthma. Prostagland Leukot Essent Fatty Acids 1989;35:69–72

7 Stenius-Aarniala B, Aro A, Hakulinen A, Ahola I, Seppala E, Vapaatalo H. Evening primrose oil and fish oil are ineffective as supplementary treatment of bronchial asthma. Ann Allergy 1989;62:534–537

8 Strong A M M, Hamill E. The effect of combined fish oil and evening primrose oil (Efamol Marine) on the remission phase of psoriasis: a 7-month double-blind randomized placebo-controlled trial. J Dermatol Treat 1993;4:33–36

9 Oliwiecki S, Burton J L. Evening primrose oil and marine oil in the treatment of psoriasis. Clin Exp Dermatol 1994;19:127–129

10 Arnold L E, Kleykamp D, Votolato N A, Taylor W A, Kontras S B, Tobin K. Gamma-linolenic acid for attention-deficit hyperactivity disorder: placebo-controlled comparison to D-amphetamine. Biol Psychiatr 1989;25:222–228

11 Aman M G, Mitchell E A, Turbott S H. The effects of essential fatty acid supplementation by Efamol in hyperactive children. J Abnorm Child Psychol 1987;15:75–90

12 Bates D, Fawcett P R W, Shaw D A, Weightman D. Trial of polyunsaturated fatty acids in non-relapsing multiple sclerosis. Br Med J 1977;2:932–933

13 Bates D, Fawcett P R W, Shaw D A, Weightman D. Polyunsaturated fatty acids in treatment of acute remitting multiple sclerosis. Br Med J 1978;2:404–405

14 Chenoy R, Hussain S, Tayob T, O'Brien P M S, Moss M Y, Morse P F. Effect of oral gamolenic acid from evening primrose oil on menopausal flushing. Br Med J 1994;308:501–503

15 Joy C B, Mumby-Croft R, Joy L A. Polyunsaturated fatty acid supplementation (fish or evening primrose oil) for schizophrenia. Cochrane Library, Oxford: Update Software, 2000

16 Haslett C, Douglas J G, Chalmers S R, Weighhill A, Munro J F. A double-blind evaluation of evening primrose oil as an antiobesity agent. Int J Obes 1983;7:549–553

17 Garcia C, Carter J, Chou A. Gamma linolenic acid causes weight loss and lower blood pressure in overweight patients with family history of obesity. Swed J Biol Med 1986;4:8–11

18 Behan P O, Behan W M H, Horrobin D. Effect of high doses of essential fatty acids on the postviral fatigue syndrome. Acta Neurol Scand 1990;82:209–216

HERBAL AND NON-HERBAL MEDICINE

19 Warren G, McKendrick M, Peet M. The role of essential fatty acids in chronic fatigue syndrome. Acta Neurol Scand 1999;99:112–116

20 Veale D J, Torley H I, Richards I M, O'Dowd A, Fitzsimons C, Belch J J, Sturrock R D. A double-blind placebo-controlled trial of Efamol Marine on skin and joint symptoms of psoriatic arthritis. Br J Rheumatol 1994;33:954–958

21 Brzeski M, Madhok R, Capell H A. Evening primrose oil in patients with rheumatoid arthritis and side effects of non-steroidal anti-inflammatory drugs. Br J Rheumatol 1991;30:370–372

22 Belch J J, Ansell D, Madhok R, O'Dowd A, Sturrock R D. Effects of altering dietary essential fatty acids on requirements for non-steroidal anti-inflammatory drugs in patients with rheumatoid arthritis: a double-blind placebo-controlled study. Ann Rheum Dis 1988;47:96–104

23 Gateley C A, Miers M, Mansel R E, Hughes L E. Drug treatments for mastalgia: 17 years experience in the Cardiff mastalgia clinic. J Roy Soc Med 1992;85:12–15

24 Gately C A, Maddox P R, Pritchard G A et al. Plasma fatty acid profiles in benign breast disorders. Br J Surg 1992;79:407–409

25 Mansel R E, Harrison B J, Melhuish J et al. A randomized trial of dietary intervention with essential fatty acids in patients with categorised cysts. Ann NY Acad Sci 1990;586:288–294

26 Jamal G A, Carmichael H, Weir A I. Gamma-linolenic acid in diabetic neuropathy. Lancet 1986;1:1098

27 Keen H, Payan J, Allawi J et al. Treatment of diabetic neuropathy with gamma-linolenic acid. Diabetes Care 1993;16:8–15

FURTHER READING

Horrobin D F. Gamma linolenic acid: an inter-mediate in essential fatty acid metabolism with potential as an ethical pharmaceutical and as a food. Rev Contemp Pharmacother 1990;1:1–41
Detailed and thoroughly referenced account of the mechanisms of GLA and effects of evening primrose oil.

FEVERFEW
(*Tanacetum parthenium* Schultz-Bip)

Synonyms	Altamisa, bachelor's buttons, *Chrysanthemum parthenium* (L), featherfew, motherherb, Mutterkraut (German).
Examples of trade names	Feverfew Glyc, Feverfew Power, Tanacet.
Source	Leaves.
Main constituents	Camphor, chrysanthemyl acetate and flavonoids. The sesquiterpene lactone parthenolide is thought to be the active principle.
Background	Feverfew is a perennial plant, native to Asia Minor. It reaches a height of 15–60 cm and is today widely naturalized throughout much of Europe, North America and Canada. Its use as an herbal remedy goes back to ancient times when it was employed for many aches and pains, in particular for conditions associated with fevers and women's ailments. Today the extract of feverfew is predominantly used for the prevention of migraine attacks and to alleviate the accompanying symptoms.
Traditional uses	Colds, fevers, headaches, rheumatism, general aches, women's ailments.

Pharmacologic action	Antimigraine, spasmolytic, antiinflammatory, antithrombotic. It has been suggested that parthenolide exerts inhibiting effects on serotonin release by human platelets in vitro. Other evidence suggests that chrysanthemyl acetate may be important. This constituent has been shown to inhibit prostaglandin synthesis in vitro and seems to possess analgesic properties.
Conditions frequently treated	Migraine. rheumatoid arthritis.
Clinical evidence	A systematic review assessed five double-blind RCTs of feverfew for migraine.[1] Three of four clinical trials report that feverfew is beneficial for the prevention of migraine in terms of attack frequency and associated symptoms such as pain and severity of nausea and vomiting.[2] One double-blind RCT of feverfew as a treatment for rheumatoid arthritis found no relevant differences for clinical or laboratory variables compared with placebo, but reports some beneficial effects for grip strength.[3]
Dosage	50–140 mg of powdered or granulated extract daily in divided doses.

Risks

Contraindications
Pregnancy, lactation, hypersensitivity to members of the *Asteraceae* family.

Precautions/warnings
Should not be used for longer than 4 months due to the lack of long-term toxicity data.

Adverse effects
Contact dermatitis, mouth ulceration and soreness, stomach complaints, 'post-feverfew syndrome' including rebound of migraine symptoms, anxiety, insomnia, muscle and joint stiffness.

Interactions
May potentiate the effects of anticoagulants.

Quality issues
The amount of active constituents may vary in and between feverfew preparations due to the lack of standardization.

Risk–benefit assessment	The available evidence is promising but at present not compelling. Given the limited number of available options for the prevention of migraine, the severity of the condition in many cases and the relative safety of feverfew, it is worth considering while carefully monitoring the patient. There are too few studies for any firm judgement on its effectiveness in rheumatoid arthritis.

HERBAL AND NON-
HERBAL MEDICINE

REFERENCES

1 Vogler B K, Pittler M H, Ernst E. Feverfew as a preventive treatment for migraine: a systematic review. Cephalalgia 1998;18:704–708

2 Pittler M H, Vogler B K, Ernst E. Efficacy of feverfew for the prevention of migraine.

Cochrane Library. Oxford: Update Software, 2000

3 Pattrick M, Heptinstall S, Doherty M. Feverfew in rheumatoid arthritis: a double-blind, placebo-controlled study. Ann Rheum Dis 1989;48:547–549

GARLIC
(Allium sativum L)

Synonyms	Ail (French), camphor of the poor, Da-Suan, Knoblauch (German), La-Juan, poor man's treacle, rustic treacle, stinking rose.
Examples of trade names	Kwai, Kyolic, Sapec.
Source	Bulb and oil from bulb.
Main constituents	Alliin, allinase, diallyl disulfide, ajoens and many others; alliin is enzymatically converted to allicin which is thought to be one of the main active ingredients and is responsible for the characteristic, sulfur-like smell.
Background	For millennia, garlic has been used as a food and spice in many countries. It has also been used in most cultures for various medicinal purposes. Its extensive scientific investigation started relatively recently but today it is one of the best-researched (and best-selling) herbal remedies.
Traditional uses	Garlic has been used both orally and topically for many purposes, most consistently perhaps to prevent and treat infections and as a way of maintaining general health.
Pharmacologic action	Antibacterial, antiviral, antifungal, antihypertensive, blood glucose lowering, antithrombotic, antimutagenic, antiplatelet. Its best-researched property is that of lowering total serum cholesterol levels; its main mechanism of action is probably the inhibition of hepatic cholesterol synthesis.
Conditions frequently treated	Hypercholesterolemia, prevention of arteriosclerosis.
Clinical evidence	Numerous RCTs published in the late 1980s and early 1990s demonstrated a significant reduction of total cholesterol and LDL cholesterol. Several systematic reviews of these data therefore arrived at positive conclusions. More recently, however, a series of negative RCTs has emerged. An updated metaanalysis

of all rigorous RCTs produced an overall result which was marginally positive when all RCTs were included (average reduction=0.41 mmol/l), but a non-significant effect on total cholesterol when only the high-quality RCTs were analyzed.[1]

The cumulative trial data on its blood pressure-lowering effects show a significant, albeit small, antihypertensive effect.[2] Some interesting, though not compelling data (e.g. [3]) suggest that, due to its broad-ranging effects on the above-mentioned and other cardiovascular risk factors, the regular intake of garlic might prevent or delay the development of arteriosclerosis. Epidemiological data indicate that the regular consumption of garlic might convey a protective effect for malignancies, in particular intestinal cancers (e.g. [4]). A recent RCT (n=100) implies that high-dose garlic consumption reduces the frequency of tick bites in a tick-endemic area.[5] All other claimed health effects, particularly those related to garlic's antimicrobial activities, are not supported by compelling evidence from sound clinical trials.

Dosage

4 g of fresh garlic daily.
8 mg of garlic oil daily.
600–900 mg of standardized extract (1.3% alliin content) daily in divided doses.

Risks

Contraindications
Pregnancy, lactation, peptic ulcers, allergies to *Liliaceae* family.

Precautions/warnings
Patients with bleeding abnormalities; before major surgery, garlic supplements should be discontinued.

Adverse effects
Breath and body odor, allergic reactions, nausea, heartburn, flatulence.

Overdose
Nausea, vomiting, risk of bleeding.

Interactions
Can increase effect of anticoagulants, could theoretically enhance hypoglycemic effects of antidiabetic medications.

Quality issues
Commercial products vary greatly in terms of concentration of active ingredients.

Risk–benefit assessment

Garlic probably does lower total cholesterol but only to a minor degree. With certain precautions. it is worth considering as an adjunct to dietary and lifestyle measures in selected patients with hypercholesterolemia. The regular intake of fresh garlic with food probably has some protective effects against intestinal cancer.

HERBAL AND NON-HERBAL MEDICINE

REFERENCES

1 Stevinson C, Pittler M H, Ernst E. Garlic for treating hypercholesterolemia: a meta-analysis of randomized clinical trials. Ann Intern Med 2000;133:420–429

2 Silagy C, Neil A. A meta-analysis of the effect of garlic on blood pressure. J Hypertension 1994;12:463–468

3 Breithaupt-Grogler K, Ling M, Boudoulas H, Belz G G. Protective effects of chronic garlic intake on elastic properties of aorta in the elderly. Circulation 1997;96:2649–2655

4 Ernst E. Can allium vegetables prevent cancer? Phytomedicine 1997;4:79–83

5 Stjernberg L, Berglund J. Garlic as insect repellent. JAMA 2000;284:831

FURTHER READING

Koch H P, Lawson L D. Garlic, 2nd edn. Baltimore: Williams and Wilkins, 1996
A comprehensive introductory text for health-care professionals.

GERMAN CHAMOMILE
(Matricaria recutita L)

Synonyms	Fleur de camomile (French), Hungarian chamomile, Kamille (German), pin heads, single chamomile, sweet false chamomile, wild chamomile.
Examples of trade names	Kamillosan, Eukamillat.
Source	Flower heads.
Main constituents	Capric acid, coumarins, flavonoids (apigenin), polysaccharides, spiroethers, tannins, terpenoid volatile oils (chamazulene, alpha-bisabolol).
Background	German chamomile is an annual herb belonging to the *Asteraceae* family. It is native to most of Europe and western Asia and naturalized throughout North America and Australia. Along with Roman or English chamomile (*Chamaemelum nobile*), it has been used for medicinal purposes since ancient times because of its reputed antiinflammatory and antispasmodic properties. Hippocrates, Dioscorides and Galen all referred to chamomile in their works. It is commonly drunk as a tea.
Traditional uses	Gastrointestinal complaints, insomnia, anxiety, teething and colic in babies, skin conditions, gum irritations.
Pharmacologic action	Antiinflammatory, antispasmodic, antibacterial.
Conditions frequently treated	Gastrointestinal complaints, skin inflammations, anxiety, insomnia.
Clinical evidence	A commercial topical preparation based on chamomile was reported to be as useful as hydrocortisone for eczema in a

HERBAL AND NON-HERBAL MEDICINE

non-randomized trial (n=161), although no statistical analysis was conducted.[1] In a subsequent RCT (n=72) the chamomile cream showed slight superiority over hydrocortisone but little difference compared with placebo.[2] Again there was no statistical analysis. Another non-randomized trial found no superiority of the same preparation over almond oil for skin damage after irradiation for breast cancer treatment.[3] A placebo-controlled RCT (n=164) found chamomile mouthwash ineffective in reducing 5-fluorouracil-induced stomatitis.[4] An RCT (n=79) found that a preparation consisting of chamomile extract and apple pectin reduced the duration of childhood diarrhea more than placebo.[5] Steam inhalation of chamomile extract was reported to have a dose-dependent effect on symptoms of the common cold in a placebo-controlled trial.[6]

Dosage

1–4 ml of liquid extract (1:1 in 45% alcohol) three times daily. 3 g of dried flowers in 150 ml hot water (chamomile tea) three times daily.

Risks

Contraindications
Pregnancy, lactation.

Precautions/warnings
Known sensitivity to other members of the *Asteraceae* family (e.g. asters, chrysanthemums, sunflowers), asthma or other allergic conditions.

Adverse effects
Allergies to chamomile species (mainly skin reactions) are documented and at least two cases of anaphylactic reactions have been reported.

Overdose
Emesis has been reported following consumption of large doses.

Interactions
Theoretically, the effects of anticoagulants could be potentiated.

Quality issues
Preparations should be standardized and authenticated as adulteration is common. Chamazulene and alpha-bisabolol are commonly used as the marker substances.

Risk–benefit assessment

There is little clinical evidence to support the therapeutic claims made for German chamomile extracts and given the risk of allergic reactions, the potential benefits do not appear to outweigh the possible risks.

REFERENCES

1 Aertgeerts P, Albring M, Klaschka F, Nasemann T, Patzelt-Wenczler R, Rauhut K, Weigl B. Comparative testing of Kamillosan cream and steroidal (0.25% hydrocortisone, 0.75% fluocortin butyl ester) and non-steroidal (5% bufexamac) dermatologic agents in maintenance therapy of eczematous diseases. Zeitschr für Hautkrankheiten 1985;60:270–277

HERBAL AND NON-HERBAL MEDICINE

2 Patzelt-Wenczler R, Ponce-Pöschl E. Proof of efficacy of Kamillosan cream in atopic eczema. Eur J Med Res 2000;5:171–175

3 Maiche A G, Grohn P, Maki-Hokkonen H. Effect of chamomile cream and almond ointment on acute radiation skin reaction. Acta Oncol 1991;30:395–396

4 Fidler P, Loprinzi C, O'Fallon J et al. Prospective evaluation of a chamomile mouthwash for prevention of 5 FU induced oral mucositis. Cancer 1996;77:522–525

5 De La Motte S, O'Reilly S, Heinisch M, Harrison F. Double-blind comparison of an apple pectin-chamomile extract preparation with placebo in children with diarrhoea. Arzeim-Forsch/Drug Res 1997;47:1247–1249

6 Saller R, Beschomer M, Hellenbrecht D, Buhring M. Dose dependency of symptomatic relief of complaints by chamomile steam inhalation in patients with common cold. Eur J Pharmacol 1990;183:728–729

FURTHER READING

Hörmann H P, Korting H C. Evidence for the efficacy and safety of topical herbal drugs in dermatology: part I: anti-inflammatory agents. Phytomedicine 1994;1(2):161–171
Includes useful information on pharmacological and clinical research into chamomile preparations.

GINGER
(*Zingiber officinale* Roscoe)

Synonyms	Ingwer (German).
Examples of trade names	Gingerall, Zintona.
Source	Rhizome.
Main constituents	Non-volatile pungent principles, non-pungent substances, volatile oil, starch, triglycerides, niacin and vitamins.
Background	Ginger is a perennial plant native to southern Asia. It has been used as food and for medicinal purposes since ancient times, particularly to treat ailments such as stomach ache, diarrhea and nausea. In the 16th century, ginger was introduced to the Caribbean and Central America by the Spanish and was later cultivated for export. Today pharmacopeias of a number of different countries list ginger extract for various conditions. German and European monographs are available and in 1997, the US Pharmacopeia approved ginger and powdered ginger monographs for inclusion in the National Formulary.
Traditional uses	Gastrointestinal complaints, dyspepsia, diarrhea, nausea, vomiting, respiratory disorders.
Pharmacologic action	Antiemetic, positive inotropic, carminative, promotes secretion of saliva and gastric juices, cholagogue.
Conditions frequently treated	Prevention of motion sickness, dyspepsia, loss of appetite.

Clinical evidence

A systematic review[1] assessed six double-blind RCTs of ginger as a treatment for nausea and vomiting. Single trials for seasickness, morning sickness due to pregnancy and chemotherapy-induced nausea collectively favor ginger over placebo. Two of three trials conducted on postoperative nausea and vomiting suggest that ginger is superior to placebo and equally effective as metoclopramide. However, another trial contradicts this finding.[2] One double-blind RCT compared ginger with placebo in the treatment of osteoarthritis and found some indication of a positive treatment effect for pain measurements.[3] There seems to be no evidence from rigorous clinical trials to support the use of ginger for other conditions.

Dosage

0.75–4.0 g of powdered extract three times daily.

Risks

Contraindications
Pregnancy, lactation. A clinical review found no scientific or medical evidence for the contraindication of ginger during pregnancy.[4] There is, however, a theoretical risk of congenital deformity in neonates.

Precautions/warnings
Children under 6 years of age; gallstones.

Adverse effects
Heartburn; mutagenic potential shown in in vitro studies requires further systematic investigations.

Interactions
Increased effects of anticoagulants; may interfere with cardiac and antidiabetic therapy.

Quality issues
The principal components of ginger may vary greatly depending on the country of origin.

Risk–benefit assessment

The available evidence suggests that ginger is potentially effective for the treatment of nausea and vomiting of various causes. The data are, however, not sufficiently convincing for firm recommendations. Given the reported low frequency of risks involved, ginger is a potential treatment option worthy of consideration except in early pregnancy.

REFERENCES

1 Ernst E. Pittler M H. Efficacy of ginger for nausea and vomiting: a systematic review of randomised clinical trials. Br J Anaesth 2000;84:367–371

2 Visalyaputra S, Petchpaisit N, Somcharoen K, Choavaratana R. The efficacy of ginger root in the prevention of postoperative nausea and vomiting after outpatient gynaecological laparoscopy. Anaesthesia 1998;53:506–510

3 Bliddal H, Rosetzky A, Schlichting P et al. A randomized, placebo-controlled, cross-over study of ginger extract and Ibuprofen in

HERBAL AND NON-HERBAL MEDICINE

osteoarthritis. Osteoarthritis Cartilage 2000;8:9–12

4 Fulder S, Tenne M. Ginger as an anti-nausea remedy in pregnancy: the issue of safety. Herbalgram 1996;38:47–50

FURTHER READING

Kommission E. Monographie Zingiberis rhizoma. Bundesanzeiger Nr 85, 5.5. 1988

German Commission E monograph on ginger.

GINKGO
(Ginkgo biloba L)

Synonyms	Duck foot tree, icho (Japanese), maidenhair tree, silver apricot.
Examples of trade names	Ginkoba, Ginkgold, Ginkopur, Gingopret, Kaveri, Rökan, Tanakan, Tebonin.
Source	Leaves.
Main constituents	Ginkgolides A, B, C, J, bilobalide, flavonoids.

Background

The ginkgo tree, native to China, Korea and Japan where ginkgo nuts are commonly eaten, is believed to be one of the most ancient trees on earth. It is the last remaining member of the *Ginkgoaceae* family, which has survived almost unchanged during the evolutionary timespan of about 200 million years and is often referred to as a 'living fossil'. Individual trees may live as long as 1000 years and grow up to a height of 40–50 meters. The unique botany of *Ginkgo biloba* is accompanied by some equally unique chemistry. The structures of the main active principles, which are thought to be flavonoids and terpene trilactones, comprising bilobalide and ginkgolides, are complex and industry-scale synthesis is still not possible. The tree is the only source and is cultivated, for instance, in the south of France and in south-eastern parts of the US. It is one of the most extensively researched medicinal plants and is the top-selling herbal remedy in the US.

Traditional uses

Asthma, hypertension, tinnitus, angina.

Pharmacologic action

Increase of microcirculatory blood flow, inhibition of erythrocyte aggregation, platelet-activating factor antagonism, free radical scavenging, edema protection. These actions suggest that there is no single mechanism of action but a complex interaction of a multitude of effects.

Conditions frequently treated

Intermittent claudication, dementia, memory impairment, tinnitus.

Clinical evidence

A metaanalysis of ginkgo for intermittent claudication assessed eight double-blind RCTs and suggested a significant but modest increase of painfree walking distance compared with placebo.[1] The majority of these studies also suggested a significant increase in maximal walking distance. Another systematic review identified nine double-blind placebo-controlled RCTs of ginkgo for the treatment of dementia and suggested that it is effective in delaying the clinical deterioration of patients or in bringing about symptomatic improvement.[2] This is corroborated by three other studies,[3-5] which include a metaanalysis assessing patients with Alzheimer's disease.[5] Ginkgo extract was also assessed for the treatment of tinnitus. A systematic review identified five RCTs and concluded that the evidence is favorable, but methodological limitations prevent firm conclusions.[6] One double-blind RCT investigated the effects of ginkgo extract in healthy individuals without cognitive impairment.[7] After 6 weeks of treatment receiving 180 mg extract or placebo daily, participants in the ginkgo group reported significant improvements in cognitive function compared with the placebo group.

Dosage

Dementia and memory impairment: 120–240 mg of standardized extract daily in divided doses.

Intermittent claudication, vertigo, tinnitus: 120–160 mg of standardized extract daily in divided doses.

Risks

Contraindications
Pregnancy, lactation, hypersensitivity to ginkgo preparations.

Precautions/warnings
Effects in children under 12 years are largely unknown.

Adverse effects
Gastrointestinal disturbances, diarrhea, vomiting, allergic reactions, pruritus, headache, dizziness, nose bleeding.

Overdose
Excessive ingestion of ginkgo seeds by children (more than 50 seeds) may cause seizures.

Interactions
Potentiation of anticoagulants.

Quality issues
Evidence in the scientific literature mostly relates to EGb761 (Schwabe, Germany), standardized to 24% ginkgo flavonol glycosides and 6% terpene lactones (3.1% ginkgolide A, B, C and 2.9% bilobalide).

Risk–benefit assessment

The available evidence suggests that ginkgo extract is an effective treatment of intermittent claudication. The size of the effect, however, is modest. In the light of its relative safety and the poor compliance with conventional treatment such as regular physical exercise and similarly modest effects of other conventional oral medications, gingko extract seems worthy of

HERBAL AND NON-HERBAL MEDICINE

consideration. For the treatment of dementia, the evidence suggests that ginkgo is an effective option. The nature and frequency of adverse events render ginkgo a reasonable therapeutic option for patients with this condition. While the evidence for tinnitus is promising, it is too weak for any firm judgement.

REFERENCES

1 Pittler M H, Ernst E. The efficacy of Ginkgo biloba extract for the treatment of intermittent claudication. A meta-analysis of randomized clinical trials. Am J Med 2000;108:276–281

2 Ernst E, Pittler M H. Ginkgo biloba for dementia. A systematic review of double-blind, placebo-controlled trials. Clin Drug Invest 1999;17:301–308

3 Wettstein A. Cholinesterase inhibitors and Ginkgo extracts – are they comparable in the treatment of dementia? Phytomedicine 2000;6:393–401

4 Kleijnen J, Knipschild P. Gingko biloba for cerebral insufficiency. Br J Clin Pharmacol 1992;34:352–358

5 Oken B S, Storzbach D M, Kaye J A. The efficacy of ginkgo biloba on cognitive function in Alzheimer's disease. Arch Neurol 1998;55:1409–1415

6 Ernst E, Stevinson C. Ginkgo biloba for tinnitus: a review. Clin Otolaryngol 1999;24:164–167

7 Mix J A, Crews W D. An examination of the efficacy of Ginkgo biloba extract EGb 761 on the neurophysiologic functioning of cognitively intact older adults. J Alt Compl Med 2000;6:219–229

FURTHER READING

DeFeudis F V. Ginkgo biloba extract (EGb 761): from chemistry to the clinic. Wiesbaden: Ullstein Medical, 1998
A thorough account of ginkgo biloba extract.
Loew D, Blume H, Dingermann T (eds). Phytopharmaka V: Forschung und klinische Anwendung. Darmstadt: Steinkopf,1999
An evidence-based approach to phytomedicine, which includes several chapters on ginkgo.

GLUCOSAMINE

Synonyms	Glukosamin (German).
Examples of trade names	Arth X Plus, Flexi-Factors, Nutri-Joint.
Source	Glucosamine is a substance that occurs naturally in cartilage. It is produced synthetically for the food supplements market.
Background	Glucosamine sulfate is the sulfate salt of 2-amino-2-deoxy-D-chitin glucopyranose which is a constituent of joint cartilage. It was therefore hypothesized that its oral supplementation might enhance cartilage repair. Glucosamine has since become a popular 'natural' treatment for arthritis.
Traditional uses	Osteoarthritis, joint pain.
Pharmacologic action	Increased mucopolysaccharide and collagen production in fibroblasts in vitro, inhibition of enzymes which break down cartilage (e.g. elastase), similar actions to chondroitin (see p 95).

Conditions frequently treated	Osteoarthritis.
Clinical evidence	Several RCTs have been conducted and most have yielded positive results. A recent systematic review[1] included 15 RCTs of glucosamine and chondroitin. Its results were cautiously positive. The overall effect size was 0.44 which was diminished by including only studies of the highest methodological quality. However, the authors pointed to several methodological weaknesses of the primary studies and suspected a degree of publication bias. Several comparative RCTs have been published. For instance, when 200 patients with gonarthrosis took either 500 mg glucosamine or 400 mg ibuprofen[2] the clinical outcome was similar in both groups and more adverse effects were noted with ibuprofen.
Dosage	500 mg of glucosamine sulfate three times daily.
Risks	**Contraindications** Pregnancy, lactation.

Precautions/warnings
Avoid use in children and diabetic patients.

Adverse effects
Constipation, diarrhea, drowsiness, dyspepsia, headache, heartburn, nausea, rash.

Interactions
None known.

Quality issues
Both glucosamine sulfate and hydrochloride are used; it is unclear which is superior.

Risk–benefit assessment	Glucosamine does seem to be superior to placebo in the treatment of osteoarthritis. A number of studies also suggest that it is similarly effective as ibuprofen but longer treatment periods are needed (e.g. 2 weeks and longer) for a clinical benefit to become manifest. The size of the clinical effect is usually moderate. No major safety problems are on record. Thus glucosamine can be recommended as an adjuvant therapy for osteoarthritis.

HERBAL AND NON-HERBAL MEDICINE

REFERENCES

1 McAlindon T E, La Valley M P, Gulin J P, Felson D T. Glucosamine and chondroitin for treatment of osteoarthritis. A systematic quality assessment and meta-analysis. JAMA 2000;283:1469–1475

2 Miller-Fabbender H, Bach G L, Haase W, Rovati L C, Setnikar I. Glucosamine sulfate compared to Ibuprofen in osteoarthritis of the knee. Osteoarthritis Cartilage 1994;2:61–69

FURTHER READING
Rapport L, Lockwood B. Glucosamine. Pharm J
2000;265:134–135
A concise overview for health-care professionals.

GRAPESEED
(Vitis vinifera)

Synonyms	Grape, *Vitis.*
Examples of trade names	Leucoselect-Phytosome.
Source	Seeds.
Main constituents	Polyphenols, flavonoids, tocopherols, tannins, fruit acids.

Background   A mounting body of (mostly epidemiological) evidence suggests that wine has a protective effect on arteriosclerotic diseases. The effect is thought to be due to polyphenols which are highly concentrated in grapeseeds. The 'French paradox', i.e. the fact that, in spite of high levels of saturated fat consumption, the cardiovascular morbidity and mortality are relatively low in France, has been explained by the regular intake of red wine.[1] Others have suggested, however, that the cardioprotective effects are not specific to red wine but relate to regular, moderate alcohol consumption (e.g. [2]). Nevertheless, grapeseed extracts are being promoted for their alleged health effects.

Traditional uses	Circulatory disorders.
Pharmacologic action	Antioxidant, antimutagenic, antiinflammatory.
Conditions frequently treated	Prevention of arteriosclerotic diseases, cancer.

Clinical evidence   A placebo-controlled preclinical RCT recently showed that the antioxidant activity in blood samples from healthy volunteers can be increased by supplementation of grapeseed extracts.[3] Rigorous trials with clinical endpoints are not available as yet.

Dosage	40–80 mg of extract once daily.
Risks	***Contraindications*** Pregnancy, lactation.

Precautions/warnings
None known.

Adverse effects
None known.

Interactions
None known.

Quality issues
Use extracts with standardized polyphenol content.

Risk–benefit assessment

Our understanding of grapeseed extract is not sufficient to attempt a risk–benefit assessment. In the absence of sound clinical data, grapeseed cannot be recommended.

REFERENCES

1 Renaud S C, Gueguen R, Siest G, Salamon R. Wine, beer and mortality in middle-age men from Eastern France. Arch Intern Med 1999;159:1865–1870
2 Rimm E B, Williams P, Fosher K, Griqui M, Stampfer M J. Moderate alcohol intake and lower risk of coronary heart disease: a meta-analysis of effects on lipids and haemostatic factors. Br Med J 1999;319:1523–1528
3 Nuttall S L, Kendall M J, Bombardelli E, Morazzoni P. An evaluation of the antioxidant activity of a standardized grape seed extract, Leucoselect®. J Clin Pharm Therapeut 1998;23:365–389

GREEN TEA
(Camellia sinensis)

Synonyms

Grüner Tee (German), matsu-cha.

Examples of trade names

Tegreen.

Source

Leaves.

Main constituents

Polyphenols (e.g. epigallocatechin and epigallocatechin-3-gallate), caffeine.

Background

The tea plant is native to East Asia. Tea has been used as a refreshing beverage for millennia. Black and green tea are made from the same plant and differ according to the curing method of the leaves. Green tea is thought to have more powerful medicinal effects. Epidemiological research suggests that regular intake is protective for a range of conditions: cancers, cardiovascular disease, kidney stones, bacterial infections and dental caries.

Traditional uses

As a stimulant and beverage.

Pharmacologic action	Antibacterial, antimutagenic, antioxidant, cholesterol lowering, inhibition of cell proliferation and tumor promotion and stimulation of the central nervous system.
Conditions frequently treated	Prevention of cancer, tumor progression, cardiovascular diseases, adjuvant treatment for AIDS.
Clinical evidence	A systematic review of its anticancer effects was based mostly on epidemiological data and included 31 human studies. Its conclusions were cautiously positive.[1] Recent epidemiological studies showed strong inverse associations of tea intake with aortic arteriosclerosis[2] and cardiovascular risk factors.[3] Similar findings have been reported repeatedly.[4] It is relevant to point out that the bulk of this evidence stems from data on drinking tea rather than consuming tea leaf supplements. The notion that green tea might be an effective adjuvant for treating AIDS is so far only hypothetical.[5]
Dosage	6–10 cups daily. 3 capsules of standardized extract daily in divided doses.
Risks	**Contraindications** Pregnancy, lactation, known allergy. **Precautions/warnings** None known. **Adverse effects** Insomnia. **Interactions** None known. **Quality issues** Standardized extracts or infusion should be used.
Risk–benefit assessment	The notion that green tea is an effective preventive agent for cancer and cardiovascular disease is based mostly on indirect evidence from epidemiological studies and has not remained unchallenged. There are no serious safety concerns. Thus, at the very least, patients who want to take green tea supplements do not need to be discouraged. It is important, however, to point out that there is no good clinical evidence for its ability to change the course of existing disease.

REFERENCES

1 Bushman J L. Green tea and cancer in humans: a review of the literature. Nutr Cancer 1998; 31:151–159
2 Geleijnse J M, Launer L J, Hofman A, Pols H A P, Witterman J C M. Tea flavonoids may protect against atherosclerosis. Arch Intern Med 1999;159:2170–2174
3 Imai K, Nakachi K. Cross sectional study of effects of drinking green tea on

cardiovascular and liver diseases. Br Med J 1995;310:693–695

4 Trevisanato S I, Kim Y-I. Tea and health. Nutr Rev 2000;58:1–10

5 McCarthy M F. Natural antimutagenic agents may prolong efficacy of human immunodeficiency virus drug therapy. Med Hypotheses 1997;48:215–220

GUAR GUM
(Cyamopsis tetragonolobus L)

Synonyms	Cyamopsis gum, Guar (German), guaran, jaguar gum.
Examples of trade names	Fat Grabbers, Fat Destroyer, Glucotard, Guarem, Guargel, Guarina, Guar Verlan, Lejguar.
Source	Seeds.
Main constituents	Galactomannan, proteins, lipids, saponins.
Background	Guar gum is a non-absorbable dietary fibre derived from the seeds of the Indian cluster bean (*Cyamopsis tetragonolobus* L). It is obtained from the grinding of the seed albumen and is a white to yellowish powder. *Cyamopsis tetragonolobus* is cultivated mainly in India and Pakistan during the months of July to December. It is also grown in Australia, South Africa and the US and is widely used by the food industry as a thickening agent.
Traditional uses	Diabetes, hyperlipidemia, weight reduction.
Pharmacologic action	Antihyperglycemic, lipid lowering.
Conditions frequently treated	Diabetes, hypercholesterolemia, obesity.
Clinical evidence	Guar gum has been the subject of a large number of RCTs. A metaanalysis of RCTs assessing its hypolipidemic effects concluded that guar gum reduces total and LDL cholesterol levels by a relatively small amount.[1] It has also been suggested as a treatment to reduce body weight. A systematic review and metaanalysis, however, concluded that the evidence does not support the use of guar gum for this indication.[2] Several relatively small double-blind RCTs suggested beneficial effects of guar gum on blood glucose levels in type II diabetic patients.[3–6] RCTs also reported positive evidence for type I diabetes, uncomplicated duodenal ulcer and dumping syndrome.[7–9]

HERBAL AND NON-HERBAL MEDICINE

Dosage 15–30 g of flour or granulated guar gum daily in divided doses.

Risks

Contraindications
Pregnancy, lactation, intestinal obstruction, oesophageal disease.

Precautions/warnings
Should be taken with adequate amounts of fluid.

Adverse effects
Flatulence, diarrhea and abdominal distension, nausea, hypoglycemic symptoms.

Interactions
May potentiate the effects of insulin, reduce absorption of acetaminophen (paracetamol), nitrofurantoin, digoxin and penicillin; may slow the absorption of oral contraceptives.

Quality issues
Composition and purity of the extract may vary.

Risk–benefit assessment Guar gum is beneficial for lowering total serum cholesterol and LDL cholesterol levels. The effect, however, is small and the possibility of adverse effects and drug interactions exists, which may outweigh its modest benefits. The clinical data for type II diabetes are encouraging but insufficient for firm recommendations. For type I diabetes, duodenal ulcer and dumping syndrome, the available evidence is not compelling. Guar gum has not been shown to be effective for the reduction of body weight so cannot be recommended as an alternative to more conventional approaches to weight reduction such as dieting or regular physical exercise.

REFERENCES

1 Brown L, Rosner B, Willet W W, Sacks F M. Cholesterol-lowering effects of dietary fiber: a meta-analysis. Am J Clin Nutr 1999;69:30–42

2 Pittler M H, Ernst E. Guar gum for body weight reduction. Meta-analysis of randomized trials. Am J Med 2001 (in press)

3 Fuessl H S, Williams G, Adrian T E, Bloom S R. Guar sprinkled on food: effect on glycaemic control, plasma lipids and gut hormones in non-insulin-dependent diabetic patients. Diabet Med 1987;4:463–468

4 Uusitupa M, Tuomilehto J, Karttunen P, Wolf E. Long term effects of guar gum on metabolic control, serum cholesterol and blood pressure levels in type 2 (non-insulin-dependent) diabetic patients with high blood pressure. Ann Clin Res 1984;16(suppl 43):126–131

5 Uusitupa M, Siitonen O, Savolainen K, Silvasti M, Penttilä I, Parviainen M. Metabolic and nutritional effects of long-term use of guar gum in the treatment of noninsulin-dependent

diabetes of poor metabolic control. Am J Clin Nutr 1989;49:345–351

6 Uusitupa M, Södervik H, Sivasti M, Karttunen P. Effects of a gel forming dietary fiber, guar gum, on the absorption of glibenclamide and metabolic control and serum lipids in patients with non-insulin dependent (type 2) diabetes. Int J Clin Pharmacol Ther Toxicol 1990; 28:153–157

7 Ebeling P, Yki-Järvinen H, Aro A, Helve E, Sinisalo M, Koivisto V A. Glucose and lipid metabolism and insulin sensitivity in type 1 diabetes: the effect of guar gum. Am J Clin Nutr 1988;48:98–103

8 Harju E J, Larmi T K. Effect of guar gum added to the diet of patients with duodenal ulcer. J Parenteral Enteral Nutr 1985;9:496–500

9 Harju E J, Larmi T K. Efficacy of guar gum in preventing the dumping syndrome. J Parenteral Enteral Nutr 1983;7:470–472

HAWTHORN
(*Crataegus* spp.)

Synonyms

Maybush, Weißdorn (German), whitethorn

Examples of trade names

Cardiplant, Crataegutt, Cratccor, Faros, Hawthorn Heart

Source

Berries, flowers and leaves of three Crataegus species: *C. Laerigata, C. monogyna, C. folium.*

Main constituents

Proanthrocyanides and flavonoids (quercetin, hyperoside, vitexin, rutin); catechin, epicatechin.

Background

About 300 Crataegus species exist which are native to temperate regions of North America, Asia and Europe. Crataegus was praised for its heart-strengthening properties by Dioscorides and Paracelsus. Systematic investigation of this plant started in the early part of the 20th century. Today it is a popular herbal cardiac medication particularly in Germany where it is marketed as a prescription medicine.

Traditional uses

For 'strengthening' the heart and other cardiovascular indications.

Pharmacologic actions

Dilation of coronary arteries, positive inotropic, dromotropic and bathmotropic effects, hypotensive, beta-blocking and ACE-inhibiting activity, anti-oxidant, cardioprotective, anti-arrhythmic, CNS depressant. The mechanism of action has shown to be similar to digitalis.

Conditions frequently treated

Congestive heart failure (NYHA I and II, possibly also III).

Clinical evidence

A systematic review[1] included eight placebo-controlled, double-blind trials published between 1983 and 1994 with a total of 433 patients suffering from congestive heart failure (NYHA I–III, but mostly II). All of these studies showed beneficial effects on objective signs or subjective symptoms. Another review summarized the more recent evidence from clinical, pre-clinical and animal studies. It concluded that these investigations demonstrated a 'beneficial effect of hawthorn on the cardiovascular system acting by several different mechanisms, with few side-effects documented.'[2] One RCT compared 900 mg hawthorn extract with 37.5 mg Captopril per day in 132 patients with NYHA II heart failure.[3] The results suggested that the regimens were similarly effective in increasing the work capacity of these patients. A large (n=3664) observational study suggested that

HERBAL AND NON-HERBAL MEDICINE

the effect amounts to roughly a 10% reduction in pressure-frequency-product both in stage I and stage II (NYHA) patients.[4] A long-term observational study confirmed this finding and additionally showed an increase in ejection fraction and signs of improved myocardial perfusion together with excellent tolerability.[5]

Dosage

900 mg standardized (2.2% flavonoids or 18.75% oligomeric procyanides) extract daily.

Risks

Contraindications
Pregnancy, lactation, allergy to plants from the *Rosaceae* family

Precautions/warnings
Sedation, hypotension or arrhythmias with high doses; hawthorn should only be used under medical supervision

Adverse effects
Nausea, dizziness, fatigue, sweating

Overdose
Respiratory failure

Interactions
Additive effects with antihypertensive drugs, nitrates, cardiac glycosides and CNS depressants

Quality issues
Only standardized products should be used.

Risk–benefit assessment

The value of hawthorn for congestive heart failure (NYHA II) is reasonably well documented and its safety profile is encouraging. There is also some preliminary evidence to show that the effect size is similar to that of conventional drugs. It can therefore be cautiously recommended for this indication in patients who insist on a herbal alternative to effective synthetic drugs. However, due to the nature of the condition, close medical supervision seems essential. Hawthorn can not be recommended for NYHA stage III and IV.

REFERENCES

1 Weihmayr Th, Ernst E. Die therapeutische Wirksamkeit von Crataegus. Fortschr Med 1996;114:27–29
2 Zapatero JM. Selections from current literature: effects of hawthorn on the cardiovascular system. Fam Pract 1999;16:534–538
3 Tauchert M, Ploch M, Hübner WD. Wirksamkeit des Weißdorn-Extraktes LI 132 im Vergleich mit Captopril – Multizentrische Doppelblindstudie bei 132 Patienten mit Herzinsuffizienz im Stadium II nach NYHA.

Münch Med Wschr 1994;136;(Suppl 136/I Feb):27–32
4 Schmidt U, Albrecht M, Podzuweit H, Ploch M, Maisenbacher J. Hochdosierte *Crataegus*-Therapie bei herzinsuffizienten Patienten NYHA-Stadium I und II. Zeitschrift für Phytotherapie 1998;19:22–30
5 Tauchert M, Gildor A, Lipinski J. Einsatz des hochdosierten Crataegusextraktes WS 1442 in der Therapie der Herzinsuffizienz Stadium. Herz 1999;24:465–474

HOP
(*Humulus lupulus* L)

Synonyms	Hopfen (German), houblon (French), humulus, lupulin, lupulus.
Source	Strobiles.
Main constituents	Flavonoids, chalcones, oleo-resin (e.g. alpha-bitter acids including humulone; beta-bitter acids including lupulone), tannins, volatile oils.
Background	A climbing perennial herb belonging to the *Cannabaceae* family, hop is found in marshy areas throughout Asia, the United States and Europe. As well as being crucial to the brewing industry, hop has a long history of use as a sedative. This potential use was first identified from observations that hop-pickers became easily fatigued, possibly from inhaling the volatile oil from the plants. Hop pillows were widely used in traditional folk medicine.
Traditional uses	Neuralgia, insomnia, excitability, restlessness, indigestion.
Pharmacologic action	Sedative, antimicrobial.
Conditions frequently treated	Insomnia, nervous tension.
Clinical evidence	A placebo-controlled RCT (n=40) of a hop and valerian combination reported subjective improvements in the sleep of healthy volunteers.[1] However, the contribution of hop to this effect is unknown. Hop is also used in herbal combinations for various indications, but no clinical trials of hop as a monotherapy for any indication were located.
Dosage	0.5–1 g of dried extract three times daily. 0.5–1 ml of liquid extract (1:1 in 45% alcohol) three times daily.
Risks	***Contraindications*** Pregnancy, lactation, depression. ***Precautions/warnings*** Disruption to menstrual cycle is considered possible. ***Adverse effects*** Allergic dermatitis, respiratory allergy and anaphylaxis have been reported following inhalation or external contact with the herb or oil.

Overdose

No information is available for humans. In animals, large parenteral doses resulted in a soporific effect followed by death and chronic administration resulted in weight loss before death.

Interactions

Theoretical interactions exist for central nervous system depressants, antipsychotics, hormonal agents and any drugs metabolized by the cytochrome P-450 system (e.g. warfarin, anticonvulsants, digoxin, theophylline, HIV protease inhibitors). Also alcohol, although a study of a hop/valerian combination reported no potentiation of alcohol.

Quality issues

Some active constituents break down during storage.

Risk–benefit assessment

There is insufficient clinical data to suggest that hop has any specific therapeutic effects. Safety information is also lacking, but some risks have been identified. A risk–benefit assessment does not therefore support the use of hop for any indication.

REFERENCE

1 Gerhard U, Linnenbrink N, Georghiadou C H, Hobi V. Effects of two plant-based remedies on vigilance. Schweizerische Rundschau für Medizin 1996;85:473–481

HORSE CHESTNUT
(Aesculus hippocastanum L)

Synonyms

Buckeye, Rosskastanie (German).

Examples of trade names

Aescorin, Catarrh cream, Noricaven, Venalot, Venostasin, Venostat.

Source

Seeds.

Main constituents

Triterpene saponins, flavonoids, tannins, quinones, sterols and fatty acids.

Background

The horse chestnut tree is native to south-east Europe and was apparently first introduced to northern Europe in 1576 by the botanist Charles de l'Écluse, from seeds brought from Constantinople. Around 1690 it was known as far as Strasbourg and during the 18th century it spread quickly over Europe. Today the tree is widely distributed all over the world. The genus name *Aesculus* derives from the Latin *esca* meaning 'food' and the Latin *hippocastanum* is reported to derive from the practice of feeding the seeds to horses with respiratory ailments.

Traditional uses

Varicose veins, hemorrhoids, respiratory diseases, diarrhea, malaria.

Pharmacologic action

Antiexudative, antiinflammatory and immunomodulatory activity. The principal active component of horse chestnut seed extract (HCSE) is the saponin escin, which has been shown to inhibit the activity of elastase and hyaluronidase, both involved in enzymatic proteoglycan degradation. Studies have shown increased levels of leukocytes in affected limbs and suggested a possible subsequent activation with release of such enzymes. Other studies reported an increased serum activity of proteoglycan hydrolases in patients with chronic venous insufficiency (CVI) which were reduced with HCSE.

Conditions frequently treated

Symptoms (pain, fatigue, pruritus, edema) or trophic changes associated with chronic venous insufficiency; hematoma.

Clinical evidence

A systematic review[1] assessed 13 double-blind RCTs of oral HCSE for the treatment of CVI. The findings of eight placebo-controlled trials suggested that HCSE is effective in reducing subjective symptoms and objective signs of CVI. Five comparative trials implied that HCSE is as effective as reference treatments such as hydroxyethylrutosides. One reviewed trial (n=240) suggested similar effects of HCSE and compression therapy.[2] For its topical use and for other indications there seems to be no evidence from rigorous clinical trials.

Dosage

Internal use: extract standardized to 100–150 mg escin daily in divided doses.
External use: apply several times daily.

Risks

Contraindications
Pregnancy, lactation, bleeding disorders.

Precautions/warnings
Open wounds, weeping eczema (external use).

Adverse effects
Pruritus, nausea, stomach complaints, bleeding, nephropathy, allergic reactions.

Interactions
Increased effects of aspirin and other anticoagulants.

Quality issues

Preparations are generally standardized to 50–75 mg escin per capsule. Quality of the extracts may vary between preparations.

Risk–benefit assessment

The available evidence suggests that HCSE is effective for the treatment of patients with CVI. Given the nature and frequency of adverse effects of oral HCSE and the relatively poor compliance with conventional treatments such as compression therapy, HCSE is worthy of serious consideration for patients with CVI.

REFERENCES

1 Pittler M H, Ernst E. Horse-chestnut seed extract for chronic venous insufficiency. A criteria-based systematic review. Arch Dermatol 1998;134:1356–1360
2 Diehm C, Trampisch H J, Lange S, Schmidt C. Comparison of leg compression stocking and oral horse-chestnut seed extract therapy in patients with chronic venous insufficiency. Lancet 1996;347:292–294

FURTHER READING

Bombardelli E, Morazzoni P, Griffini A. *Aesculus hippocastanum* L. Fitoterapia 1996;67:483–511
A comprehensive review on horse chestnut with an emphasis on botanical aspects.
Loew D, Blume H, Dingermann T (eds). Phytopharmaka V: Forschung und klinische Anwendung. Darmstadt: Steinkopf, 1999
An evidence-based approach to phytomedicine with several chapters devoted to horse chestnut seed extract.

KAVA KAVA
(*Piper methysticum* Forster)

HERBAL AND NON-HERBAL MEDICINE

Synonyms

Intoxicating pepper, kava, kawa, kawa pepper, Rauschpfeffer (German), yangona.

Examples of trade names

Antares, Antiglan, Kavatino, Kavosporal, Laitan, Potter's Antigian Tablets, Viocava.

Source

Rhizome.

Main constituents

Kavapyrones including kavain, methysticin, desmethoxyyangonin, yangonin, dihydrokavain, dihydromethysticin.

Background

Kava is the beverage prepared from the rhizome of the kava plant (*Piper methysticum* Forster). Native to the islands of the South Pacific, kava has long been used for medicinal and recreational purposes. The name kava kava derives from the Polynesian word *awa* or *kava* meaning bitter and refers to the characteristic taste of the beverage. Probably the first Europeans who came into contact with kava sailed on Captain James Cook's first voyage to the South Pacific (1768–71). The first detailed botanical description of the plant, however, was by Johann Georg Forster in 1777, who sailed on Cook's second voyage.

At the beginning of the 19th century the knowledge of kava as a medicinal plant spread to Europe, which led to its usage as a treatment particularly for venereal diseases. At the beginning of the 20th century scientists isolated a series of compounds which were called kavapyrones and are now thought to be the active principle of kava.

Traditional uses Gonorrhea, syphilis, chronic cystitis, weight reduction, muscle relaxation, sleep induction.

Pharmacologic action Anxiolytic, sedative, anesthetic, muscle relaxant. Studies suggest that kavapyrones, the pharmacologically active components, act on the central nervous system. Kavapyrones are thought to mediate effects on $GABA_A$ receptors, particularly in the hippocampus and amygdala complex. Central nervous effects of kavain and kava extract have also been demonstrated in studies on human volunteers using EEG measurements.

Conditions frequently treated Anxiety, insomnia.

Clinical evidence A systematic review and metaanalysis[1] assessed seven randomized, double-blind trials of kava for anxiety. This study suggested a significant beneficial effect compared with placebo. Comparative studies indicate no significant difference between benzodiazepines and kavain or kava extract.[2,3] For the treatment of insomnia, only limited evidence exists. The suggested mechanism of action and data from animal experiments, however, support the notion that the extract may be helpful for this condition. One RCT reported improved quality of sleep after a single dose of 300 mg kava extract.[4]

Dosage 300 mg of standardized extract (210 mg kavapyrones) daily in divided doses.

Risks

Contraindications
Pregnancy, lactation, endogenous depression.

Precautions/warnings
The extract can cause visual disturbances and may affect reaction time. Care must be taken when driving or operating machinery. Avoid long-term use.

Adverse effects
Stomach complaints, restlessness, mydriasis, allergic skin reactions, dermatomyositis, hepatitis.

Interactions
Potentiation of drugs acting on the central nervous system such as alcohol, benzodiazepines and barbiturates. May reduce the effects of levodopa.

HERBAL AND NON-
HERBAL MEDICINE

HERBAL AND NON-HERBAL MEDICINE

Quality issues

The extract is generally standardized to kavapyrone content. The quality of the extracts may vary between preparations.

Risk–benefit assessment

The available evidence suggests that kava extract is superior to placebo for the treatment of anxiety. In the light of its suggested effectiveness compared with conventional anxiolytic drug treatment and the nature and frequency of adverse effects recognized so far, kava is worthy of consideration. It may be beneficial for the treatment of insomnia in some patients, but the evidence is as yet insufficient.

REFERENCES

1 Pittler M H, Ernst E. Efficacy of kava for treating anxiety: systematic review and meta-analysis. J Clin Psychopharmacol 2000; 20:84–89

2 Lindenberg D, Pitule-Schödel H. D,L-Kavain im Vergleich zu Oxazepam bei Angstzuständen. Fortschr Med 1990;108:31–34

3 Woelk H, Kapoula O, Lehrl S, Schröter K, Weinholz P. Behandlung von Angst-Patienten. Z Allg Med 1993;69:271–277

4 Emser W, Bartylla K. Verbesserung der Schlafqualität. Zur Wirkung von

Kava-Extrakt WS1490 auf das Schlafmuster bei Gesunden. TW Neurologie Psychiatrie 1991;5:636–642

FURTHER READING

Singh Y N, Blumenthal M. Kava, an overview. Herbalgram 1998;39:33–55
A review emphasizing ethnobotanical aspects of kava, its pharmacology and medicinal use.

LAVENDER
(*Lavandula angustifolia* Miller)

Synonyms

Aspic, English lavender, lavanda, lavande commun (French), Lavendel (German), true lavender.

Source

Flowering tops.

Main constituents

Volatile oil (linrayl acetate, linalool), tannins, hydroxy-coumarins.

Background

Native to the Mediterranean and common in southern Europe, lavender is widely cultivated in domestic gardens and for use in perfumes and toiletries. It has been used for centuries to treat various ailments.

Traditional uses

Insomnia, migraines, neuralgia, functional abdominal complaints, appetite stimulant, cuts, bruises, burns.

Pharmacologic action

Astringent, sedative, anticonvulsant.

Conditions frequently treated

Insomnia, headaches.

Clinical evidence

A large RCT (n=635) of postnatal perineal discomfort found no difference between lavender essential oil, synthetic lavender oil and an inert substance added to a bath.[1] A small (n=20) RCT found no effect of lavender oil aromatherapy on recovery from exercise compared with no intervention.[2] A very small RCT (n=10) reported that the addition of lavender essential oil to a footbath was associated with delayed changes in autonomic activity relative to a footbath without essential oil, indicating greater relaxation.[3] An observational study of four geriatric patients with impaired sleep due to discontinuation of benzodiazepines reported that lavender oil aromatherapy increased sleep time.[4] A study with healthy volunteers (n=40) reported increased relaxation, less depressed mood and faster, more accurate mathematic computations following lavender oil aromatherapy.[5]

Dosage

1–2 teaspoons of dried flowers in 150 ml of hot water (lavender tea). 1–2 drops of oil taken with a sugar cube.

Risks

Contraindications
Pregnancy, lactation.

Precautions/warnings
The essential oil should be regarded as potentially poisonous if more than a few drops are taken internally.

Adverse effects
Nausea, vomiting, headache and chills have been reported following inhalation or absorption through the skin. Contact allergy and phototoxicity are also possible.

Overdose
Large doses are reported to exert 'narcotic-like' effects.

Interactions
Theoretically could potentiate effects of central nervous system depressants.

Quality issues
Standardized preparations of the herb are rare, but lavender oil is often an ingredient in external rubs and massage oils and the essential oil is widely available.

Risk–benefit assessment

Clinical trial evidence is limited and does not tend to suggest that lavender has specific therapeutic effects. Taken in conjunction with the possible risks associated with its use, lavender cannot be recommended for medicinal purposes.

HERBAL AND NON-HERBAL MEDICINE

REFERENCES

1 Dale A, Cornwell S. The role of lavender oil in relieving perineal discomfort following childbirth: a blind randomised clinical trial. J Adv Nurs 1994;19:89–96

2 Romine I J, Bush A M, Geist C R. Lavender aromatherapy in recovery from exercise. Percept Mot Skills 1999;88: 756–758

3 Saeki Y. The effect of foot-bath with or without the essential oil of lavender on the autonomic nervous system: a randomised trial. Compl Ther Med 2000;8:2–7

4 Hardy M, Kirk-Smith M D, Stretch D D. Replacement of drug treatment for insomnia by ambient odour. Lancet 1995;346:701

5 Diego M A, Jones N A, Field T et al. Aromatherapy positively affects mood, EEG patterns of alertness and math computations. Int J Neurosci 1998; 96:217–224

MELATONIN

Synonyms	N-acetyl-5-methoxytryptamine.
Examples of trade names	Bevitamel, Tranzone.
Source	Melatonin exists in the pineal gland, retina and gut as well as some plants and foods. Commercial melatonin products are usually produced synthetically.
Background	Melatonin is a neurohormone synthesized from tryptophan and secreted by the pineal gland. Release is stimulated by darkness and suppressed by light. Melatonin is involved in the regulation of bodily rhythms such as temperature and sleep. Serum concentrations increase 10–50 fold 1–2 hours before bedtime, reaching a peak at about midnight. Melatonin has a half-life of about 20–50 minutes.
Pharmacologic action	Synchronizing hormone secretion, sedative, antioxidative, immune stimulating, antiproliferative, free radical scavenging.
Conditions frequently treated	Insomnia, jet lag.
Clinical evidence	Several small placebo-controlled RCTs suggest melatonin may be helpful for insomnia[1–3] but negative results have also been reported.[4,5] Similarly with shift work disorder, recent RCTs with negative outcomes[6,7] have contradicted earlier findings.[8,9] For jet lag, several trials have demonstrated beneficial effects (e.g. [10,11]) and one negative result has been reported.[12] However, in this study involving doctors returning to Norway after 5 days in New York, it is possible that circadian rhythms had not fully adjusted to New York time. One small RCT found a prophylactic effect of melatonin on cluster headaches.[13] Studies involving cancer patients have not produced convincing results.[14,15]
Dosage	*Insomnia:* 0.3–10 mg (0.3–1 mg initially) 2 hours before bedtime.

Jet lag: 5 mg 22–2300 hrs local time on arrival for 4 days.

Risks

Contraindications
Pregnancy, lactation, prepubertal children, autoimmune disease, hepatic insufficiency, cerebrovascular or neurologic disorders, patients taking immunosuppressants or corticosteroids.

Precautions/warnings
Driving or operating machinery should be avoided for 4–5 hours following melatonin administration.

Adverse effects
Abdominal cramps, fatigue, dizziness, headache, irritability. Hangover effects are unlikely due to the short half-life of melatonin.

Overdose
Large doses (1200 mg) have been associated with depression.

Interactions
May potentiate the anxiolytic effects of benzodiazepines.

Quality issues
Most commercial melatonin is synthesized. Extracts from animal preparations should not be used due to possible contaminants. Melatonin is not available for sale over the counter in the UK or Germany.

Risk–benefit assessment

The effectiveness of melatonin for any indication is undetermined. However, at physiologic doses it appears to have few risks, so may be worth considering for jet lag and insomnia.

HERBAL AND NON-HERBAL MEDICINE

REFERENCES

1 Garfinkel D, Laudon M, Zisapel N. Improvement of sleep quality by controlled-release melatonin in benzodiazepine-treated elderly insomniacs. Arch Gerontol Geriat 1997;24:223–231

2 Garfinkel D, Laudon M, Nof D, Zisapel N. Improvement of sleep quality in elderly people by controlled-release melatonin. Lancet 1995; 346:541–544

3 Haimov I, Lavie P, Laudon M, Herer P, Vigder C, Zisapel N. Melatonin replacement therapy of elderly insomniacs. Sleep 1995;18:598–599

4 Dawson D, Rogers N L, Van Den Heuvel C, Kennaway D J, Lushington K. Effect of sustained nocturnal transbuccal melatonin administration on sleep and temperature in elderly insomniacs. J Biol Rhythms 1998; 13:532–538

5 Ellis C M, Lemmens G, Parkes J D. Melatonin and insomnia. J Sleep Res 1996;5:61–65

6 Wright S W, Lawrence L M, Wrenn K D, Haynes M L, Welch L W, Schlack H M. Randomized clinical trial of melatonin after night-shift work: efficacy and neuropsychologic effects. Ann Emerg Med 1998;32:334–340

7 James M, Tremea M O, Jones J S, Krohmer J R. Can melatonin improve adaption to night shift? Am J Emerg Med 1998;16:367–370

8 Folkard S, Arendt J, Clark M. Can melatonin improve shift workers' tolerance of the night shift? Some preliminary findings. Chronobiol Int 1993;10:315–320

9 Dawson D, Encel N, Lushington K. Improving adaptation to simulated night shift: timed exposure to bright light versus daytime melatonin administration. Sleep 1995; 18:11–21

10 Petrie K, Conaglen J V, Thompson L, Chamberlain K. Effect of melatonin on jet lag

after long haul flights. Br Med J 1989; 298:705–707

11 Suhner A, Schlagenhauf P, Johnson R, Tschopp A, Steffen R. Comparative study to determine the optimal melatonin dosage form for the alleviation of jet lag. Chronobiol Int 1998;15:655–666

12 Spitzer R L, Terman M, Williams J B, Terman J S, Malt U F, Singer F, Lewy A J. Jet lag: clinical features, validation of a new syndrome-specific scale and lack of response to melatonin in a randomized, double-blind trial. Am J Psychiatr 1999;156:1392–1396

13 Leone M, D'Amico D, Moschiano F, Fraschini F, Bussone G. Melatonin versus placebo in the prophylaxis of cluster headache: a double-blind pilot study with parallel groups. Cephalalgia 1996;16:494–496

14 Lissoni P, Paolorossi F, Tancini G et al. Is there a role for melatonin in the treatment of neoplastic cachexia? Eur J Cancer 1996; 32A:1340–1343

15 Lissoni P, Giani L, Zerbini S, Trabattoni P, Rovelli F. Biotherapy with the pineal immunomodulating hormone melatonin versus melatonin plus aloe vera in untreatable advanced solid neoplasms. Nat Immun 1998; 16:27–33

FURTHER READING

Avery D, Lenz M, Landis C. Guidelines for prescribing melatonin. Ann Med 1998; 30:122–130
Review of pharmacological and clinical research findings with melatonin.

MILK THISTLE
(Silybum marianum L)

Synonyms	Cardus marianus, holy thistle, lady's thistle, Mariendistel (German), Marian thistle, Mary thistle.
Examples of trade names	Legalon, Silymarit, Milk Thistle Phytosol.
Source	Seeds.
Main constituents	Flavoligans, silybin A and B, silydistin, silydianin.
Background	Milk thistle belongs to the *Compositae* (*Asteraceae*) family. Its common name stems from the legend that the white veins in the plant leaves come from a drop of the Virgin Mary's milk. Milk thistle is native to the Mediterranean but also grows in North and South America. It was used in ancient Greece for medicinal purposes.
Traditional uses	Tonic for nursing mothers, antidote after mushroom poisoning, psoriasis, 'liver cleansing' agent.
Pharmacologic action	Alters the membrane structure of liver cells so that toxins are hindered from entering hepatocytes, increases their regenerative capacity, competes with binding sites for liver toxins, acts as free radical scavenger and possibly cholesterol-lowering agent.
Conditions frequently treated	Liver diseases, in particular hepatitis and (alcoholic) cirrhosis.

Clinical evidence

A systematic review[1] included 14 placebo-controlled, double-blind RCTs and 15 RCTs with non-placebo controls in a variety of liver diseases. Twelve of these studies used the standardized German preparation Legalon. Of seven studies in chronic alcoholic liver disease, five reported significant improvements in at least one outcome variable. For viral hepatitis (four studies), the data were highly contradictory. For liver cirrhosis (four studies), two trials showed a positive trend and two studies demonstrated a significant effect.

Dosage

200 mg of standardized extract (70% silymarin) three times daily.

Risks

Contraindications
Pregnancy, lactation.

Precautions/warnings
Milk thistle should not be used as a justification for continuing alcohol abuse.

Adverse effects
Diarrhea.

Interactions
Theoretically, improvement of liver function could increase metabolism of some medications which are metabolized in the liver.

Quality issues
Products are generally standardized to 70% silymarin content.

Risk–benefit assessment

Milk thistle is likely to convey some benefit, particularly for patients suffering from chronic alcoholic liver disease. However, to date, the evidence is not fully conclusive. No serious risks exist. Thus milk thistle is worth considering when no other effective treatments are available or in conjunction with conventional treatments.

REFERENCE

1 Mulrow C, Lawrence V. Report on milk thistle:
effects on liver disease and cirrhosis and
clinical adverse effects. Evidence
Report/Technology Assessment 2000
(unpublished)

MISTLETOE
(*Viscum album* L)

Synonyms

All heal, bird lime, devil's fuge, golden bough, viscum.

Examples of trade names

Eurixor, Helixor, Iscador.

HERBAL AND NON-HERBAL MEDICINE

Source	Leaves, branches and berries.
Main constituents	Mistletoe lectins, phoratoxins and viscotoxins, amines, choline, histamine, flavonoids, terpenoids, alkaloids and tannins.
Background	*Viscum album* (and related species such as *Viscum abietis* and *Viscum austriacum* which are native to Europe and Asia) is a semiparasitic plant that lives in tree species such as oak, pine, elm and apple. The medicinal use of mistletoe goes back to early Celtic times. Rudolf Steiner (1861–1925), the founder of anthroposophy, believed the parasitic nature of mistletoe was similar to the nature of malignant growth and thus hypothesized that mistletoe could be used therapeutically for cancer. Based on anecdotal reports of cancer improvement, mistletoe became a popular anthroposophical 'cancer cure' in Europe and its use has now spread to the US and beyond. Anthroposophical products are usually fermented while phytotherapeutic preparations are conventional extracts. In addition, a pure mistletoe lectin product has recently become available.
Traditional uses	Because of its toxicity, mistletoe has relatively few traditional uses; they include hypertension, epilepsy, insomnia and depression.
Pharmacologic actions	Cytotoxic, immunomodulatory.
Conditions frequently treated	All types of cancer. The treatment is promoted both for reducing tumor burden and for increasing quality of life in palliative cancer care. The immunomodulatory effect is also invoked for promoting mistletoe as a treatment for AIDS.
Clinical evidence	Several clinical studies have indicated improvements in immune function, quality of life and survival rate of cancer patients[1] yet the evidence is far from uniform. An independent and authoritative systematic review[2] included 11 CCTs (bronchial carcinoma, colorectal carcinoma, breast cancer, gastric cancer and ovarian cancer). All except one (the most rigorous) of these studies yielded results or trends in favor of mistletoe. Because of the methodological weaknesses of these trials, the authors conclude that 'Mistletoe preparations cannot be recommended in the treatment of cancer patients except in clinical trials'.[2] The most recent trial[3] is probably also the most rigorous study on the subject to date; 477 patients with resected head and neck cancers were randomized to receive either standard treatment alone or with additional subcutaneous mistletoe injections. After an average follow-up period of 4 years there were no

intergroup differences in disease-free survival or any other outcomes.

Dosage

2–6 g of dried leaves orally three times daily. 1–3 ml of liquid extract (1:1 solution in 25% alcohol) three times daily. 0.5 ml of tincture (1:5 solution in 45% alcohol) three times daily.
Solutions for injection: as instructed by the manufacturer.

Risks

Contraindications
Pregnancy, lactation.

Precautions/warnings
Patients should be monitored for dehydration and electrolyte imbalances and warned about the toxicity of mistletoe; cancer patients should be advised not to discontinue their conventional therapies.

Adverse effects
Bradycardia, dehydration, delirium, diarrhea, gastroenteritis, hallucinations, hepatitis, hypo- and hypertension, fever, leukocytosis, mydriasis, myosis, nausea, seizures, vomiting. Several fatalities have been reported. Local reactions at the site of injection are common.

Overdose
Adverse effects as above.

Interactions
Can enhance or potentiate effects of antihypertensive drugs, cardiac depressants and central nervous system depressants.

Quality issues
Only standardized preparations with standardized lectin content should be used.

Risk–benefit assessment

Mistletoe preparations may turn out to have some beneficial effects (e.g. on quality of life) in the treatment of cancer. However, the size of the effect is almost certainly small. They are also associated with considerable risks. Thus, on the basis of the data currently available, they should be obsolete as a sole cancer treatment and used with caution as an adjunctive cancer therapy.

HERBAL AND NON-HERBAL MEDICINE

REFERENCES

1 Kaegi E. Unconventional therapies for cancer: 3. Iscador. Canad Med Assoc J 1998;158:1157–1159

2 Kleijnen J, Knipschild P. Mistletoe treatment for cancer. Review of controlled trials in humans. Phytomedicine 1994; 1:255–260

3 Steuer Vogt M K, Bonkowsky V, Ambrosch P et al. The effect of an adjuvant mistletoe treatment programme in resected neck cancer patients. Eur J Cancer 2001 (in press)

NETTLE
(*Urtica dioica* L)

Synonyms	Brennessel (German), common nettle, stinging nettle.
Examples of trade names	Bazoton, Fragador, Hostid, Kleer, Prostaforton, Prostagalen.
Source	Leaves and roots.
Main constituents	*Leaf*: minerals, amines, flavonoids, sterols, tannins, vitamins, volatile oil. *Root*: polysaccharides, sterols, lectins, lignans, fatty acids, tannins, terpenes, coumarin.
Background	Stinging nettle is a perennial herb growing to a height of about 1.5 meters. It grows throughout much of the temperate zones of both hemispheres. The genus name *Urtica* derives from the Latin verb *urere* ('to burn'), while the species name *dioica* (two houses') refers to the flowers bearing male and female on separate plants. Nettle is considered a weed and causes a characteristic itching rash upon contact with the skin. It has enjoyed a long history of medicinal use. Galen (129–199 AD) reported its beneficial medicinal effects in a number of conditions such asthma and disorders of the spleen.
Traditional uses	Rheumatism, asthma, kidney disorders, bleeding conditions, infantile and psychogenic eczema, muscle relaxant during childbirth.
Pharmacologic action	Diuretic, antihypertensive, immunostimulatory and antiinflammatory.
Conditions frequently treated	*Leaf*: rheumatism, inflammatory diseases of the lower urinary tract, kidney gravel. *Root*: micturition disorders in benign prostatic hyperplasia.
Clinical evidence	A number of RCTs have investigated nettle root extract for the treatment of benign prostatic hyperplasia.[1-4] These report improvements in symptom scores and urinary flow compared with placebo. Other positive evidence comes from double-blind RCTs investigating preparations containing nettle root in combination with extract of *Pygeum africanum*[5] or saw palmetto extract.[6] Stinging nettle herb has also been the subject of RCTs reporting positive effects in patients with allergic rhinitis[7] and acute arthritis.[8] One RCT investigated the effects of stinging nettle leaves for osteoarthritic pain of the base of the thumb or index finger and reported beneficial effects for pain and disability scores compared with deadnettle (*Laminum album*).[9]

Dosage   *Leaf*: 0.6–2.1 g of dry extract daily in divided doses.
                    Root: 0.7–1.3 g of dry extract daily in divided doses.

Risks   ***Contraindications***
                    Pregnancy, lactation.

                    Precautions/warnings
                    Children under the age of 2 years.

                    Adverse effects
                    Gastrointestinal complaints, allergic reactions, urticaria, pruritus, oedema, decreased urine volume.

                    Interactions
                    May potentiate the effects of diuretic and antihypertensive agents.

Risk–benefit assessment   The evidence of nettle root extract for benign prostatic hyperplasia is encouraging but not compelling. The available data on the nature and frequency of its adverse effects, however, indicate that it may be worthy of consideration. For other interventions such as saw palmetto extract, the evidence is relatively stronger. There is little evidence of the efficacy of nettle root extract for any other condition. For nettle leaf, encouraging findings are emerging for its use in arthritis yet the evidence is not sufficiently strong to allow any firm recommendation.

REFERENCES

1 Engelmann U, Boos G, Kres H. Therapie der benignen Prostatahyperplasie mit Bazoton Liquidum. Urologe B 1996;36:287–291
2 Fischer M, Wilbert D. Wirkprüfung eines Phytopharmakons zur Behandlung der benignen Prostatahyperplasie. In: Rutishauser G (ed) Benigne Prostatahyperplasie III. München: Zuckerschwerdt, 1992, p 79
3 Dathe G, Schmid H. Phytotherapie der benignen Prostatahyperplasie (BPH). Doppelblindstudie mit Extraktum Radicis Urticae (ERU). Urologe B 1987;27:223–226
4 Vontobel H P, Herzog R, Rutishauser G, Kres H. Ergebnisse einer Doppelblindstudie über die Wirksamkeit von ERU-Kapseln in der konservativen Behandlung der benignen Prostatahyperplasie. Urologe A 1985; 24:49–51
5 Krzeski T, Kazon M, Borkowski A, Witeska A, Kuczera J. Combined extract of Urtica dioica and Pygeum africanum in the treatment of benign prostatic hyperplasia: double-blind comparison of two doses. Clin Therapeut 1993;15:1011–1020
6 Sökeland J, Albrecht J. Combined sabal and urtica extract versus finasteride in BPH (Aiken stage I–II). Urologe A 1997;36:327–333
7 Mittman P. Randomized, double-blind study of freeze-dried Urtica dioica in the treatment of allergic rhinitis. Planta Med 1990;56:44–47
8 Chrubasik S, Enderlein W, Bauer R, Grabner W. Evidence of antirheumatic effectiveness of Herba Urticae dioicae in acute arthritis. A pilot study. Phytomedicine 1997;4:105–108
9 Randall C. Randall H, Dobbs F, Hutton C, Sanders H. Randomised controlled trial of nettle sting for treatment of base-of-thumb pain. J Roy Soc Med 2000;93:305–309

FURTHER READING

Bombardelli E, Morazzoni P. Urtica dioica L. – review. Fitoterapia 1997;68:387–401
A comprehensive review on nettle with an emphasis on botanical aspects.

HERBAL AND NON-HERBAL MEDICINE

PASSION FLOWER
(Passiflora incarnata L)

Synonyms	Apricot vine, fleur de la passion (French), grenadille, Maypops, Passionsblume (German), passion vine, purple passion flower, wild passion flower.
Examples of trade names	Natracalm, Naturest, Passedan, Passiflorin.
Source	Aerial parts, particularly leaves.
Main constituents	Alkaloids, flavonoids, maltol, fatty acids.
Background	A member of the *Passifloraceae* family, passion flower is a perennial vine native to the southern United States. Its Latin name is connected to Christ, *passio* meaning suffering and *incarnata* meaning incarnate, with its flowered fringe thought to represent the crown of thorns and its five anthers representing the five stigmata. Historically, it has been used as a sedative at least as far back as the Aztecs.
Traditional uses	Neuralgia, generalized seizures, hysteria, insomnia.
Pharmacologic action	Sedative, anxiolytic.
Conditions frequently treated	Insomnia, tension.
Clinical evidence	No studies of passion flower monotherapy were located. In combination with hawthorn, improvements were demonstrated in the physical exercise capacity of patients (n=40) with dyspnea in a double-blind, placebo-controlled RCT.[1] Two RCTs of herbal combinations including passion flower reported reduced anxiety in patients with adjustment disorder with anxious mood[2] and sedative effects on healthy volunteers.[3] The role of passion flower in these effects is unknown, however.
Dosage	0.5–1 ml of liquid extract (1:1 in 25% alcohol) three times daily.
Risks	***Contraindications*** Pregnancy, lactation. ***Precautions/warnings*** Ability to drive or operate machinery may be impaired after taking passion flower.

Adverse effects
Nausea, vomiting, drowsiness and ventricular tachycardia have been reported.

Overdose
Excessive doses may cause sedation.

Interactions
Theoretically potentiation of CNS depressants is possible.

Quality issues
Passion flower is often combined with other herbs in commercial preparations for insomnia. Its active principles have not been identified, although flavonoids are generally used for standardization.

Risk–benefit assessment   There is little clinical data to support the medicinal use of passion flower. Information on its safety is also lacking. Its use as a monopreparation cannot therefore be recommended since there is insufficient evidence to assess the relative risks and benefits.

REFERENCES
1 Von E M, Brunner H, Haegeli A, Kreuter U, Martina B, Meier B, Schaffner W. Hawthorne/passion flower extract and improvement in physical exercise capacity of patients with dyspnoea class II of the NYHA functional classification. Acta Ther 1994;20:47–66
2 Boutin R N, Bouhrtol T, Guitton B, Broutin E. A combination of plant extracts in the treatment of outpatients with adjustment disorder with anxious mood: controlled study versus placebo. Fundament Clin Pharmacol 1997;11:127–132
3 Gerhard U, Hobi V, Kocher R, Konig C. Acute sedative effect of a herbal relaxation tablet as compared to that of bromazepam. Schweiz Rundsch Med Prax 1991;80:1481–1486

PEPPERMINT
(Mentha x piperita L)

Synonyms   Brandy mint, Katzenkraut (German), lamb mint, Pfefferminz (German).

Examples of trade names   Ben-Gay, Colpermin, Kiminto, Mentacur, Mintec, Rhuli Gel, SX Mentha.

Source   Leaves and essential oil.

Main constituents   *Leaf*: luteolin, hesperidin, rutin, caffeic, chlorogenic and rosmarinic acids, volatile oil.
Essential oil: menthol, menthone, menthyl acetate, cineol, isomenthone, menthofuran, limonene.

Background   Peppermint is a perennial aromatic herb growing to a height of about 1 meter. It grows along stream banks and moist wastelands throughout much of Europe and North America and is characterized by its smell and its square stem, which is typical for members of the mint family. It is a natural hybrid of water mint

(*Mentha aquatica*) and spearmint (*Mentha spicata*). Peppermint has a long history of medicinal use as indicated by records from Roman and Greek periods. Its genus name, *Mentha*, is derived from the Greek mythical nymph *Mintha*, who metamorphosed into this plant. Today, peppermint is listed in the national pharmacopeias of the UK, Austria, France, Hungary, Russia and Germany. The leading producer of peppermint oil is the US.

Traditional uses

Leaf: gastrointestinal disorders, complaints of the gallbladder and bile duct, flatulence.
Essential oil: irritable bowel syndrome, common cold, inflammation of the oral mucosa, myalgia, neuralgia.

Pharmacologic action

Antispasmodic, carminative, cholagogue, antiseptic, cooling. The principal active constituent of peppermint oil is thought to be menthol, a cyclic monoterpene with calcium channel-blocking activity.

Conditions frequently treated

Leaf: complaints of the gastrointestinal tract.
Essential oil: irritable bowel syndrome, common cold, myalgia.

Dosage

Leaf: 3–6 g as infusion daily.
0.8–1.8 g of dry extract daily in divided doses.
Essential oil: 0.6–1.2 ml in enteric-coated capsules.
3–4 drops in hot water (as inhalant) internally.
Apply as needed externally.

Clinical evidence

A systematic review and metaanalysis[1] of eight RCTs assessing peppermint oil (mostly enteric-coated capsules) for irritable bowel syndrome reported that, although the majority of trials report beneficial effects, methodological limitations prevent firm conclusions. Two RCTs from the same research group suggested positive effects of externally applied peppermint oil in healthy volunteers and for patients with tension-type headache.[2,3] Positive effects have also been reported for peppermint in a combination preparation for patients with functional dyspepsia.[4] An RCT suggested peppermint tea as a possible adjuvant treatment for urinary tract infection.[5]

Risks

Contraindications
Pregnancy and lactation, children under the age of 12 years, obstruction of the bile duct, cholecystitis.

Precautions/warnings
Individuals with glucose-6 phosphate dehydrogenase deficiency; gallstones, hiatal hernia.

Adverse effects
Allergic reactions, laryngeal or bronchial spasm, mouth ulceration, heartburn, perianal burning, gastrointestinal complaints, headache, dizziness, pruritus.

Overdose

The fatal dose of menthol in humans is estimated to be 1 g per kg body weight.

Interactions

None known.

Risk–benefit assessment

Although RCTs of peppermint oil for irritable bowel syndrome report positive effects, the evidence is not convincing. The possibility of adverse effects exists, which may outweigh any possible benefits. For functional dyspepsia and tension-type headache, the effectiveness of peppermint oil is promising but not established beyond reasonable doubt. For the latter condition and most other external applications peppermint oil can be · considered safe. The use of peppermint in teas and as an inhalant is not backed by data from rigorous trials but can be considered safe.

REFERENCES

1 Pittler M H, Ernst E. Peppermint oil for irritable bowel syndrome: a critical review and meta-analysis. Am J Gastroenterol 1998;93:1131–1135

2 Göbel H, Schmidt G, Soyka D. Effect of peppermint and eucalyptus oil preparations on neurophysiological and experimental algesimetric headache parameters. Cephalalgia 1994;14:228–234

3 Göbel H, Fresenius J, Heinze A, Dworschak M, Soyka D. Effectiveness of peppermint oil and paracetamol in the treatment of tension type headache. Nervenarzt 1996;67:672–681

4 Madisch A, Heydenreich C J, Wieland V, Hufnagel R, Hotz J. Treatment of functional dyspepsia with a fixed peppermint oil and caraway oil combination preparation as compared to cisapride: a multicenter, reference-controlled double-blind equivalence study. Arzneim-Forsch/Drug Res 1999;49:925–932

5 Ebbinghaus K D. A 'tea' containing various plant products as adjuvant to chemotherapy of urinary tract infections. Therapiewoche 1985;35:2041–2051

HERBAL AND NON-HERBAL MEDICINE

PHYTOESTROGENS

Examples of trade names

Promensil, Soyselect.

Source

Plants, fruits, vegetables, grains.

Main constituents

Coumestans (coumestrol), lignans (enterodiol, enterolactone), isoflavones (genistein, diadzein).

Background

Phytoestrogens are non-steroidal plant-derived compounds with diverse chemical structures possessing weak estrogenic activity. It has been suggested that the high consumption of dietary phytoestrogens of Asian populations is associated with a low incidence of hormone-related disease. Soy isoflavones are a common dietary source of phytoestrogens.

Pharmacologic action	Estrogenic, antiestrogenic, anticarcinogenic, antimutagenic, antiproliferative, antioxidative, mild antiinflammatory.
Conditions frequently treated	Menopausal symptoms, prevention of heart disease, breast cancer and osteoporosis in menopausal women.
Clinical evidence	A number of case-control studies suggest a link between soy phytoestrogen consumption and reduced risk of breast and other cancers (e.g. [1]). A metaanalysis of 38 controlled trials reported that consumption of soy protein rather than animal protein significantly decreased serum concentrations of total cholesterol, LDL cholesterol and triglycerides.[2] Whether these effects on lipids could be attributed to the phytoestrogen content of soy has been questioned, however.[3] Several RCTs reported a reduction of menopausal symptoms, particularly hot flushes, with dietary linseed and wheat, soy products and isoflavones derived from red clover,[4-11] but these results are not fully convincing. In one RCT relating to osteoporosis, consumption of soy protein over 6 months increased bone mineral density and content in the lumbar spine but not other skeletal areas, compared with casein.[12] A crossover RCT reported that compared with sunflower seed, consumption of flaxseed for 6 weeks reduced the rate of bone resorption of postmenopausal women.[13] A number of trials have shown that ipriflavone, a synthetic isoflavone, prevents postmenopausal bone loss (e.g. [14]).
Dosage	40–100 mg of isoflavones daily.
Risks	*Contraindications* None known for phytoestrogens consumed as part of diet. Concentrated isoflavone supplements should not be taken during pregnancy or lactation, by children or those with hormone-dependent tumors. *Precautions/warnings* Duration of the menstrual cycle may be affected. *Adverse effects* Flatulence. *Overdose* Effects of large quantities of phytoestrogens, as consumed by infants fed soy milk or individuals taking concentrated supplements, are not known. Impairments to the reproductive system are considered possible, but have not been reported. *Interactions* None known.

Quality issues
Soy products may be genetically modified.

Risk–benefit assessment

The available evidence suggests that increasing consumption of phytoestrogens in the diet has few risks and various potential health benefits. It seems unlikely that even when taken as a concentrated supplement, effects can match those of hormone replacement therapy. The adverse effect profile may prove to be more favorable, however.

REFERENCES

1 Ingram D, Sanders K, Kolybaba M, Lopez D. Case-control study of phytoestrogens and breast cancer. Lancet 1997;350:990–994

2 Anderson J W, Johnstone B M, Cook-Newell M E. Meta-analysis of the effects of soy protein intake on serum lipids. New Engl J Med 1995;333:276–282

3 Sirtori C R. Dubious benefits and potential risk of soy phytoestrogens. Lancet 2000;355:849

4 Murkies A L, Lombard C, Strauss B J, Wilcox G, Burger H G, Morton M S. Dietary flour supplementation decreases post-menopausal hot flushes: effect of soy and wheat. Maturitas 1995;21:189–195

5 Dalais F S, Rice G E, Wahlqvist M L et al. Effects of dietary phytoestrogens in postmenopausal women. Climacteric 1998;l:124–129

6 Washburn S, Burke G L, Morgan T, Anthony M. Effect of soy protein supplementation on serum lipoproteins, blood pressure and menopausal symptoms in perimenopausal women. Menopause 1999;69:7–13

7 Albertazzi P, Pansini F, Bonaccorsi G, Zanotti L, Forini E, De Aloysio D. The effect of dietary soy supplementation on hot flushes. Obstet Gynecol 1998;91:6–11

8 Scambia G, Mango D, Signorile P G et al. Clinical effects of a standardized soy extract in postmenopausal women: a pilot study. Menopause 2000;7:105-111

9 Brezinski A, Adlercreutz H, Rosler A et al. Short term effects of phytoestrogen-rich diet on postmenopausal women. Menopause 1997;4:89–90

10 Baber R J, Templeman C, Morton T, Kelly G E, West L. Randomised placebo-controlled trial of an isoflavone supplement and menopausal symptoms in women. Climacteric 1999;2:85–92

11 Knight D C, Howes J B, Eden J A. The effect of Promensil, an isoflavone extract, on menopausal symptoms. Climacteric 1999;2:79–84

12 Potter S M, Baum J A, Teng H, Stillman R J, Shay N F, Erdman J W. Soy protein and isoflavones: their effects on blood lipids and bone density in postmenopausal women. Am J Clin Nutr 1998; 68 (suppl):1375–1379

13 Arjmandi B H, Juma S, Lucas E A, Wei L, Venkatesh S, Khan D A. Flaxseed supplementation positively influences bone metabolism in postmenopausal women. J Am Nutraceutical Assoc 1998; 1:27–32

14 Gennari C, Agnusdei D, Crepaldi G et al. Effect of ipriflavone – a synthetic derivative of natural isoflavones – on bone mass loss in the early years after menopause. Menopause 1998;5:9–15

FURTHER READING

Anderson J J B, Anthony M S, Cline J M, Washburn S A, Garner S C. Health potential of soy isoflavones for menopausal women. Public Health Nutr 1999;2:489–504

Comprehensive review of in vitro, animal and human studies of the beneficial effects of soy isoflavones.

PROPOLIS

Synonyms

Bee glue, Bienenharz (German).

Examples of trade names

Propolis Immuntinktur.

Source	Beehives.
Main constituents	Flavonoid aglycones, hydroxycinammic acids.
Background	Propolis is a resinous material made by bees, produced by combining resin from the buds of various trees, particularly *Populus* species, with other substances such as salivary secretions and bee wax. It has antimicrobial properties and the bees primarily use it to apply a thin layer on the internal walls of their hives, in particular the brood chambers. Propolis is responsible for the relatively low rate of bacterial contamination and moulds in the hive or other cavities that bees inhabit. The material is also used to disinfect incoming bees at the entrance to the hive. This is reflected by the meaning of the term propolis, which is derived from the Greek *pro* ('before') and *polis* ('town').
Traditional uses	Laryngitis, duodenal ulcers, gastric disturbances, dermatitis (it was also used for varnishing Stradivarius violins).
Pharmacologic action	Antibacterial, antifungal, antiviral, antiinflammatory.
Conditions frequently treated	Propolis is sometimes a constituent of mouthwash liquids.
Clinical evidence	A non-randomized, double-blind, placebo-controlled trial assessed the effects of a mouthrinse containing propolis in 100 individuals.[1] It reported some positive effects on the Silness & Löe plaque index after 4 weeks of treatment. In a subsequent double-blind RCT (n=42) patients were instructed to rinse twice daily with 10% propolis in ethanol for 5 days. There were no significant differences on the plaque index compared with placebo.[2] Toothpaste containing propolis was tested in a non-randomized, double-blind trial (n=103) which reported no beneficial effects on caries and plaque formation compared with placebo toothpaste.[3] Double-blind, placebo-controlled RCTs exist for ulcerative colitis and Crohn's disease, reporting negative results,[4] and acute uterine cervicitis, reporting some positive findings.[5] Beneficial effects for rheumatic disorders are reported in a non-randomized, single-blind, placebo controlled trial (n=190).[6] A multicenter RCT which assessed propolis for genital herpes[7] found some antiviral activity, corroborating the results of another study,[8] and concluded that propolis appeared to be more effective than acyclovir and placebo in healing lesions and reducing local symptoms.

Dosage   *Mouthrinse*: apply several times daily.

Risks

Contraindications
Allergic predisposition to bee stings.

Precautions/warnings
Other allergic predispositions.

Adverse effects
None known.

Interactions
None known.

Quality issues
Depending on the plant sources and the geographic origin, the chemical composition will vary.

Risk–benefit assessment   There are too few rigorous clinical studies of propolis for any condition to make firm recommendations. Some positive findings exist for acute rheumatic disorders, uterine cervicitis and genital herpes. Whether it has beneficial effects as a constituent in mouthwashes is unclear. Propolis seems relatively safe but in the light of the costs involved and the availability of other conventional treatment approaches, these should be preferred.

REFERENCES

1 Schmidt H, Hampel C-M, Schmidt G, Riess E, Rödel C. Doppelblindversuch über den Einfluß eines propolishaltigen Mundwassers auf die entzündete und gesunde Gingiva. Stomatol der DDR 1980;30:491–497
2 Murray M C, Worthington H V, Blinkhorn A S. A study to investigate the effect of a propolis-containing mouthrinse on the inhibition of de novo plaque formation. J Clin Periodontol 1997;24:796–798
3 Poppe B, Michaelis H. Ergebnisse einer zweimal jährlich kontrollierten Mundhygienaktion mit propolishaltiger Zahnpasta (Doppelblindstudie). Stomatol der DDR 1986;36:195–203
4 Danø A P, Hylander Møller E, Jarnum S. Effekten af naturstoffet propolis ved colitis ulcerosa og Crohn's sygdom. Ugeskr Læg 1979;141:1888–1890
5 Santana Pérez E, Lugones Botell M, Pérez Stuart O, Castillo Brito B. Parasitisimo vaginal y cervicitis aguda: tratamiento local con propoleo. Informe preliminar. Rev Cubana Enfermer 1995;11:51–56

6 Béla S, Sándor S, Béla L, György M, Ede S. Local treatment of rheumatic disorders by propolis. Orvosi Hetilap 1996;137:1365–1370
7 Vynograd N, Vynograd I, Sosnowski Z. A comparative multi-centre study of the efficacy of propolis, acyclovir and placebo in the treatment of genital herpes (HSV). Phytomedicine 2000;7:1–6
8 Szmeja Z, Sosnowski Z. Therapeutic value of flavonoid in rhinovirus infections. Otolaryngol Pol 1989;43:180–184

FURTHER READING
Bankova V S, De Castro S L, Marcucci M C. Propolis: recent advances in chemistry and plant origin. Apidologie 2000;31:3–15
An overview of information published since 1995 on propolis constituents.

American Apitherapy Society: www.apitherapy.org
A useful website for more information on propolis.

RED CLOVER
(*Trifolium pratense* L)

Synonyms	Ackerklee (German), beebread, cow clover, meadow clover, purple clover, Rotklee (German), trefoil, trèfle des prés (French), wild clover.
Examples of trade names	Promensil.
Source	Flower heads.
Main constituents	Flavonoids, isoflavonoids, coumarins, carbohydrates, saponins, volatile oil.
Background	A member of the *Leguminosae* family, red clover is native to most of Europe and naturalized in the US. It has a long history in agriculture and religion and was considered a charm against witchcraft in the Middle Ages. It has long been used by traditional Chinese physicians and Russian folk healers for various medicinal purposes.
Traditional uses	Chronic skin disease, whooping cough, cancer, tuberculosis.
Pharmacologic action	Estrogenic.
Conditions frequently treated	Menopausal symptoms, eczema, psoriasis, cough.
Clinical evidence	Two RCTs of an isoflavone supplement derived from red clover have found no superiority over placebo for any menopausal symptoms and no endometrial changes.[1,2] However, in both trials the authors suggested that isoflavone ingestion in the placebo group may have masked any effect of red clover. Clinical trials in other indications were not located.
Dosage	500 mg extract daily standardized to 40 mg isoflavones. 1.5–3 ml of liquid extract (1:1 in 25% alcohol) three times daily.
Risks	***Contraindications*** Pregnancy, lactation, infants. ***Precautions/warnings*** Bleeding disorders. ***Adverse effects*** Breast tenderness, menstruation changes, weight gain.

Interactions

Theoretically red clover may interfere with anticoagulants and hormonal therapies.

Quality issues

Red clover may appear in products combined with other herbs.

Risk–benefit assessment

There is little clinical evidence to support the use of red clover and limited information on its safety, so the risk–benefit ratio is difficult to determine. From existing evidence it appears that there are few risks, but also few specific benefits.

REFERENCES

1 Baber R J, Templeman C, Morton T, Kelly G E, West L. Randomized, placebo-controlled trial of an isoflavone supplement and menopausal symptoms in women. Climacteric 1999;2:85–92

2 Knight D C, Howes J B, Eden J A. The effect of Promensil™, an isoflavone extract, on menopausal symptoms. Climacteric 1999;2:79–84

SAW PALMETTO
(Serenoa repens Bartram)

Synonyms

American dwarf palm tree, cabbage palm, sabal, *Sabal serrulata*, Sägepalme (German), Zwergsägepalme (German).

Examples of trade names

Permixon, Propalmex, Prostagutt, Prosta Urgenin Uno, Remoprostan, Strogen, SX Sabal.

Source

Fruits.

Main constituents

Fatty acids, phytosterols, flavonoids and polysaccharides.

Background

Saw palmetto, the only surviving species of the genus *Serenoa*, is a dwarf palm native to the coastal regions of the southern states in North America, particularly South Carolina and Florida. In traditional American medicine it was used as an extract for conditions such as bladder or urethral irritations. The fruits of saw palmetto were also employed as a tonic in cases of consumption or bronchitis. Between 1906 and 1950 the US Pharmacopeia and the National Formulary included tea of saw palmetto for urogenital ailments. Today, commercially available preparations contain the lipophilic fraction, extracted with hexane or liquid carbon dioxide. It is a popular herbal remedy, particularly in Germany, where it is frequently used for the urinary symptoms of benign prostatic hyperplasia.

Traditional uses

Cystitis, testicular atrophy, to increase sexual vigor, dysentery, hirsutism.

HERBAL AND NON-HERBAL MEDICINE

Pharmacologic action	Inhibition of 5-alpha-reductase, inhibitory effects on the binding of dihydrotestosterone to androgen receptors in the prostate, antiinflammatory, prolactin inhibition.
Conditions frequently treated	Benign prostatic hyperplasia.
Dosage	320 mg of liposterolic extract daily in divided doses.
Clinical evidence	A systematic review[1] assessed 18 RCTs of saw palmetto for the treatment of benign prostatic hyperplasia. It concluded that *Serenoa repens* significantly improves urologic symptoms and flow measures compared with placebo. Compared with finasteride, *Serenoa repens* produces similar improvements of urinary tract symptoms and urinary flow measures, with fewer adverse effects. These results are largely corroborated by more recently conducted double-blind RCTs.[2–5] A double-blind RCT also reports beneficial effects of saw palmetto for androgenic alopecia.[6] There seems to be no evidence to support the notion that it decreases prostate volume.
Risks	**Contraindications** Pregnancy, lactation. **Precautions/warnings** Should be used cautiously in conditions other than benign prostatic hyperplasia due to the lack of data. **Adverse effects** Gastrointestinal complaints, constipation, diarrhea, dysuria, decreased libido. **Interactions** May interact with hormone replacement therapy, oral contraceptives. **Quality issues** The quality of the extracts may vary between preparations.
Risk–benefit assessment	There is good evidence for the effectiveness of saw palmetto for benign prostatic hyperplasia. It seems to improve the symptoms and objective signs of benign prostatic hyperplasia to the same extent as finasteride. The encouraging safety profile of saw palmetto extract renders it an attractive option for patients with this condition. Data from long-term clinical studies are, however, not available. There is no compelling evidence for any other condition.

REFERENCES

1 Wilt T J, Ishani A, Stark G, MacDonald R, Lau J, Mulrow C. Saw palmetto extracts for treatment of benign prostatic hyperplasia. JAMA 1998;280:1604–1609

2 Marks L S. Partin A W, Epstein J I et al. Effects of a saw palmetto herbal blend in men with symptomatic benign prostatic hyperplasia. J Urol 2000;163:1451–1456

3 Mohanty N K, Jha R J, Dutt C. Randomized double-blind controlled clinical trial of Serenoa repens versus placebo in the management of patients with symptomatic grade I to grade II benign prostatic hyperplasia. Indian J Urol 1999;16:26–31

4 Bauer H W, Casarosa C, Cosci M, Fratta M, Blessmann G. Sabalfrucht Extrakt zur Behandlung der benignen Prostatahyperplasie. Münch Med Wochenschr 1999;141(25):62

5 Stepanov V N, Siniakova L A, Sarrazin B, Raynaud J P. Efficacy and tolerability of the lipidosterolic extract of Serenoa repens in benign prostatic hyperplasia. A double-blind comparison of two dosage regimens. Adv Ther 1999;16:231–241

6 Morganti P, Fabrizi G, James B, Bruno C. Effect of gelatine-cystine and Serenoa repens extract on free radicals levels and hair growth. J Appl Cosmetol 1998;16:57–64

FURTHER READING

Bombardelli E, Morazzoni P. Serenoa repens (Bartram) J.K. Small. Fitoterapia 1997;68:99–113
A comprehensive review on saw palmetto with an emphasis on botanical aspects.

Plosker G L, Brogden R N. Serenoa repens (Permixon). Drugs Aging 1996;9:379–391
A thorough review, particularly on the pharmacology of saw palmetto.

SHARK CARTILAGE

Synonyms   Haifischknorpel (German).

Examples of trade names   Arthrelan, Carticin, GNC Liquid Shark Cartilage.

Source   Cartilage from the fin of the hammerhead shark (*Sphyrna lewini*) and the spiny dogfish shark (*Squalus acanthias*).

Main constituents   Sphyrastatin 1 and 2 (glycoproteins).

Background   Based on the assumption that sharks never get cancer, it was hypothesized that shark cartilage might have anticancer properties in humans. Due to much publicity and clever marketing, shark cartilage became a popular food supplement in the 1990s. The debate over whether or not shark cartilage is associated with health benefits has developed into an ongoing, at times emotional controversy.[1–3]

Pharmacologic action   Antiangiogenic (starving tumors of essential nutrients) effects have been well documented in various test models and constitute the postulated mechanism of action. However, it seems debatable whether this is applicable to oral administration in humans because large macromolecules like sphyrastatins are not usually absorbed in sufficiently large quantities by the intestinal tract.

HERBAL AND NON-HERBAL MEDICINE

Conditions frequently treated	Cancer, arthritis.
Clinical evidence	Early reports that shark cartilage cured cancer, prolonged patients' lives or improved their quality of life were based on anecdotes or uncontrolled studies.[4] One such trial reported that 10 out of 20 patients experienced a partial or complete response after 8 weeks of shark cartilage therapy.[2] Interpretable studies found no reliable evidence that shark cartilage conveys any beneficial effects to cancer patients.[5] No rigorous studies for other indications exist. The debate continues about the bioavailability of the large glycoproteins from shark cartilage taken orally.
Dosage	Depending on the purity of the supplement, 500–4500 mg daily in divided doses.
Risks	**Contraindications** Pregnancy, lactation. **Precautions/warnings** Liver diseases. **Adverse effects** Hepatitis. **Interactions** None known. **Quality issues** Large variations in the purity of commercially available preparations exist.
Risk–benefit assessment	According to the most reliable evidence to date, shark cartilage is not an effective cure for cancer. Serious safety concerns have been repeatedly voiced (e.g. [5,6]). For all other alleged indications there is a total absence of reliable clinical data. Its use should be discouraged unless data to the contrary emerge.

REFERENCES

1 Lane I W, Comac L. Sharks don't get cancer. How shark cartilage can save your life. New York: Avery, 1992

2 Mathews J. Media feeds frenzy over shark cartilage as a cancer treatment. J Natl Cancer Inst 1993;85:1190–1191

3 Folkman J. What is the evidence that tumors are angiogenesis dependent? J Natl Cancer Inst 1990;82:2–4

4 Miller D R. Phase I/II trial of the safety and efficacy of shark cartilage in the treatment of advanced cancer. J Clin Oncol 1998; 16:3649–3655

5 Ashar B, Vargo E. Shark cartilage-induced hepatitis. Ann Intern Med 1996;125:780–781

6 Hunt T J, Conelly J F. Shark cartilage for cancer treatment. Am J Health-Syst Pharm 1995;52:1756–1760

SIBERIAN GINSENG
(*Eleutherococcus senticosus* Maxim)

Synonyms	Devil's shrub, eleuthero ginseng, ninjin (Japanese), Russian ginseng, touch-me-not.
Examples of trade names	Elagen, Eleutherococcus Lomapharm, Konstitutin Forte, Lebensenergie-Kapseln, Vigoran, Vital-Kapseln-ratiopharm.
Source	Root.
Main constituents	Eleutherosides (A–G), starch, vitamin A.
Background	Siberian ginseng is a slender shrub native to Siberia and northern China, which grows to a height of about 2–3 meters. It belongs to the same family (*Araliaceae*) as Asian ginseng (*Panax ginseng* C A Meyer) but is of a different genus and therefore not considered a true ginseng. It was tested in the former Soviet Union during the 1960s as a substitute for ginseng. In pharmacological studies it was found to exert similar effects to *Panax ginseng* root. Subsequently it was integrated into the Russian Pharmacopeia where it is listed as a tonic.
Traditional uses	To increase endurance and stress tolerance, to counteract weakness and fatigue, to improve general health and appetite and aid memory.
Pharmacologic action	Immunostimulatory, cytostatic, hypoglycemic, inhibition of platelet aggregation.
Conditions frequently treated	Cancer, cardiovascular diseases, sexual function; also commonly used to boost vitality, exercise performance and immune function.
Clinical evidence	A systematic review assessed all available double-blind RCTs of Siberian ginseng root extract for any indication.[1] Only three trials relating to physical performance, psychomotor performance and cognitive function and herpes simplex type II infections were identified. Single RCTs reported positive effects on psychomotor performance and cognitive function and herpes simplex type II infections.[2,3] One study administered 3.4 ml once daily for 6 weeks and reported no intergroup differences on measures of physical performance.[4] Overall, the review concluded that the effectiveness of Siberian ginseng root extract is not established beyond reasonable doubt for any indication. This finding is largely corroborated for physical performance.[5]

HERBAL AND NON-HERBAL MEDICINE

Dosage   100–200 mg of solid (20:1) extract daily in divided doses.

Risks

Contraindications
Hypertension, pregnancy and lactation, children under the age of 12 years.

Precautions/warnings
Premenopausal women, fever, mania, schizophrenia, asthma, diabetes, cardiac disorders.

Adverse effects
Diarrhea, dizziness, hypertension, pericardial pain, tachycardia, extrasystoles, insomnia, headaches.

Overdose
'Ginseng abuse syndrome' (dose approximately 3 g daily) has been reported for Asian ginseng (*Panax ginseng*). It may be sold in combination preparations including Siberian ginseng. Symptoms include hypertension, sleeplessness, skin eruptions, morning diarrhea, agitation. Doses of 15 g daily and over were associated with depersonalization, confusion and depression.

Interactions
May interact with anxiolytic or sedative agents, with cardiac, hypo- and hypertensive, anticoagulant and hypoglycemic agents; may increase serum digoxin levels.

Quality issues
Evidence in the scientific literature relates mostly to Elagen standardized ginseng extract from *Eleutherococcus senticosus* (eleutherosides B, E) and ESML *Eleutherococcus senticosus* Maxim L extract (including eleutherosides B, E and ethanol 30–34%).

Risk–benefit assessment   The available trial evidence suggests that the effectiveness of Siberian ginseng root extract for any indication is not established beyond reasonable doubt. Thus, considering the possibility of potentially serious adverse effects (and contrary to the opinion of the Commission E), the use of Siberian ginseng as a therapeutic intervention cannot, at present, be recommended.

REFERENCES

1 Vogler B K, Pittler M H, Ernst E. The efficacy of ginseng. A systematic review of randomised clinical trials. Eur J Clin Pharmacol 1999; 55:567–575

2 Winther K, Ranløv C, Rein E, Mehlsen J. Russian root (Siberian Ginseng) improves cognitive functions in middle-aged people, whereas Ginkgo biloba seems effective only in the elderly. J Neurol Sci 1997;150:S90

3 Williams M. Immuno-protection against herpes simplex type II infection by eleutherococcus root extract. Int J Alt Compl Med 1995;13(7):9–12

4 Dowling E A, Redondo D R, Branch J D, Jones S, McNabb G, Williams M H. Effect of Eleutherococcus senticosus on submaximal and maximal exercise performance. Med Sci Sports Exerc 1996;28:482–489

5 Bahrke M S, Morgan W P. Evaluation of the ergogenic properties of ginseng. Sports Med 2000;29:113–133

ST JOHN'S WORT
(*Hypericum perforatum* L)

Synonyms	Amber touch-and-heal, devil's scourge, goatweed, hypericum, Johanniskraut (German), Klamath weed, millepertuis (French), rosin rose, Tipton weed, witch's herb.
Examples of trade names	Hypercalm, Hyperforat, Hyperiforce, Jarsin, Kira, Nutri Zac, Psychotonin.
Source	Aerial parts.
Main constituents	Naphthodianthrones (e.g. hypericin, pseudohypericin), flavonoids, bioflavonoids, phloroglucinols (e.g. adhyperforin, hyperforin), tannins, volatile oils, xanthones.
Background	A member of the *Hypericaceae* family, St John's wort is a herbaceous, yellow-flowered perennial growing on woodland, heathland and roadsides. It is native to most of Europe, Asia and northern Africa and naturalized in the US and Australia by European colonists. The Latin name *hypericum* derives from the two Greek words *hyper* and *eikon* meaning 'over' and 'icon', as in 'over an apparition', referring to the belief that it had the power to ward off evil spirits. The common name St John's wort is thought to derive from associations with St John the Baptist – the flowers tend to bloom around the time of his feast day (June 24th) and the red pigments in the buds and flowers were associated with his blood. St John's wort has been used for medicinal purposes since the classical period. The texts of Hippocrates, Pliny, Dioscorides and Galen all mention the herb as a tonic for a wide range of conditions.
Traditional uses	Wound healing, diuretic, melancholy, pain relief and many others as diverse as snake bites, bedwetting in children, malaria and insanity.
Pharmacologic action	Antiretroviral, antidepressant. The mechanism is unclear but possibilities include inhibition of serotonin reuptake, noradrenaline and dopamine, modulation of interleukin-6 activity and GABA receptor binding; suggestions that MAO inhibition is responsible have been disproved.
Conditions frequently treated	Depression, low mood.
Clinical evidence	The efficacy of St John's wort in treating mild to moderate depressive disorders has been demonstrated in a number of double-blind, placebo-controlled RCTs and confirmed by metaanalysis.[1] There are also several comparative RCTs (e.g. [2–5])

HERBAL AND NON-HERBAL MEDICINE

indicating that it may be as effective as conventional antidepressants, including one with severely depressed patients.[6] Results from two trials suggest that St John's wort may be as effective as light therapy for seasonal affective disorder.[7,8] An open-label dose-controlled study of intravenous hypericin reported no antiretroviral effects in HIV-infected patients.[9] Positive results from uncontrolled trials exist for premenstrual syndrome,[10] menopausal symptoms[11] and fatigue.[12]

Dosage

300–900 mg of standardized dried extract (0.3% hypericin content) daily in divided doses.

Risks

Contraindications
Pregnancy, lactation.

Precautions/warnings
Photosensitization is possible, particularly in fair-skinned individuals.

Adverse effects
Most common reports are of gastrointestinal symptoms, allergic reactions, fatigue and anxiety. Several cases of mania and one of subacute toxic neuropathy have been reported.

Overdose
No cases have been reported in humans so consequences are unknown. Data from animal and preclinical studies suggest that the usual therapeutic doses are about 30–40 times below the level of phototoxicity.

Interactions
Concomitant use with serotonin reuptake inhibitors has resulted in cases of serotonin syndrome. Breakthrough bleeding has been reported for combined oral contraceptives. Acute rejection in transplant patients has been reported for cyclosporins. Other case reports and clinical investigations suggest reduced plasma levels of medications metabolized by hepatic cytochrome P450 microsomal oxidase enzymes (e.g. warfarin, anticonvulsants, digoxin, theophylline, HIV protease inhibitors). An RCT has demonstrated no interaction with alcohol.

Quality issues
Since the active constituents are not established, the whole extract must be considered necessary for a therapeutic effect. Hypericin is used as a marker substance in most standardized preparations although some products are standardized to hyperforin.

Risk–benefit assessment

There is evidence suggesting that St John's wort is as effective as conventional antidepressants for treating mild to moderate depression and is associated with fewer adverse effects. As a monotherapy, therefore, it may be an appropriate alternative to synthetic drugs for mildly or moderately depressed patients. For severe depression and other conditions there is insufficient evidence to recommend the use of St John's wort.

REFERENCES

1　Linde K, Ramirez G, Mulrow C D, Pauls A, Weidenhammer W, Melchart D. St John's wort for depression – an overview and meta-analysis of randomised clinical trials. Br Med J 1996; 313:253–258

2　Harrer G, Schmidt U, Kuhn U, Biller A. Comparison of equivalence between the St. John's wort extract LoHyp-57 and fluoxetine. Drug Res 1999;49:289–296

3　Philipp M, Kohnen R, Hiller K O. Hypericum extract versus imipramine or placebo in patients with moderate depression: randomised multicentre study of treatment for eight weeks. Br Med J 1999;319:1534–1538

4　Schrader E. Equivalence of St. John's wort extract (Ze 117) and fluoxetine: a randomized, controlled study in mild-moderate depression. Int Clin Psychopharm 2000;15:61–68

5　Woelk H. Comparison of St. John's wort and imipramine for treating depression: randomised controlled trial. Br Med J 2000;421:536–539

6　Vorbach E U, Arnoldt K H, Hubner W D. Efficacy and tolerability of St. John's wort extract LI 160 versus imipramine in patients with severe depressive episodes according to ICD-10. Pharmacopsychiatr 1997;30(suppl):81–85

7　Wheatley D. Hypericum in seasonal affective disorder (SAD). Cur Med Res Opin 1999;15:33–37

8　Kasper S. Treatment of seasonal affective disorder (SAD) with Hypericum extract. Pharmacopsychiatr 1997;30:89–93

9　Gulick R M, McAuliffe V, Holden-Wiltse J et al. Phase 1 studies of hypericin, the active compound in St. John's wort, as an antiretroviral agent in HIV-infected adults. Ann Intern Med 1999;130:510–514

10　Stevinson C, Ernst E. Hypericum for premenstrual syndrome: a pilot study. Br J Obst Gynecol 2000;107:870–876

11　Grube B, Walper A, Wheatley D. St. John's wort extract: efficacy for menopausal symptoms of psychological origin. Adv Ther 1999;16:177–186

12　Stevinson C, Dixon M, Ernst E. Hypericum for fatigue – a pilot study. Phytomedicine 1998;5:443–447

FURTHER READING

Bombardelli E, Morazzoni P. Hypericum perforatum. Fitoterapia 1995;LXVI:43–68
Thorough description of the history, botany, chemistry and pharmacology of St John's wort.

HERBAL AND NON-HERBAL MEDICINE

TEA TREE
(Melaleuca alternifolia)

Synonyms　　Melaleuca, Teebaum (German).

Source　　Essential oil from leaves and branches.

Main constituents　　Terpenes (pinene, terpinene, symene), cineole and numerous other compounds.

Background　　A member of the myrtle family (*Myrtaceae*), the tea tree is native to the coastal areas of Australia. Apparently, early European settlers made a tea from its leaves and thus the name was derived. Tea tree oil has become immensely popular as a topical antiseptic agent. Today it is included in many cosmetic products and commercial Australian production has risen from 20 tonnes per year in 1990 to 140 tonnes currently.

Traditional uses   Australian aborigines used it for burns, cuts and insect bites. It is sometimes advocated for eczema, lice infestation and psoriasis. Most of its present usage is for its antimicrobial action.

Pharmacologic action   Antifungal, antibacterial, antiviral.

Conditions frequently treated   Skin infections and associated conditions.

Clinical evidence   A recent systematic review found only four RCTs.[1] They yielded some evidence that tea tree oil may be effective in treating non-inflamed acne, tinea pedis and onychomycosis. This evidence was deemed encouraging but not ultimately compelling.

Dosage   5–100% tea tree oil preparations applied several times daily.

Risks   *Contraindications*
Pregnancy, lactation, allergy to tea tree oil.

Precautions/warnings
None for oral use; not for external use on mucous membranes.

Adverse effects
Allergy (frequent), mild skin irritation, toxic when taken orally.

Interactions
None known.

Quality issues
According to a 1995 Australian standard, tea tree oil should contain at least 30% terpinen-4-ol and less than 15% cineole.

Risk–benefit assessment   There are few risks associated with the proper use of tea tree oil. In vitro experiments demonstrate its antimicrobial activity but clinical evidence is scarce. Thus the balance of evidence is mildly in favor of tea tree oil.

REFERENCE

1 Ernst E. Huntley A. Tea tree oil: a systematic review of randomised clinical trials. Forsch   Komplementärmed Klass Naturheilkd 2000;7:17–20

THYME
(*Thymus vulgaris* L)

Synonyms   Common garden thyme, rubbed thyme, thyme, thymi herba, Thymian (German).

Examples of trade names	Aspecton, Bronchicum, Bronchipret, Olbas, Pertussin, Sinupret, Thyminpion.
Source	Leaves and flowers.
Main constituents	Phenols (thymol, carvacrol), camphene, eugenol, rosmarinic acid.
Background	*Thymus vulgaris* is in the same genus as mint. It is native to Italy and Spain and is cultivated throughout the world. Thyme has been used for culinary and medicinal purposes for millennia. Many subspecies exist; *Thymus vulgaris* and *Thymus zygis* are used interchangeably for medicinal purposes.
Traditional uses	Disinfection of skin (topical use) and mucous membranes, (whooping) cough, dyspepsia, upper respiratory tract infections, dental hygiene (oral use).
Pharmacologic actions	Antimicrobial, antiseptic, carminative, expectorant, antitussive, diaphoretic, antimutagenic, spasmolytic, antiflatulent, antihelminthic, antioxidant and antiinflammatory.
Conditions frequently treated	Cough, upper respiratory tract infections, bronchitis and as a dental antiseptic.
Clinical evidence	No compelling trial evidence exists for thyme given on its own. Encouraging data have been reported for chronic bronchitis treated by thyme in combination with other herbs in large (n > 3000) comparative clinical trials (e.g. [1]).
Dosage	1–2 g of extract daily in divided doses.
Risks	*Contraindications* Pregnancy, lactation, gastritis, enterocolitis, allergy to *Labiatae* family, congestive heart failure. *Precautions/warnings* Patients with gastrointestinal problems. *Adverse effects* Nausea, vomiting, diarrhea, headache, dizziness, respiratory distress, bradycardia, dermatitis (topical use). *Overdose* Effects on humans not known but loss of reflexes has been reported in animal studies. *Interactions* None known.

HERBAL AND NON-HERBAL MEDICINE

Quality issues
Use standardized extracts with 0.6–1.2% volatile oil and 0.5% phenol content.

Risk–benefit assessment

Lack of data regarding thyme as a monotherapy prevents a conclusive evaluation. Combination products have been shown to do more good than harm. Large comparative trials have suggested that they are superior to synthetic medications for bronchitis.

REFERENCE

1 Ernst E, März R, Sieder C. A controlled multi-centre study of herbal versus synthetic secretolytic drugs for acute bronchitis. Phytomedicine 1997;4:287–293

FURTHER READING

Van Den Broucke C O, Lemli J A. Pharmacological and chemical investigation of thyme liquid extracts. Planta Med 1981;41:129–135

VALERIAN
(*Valeriana officinalis* L)

Synonyms

All-heal, amantilla, Baldrian (German), fragrant valerian, heliotrope, herbe aux chats (French), wild valerian.

Examples of trade names

Valerina, Natrasleep, Valdispert Forte, Sedonium, Benedorm.

Source

Rhizome.

Main constituents

Amino acids (gamma-aminobutyric acid; GABA), alkaloids, iridoids/valepotriates, volatile oils, phenylpropanoids, sesquiterpenoids.

Background

Valeriana officinalis is one of over 200 members of the *Valerianaceae* family. A herbaceous perennial, it is native to most of Europe and Asia and grows in damp swampy areas. The name *Valeriana* derives from the Latin word *valere* meaning well-being. Its use as a medicinal herb dates back to the times of Hippocrates and Dioscorides.

Traditional uses

Digestive problems, flatulence, urinary tract disorders.

Pharmacologic action

Sedative, anxiolytic. Mechanisms are unclear, but GABA receptors may be involved.

Conditions frequently treated

Insomnia, anxiety.

Clinical evidence

The hypnotic effects of valerian have been investigated in several double-blind placebo-controlled RCTs. Improvements following single doses have been reported (e.g. [1]) as well as with repeated administration (e.g. [2]). A systematic review of the subject concluded that the evidence was promising but not conclusive, due to inconsistent results and methodological limitations.[3] An RCT published subsequently found valerian to be as effective as oxazepam in enhancing the sleep quality of insomniacs after 4 weeks.[4] One RCT (n=48) suggested valerian may reduce situational anxiety in healthy adults.[5]

Dosage

400–900 mg of extract 30–60 minutes before bedtime.

Risks

Contraindications
Pregnancy, lactation, known allergy, hepatic impairment.

Precautions/warnings
Care should be taken if driving or operating machinery when taking valerian.

Adverse effects
Headache and gastrointestinal symptoms occasionally reported. Morning hangover reported occasionally although RCTs investigating safety factors have found no impairment of reaction time or alertness the morning after intake. Hepatotoxicity has been reported from herbal preparations in which valerian was combined with other herbs, including skullcap.

Overdose
Symptoms of tachycardia, nausea, vomiting, dilated pupils, drowsiness, confusion, visual hallucinations, blurred vision, cardiac disturbance, excitability, headache, hypersensitivity reactions and insomnia have been reported following acute overdoses, with full recoveries made in all cases.

Interactions
Theoretically, potentiation of the effects of sedatives, hypnotics or other central nervous system depressants is possible at high doses. RCTs have shown no potentiation of alcohol.

Quality issues
Composition and purity of extracts vary greatly. Standardized extracts often use valepotriates as the marker substance although valerenic acid is considered more reliable due to its stability. Aqueous extracts are devoid of valepotriates.

Risk–benefit assessment

Neither the efficacy nor safety of valerian has been established beyond reasonable doubt. However, the preliminary evidence for both are promising and valerian may be worth considering as a monotherapy for promoting sleep.

HERBAL AND NON-HERBAL MEDICINE

HERBAL AND NON-HERBAL MEDICINE

REFERENCES

1 Leathwood P D, Chauffard F, Heck E, Munoz-Box R. Aqueous extract of valerian root (*Valeriana officinalis* L) improves sleep quality in man. Pharmacol Biochem Behav 1982;17:65–71

2 Vorbach E U, Gortelmeyer R, Bruning J. Therapie von Insomnien: Wirksamkeit und Verträglichkeit eines Baldrianpräparats. Psychopharmakotherapie 1996;3:109–115

3 Stevinson C, Ernst E. Valerian for insomnia: systematic review of randomized placebo-controlled trials. Sleep Med 2000;1:91–99

4 Dorn M. Baldrian versus oxazepam: efficacy and tolerability in non-organic and non-psychiatric insomniacs: a randomized, double-blind, clinical comparative study. Forsch Komplementärmed Klass Naturheilkd 2000;7:79–84

5 Kohnen R, Oswald W D. The effects of valerian, propranolol and their combination on activation, performance and mood of healthy volunteers under social stress conditions. Pharmacopsychiatry 1988;21:447–448

FURTHER READING

Bos R, Woerdenbag H J, De Smet P A G M, Scheffer J J C. Valeriana species. In: De Smet P A G M, Keller K, Hänsel R, Chandler R F (eds) Adverse effects of herbal drugs, volume 3. Berlin: Springer 1997
Thorough overview of safety information on valerian.

WILLOW
(Salix spp.)

Synonyms
Brittle willow, purple willow, Silberweide (German), white willow.

Examples of trade names
Assalix Assplant, Rheumakaps.

Source
Bark.

Main constituents
Derivatives of salicin, mainly salicortin, tremulacin, tannins.

Background
Dioscorides (50 AD) recommended willow bark as a remedy for inflammatory joint diseases and gout. The English clergyman Edward Stone rediscovered willow bark extracts as a remedy against fever and pain. Salicin was isolated as an active compound from the extract by the French pharmacist Leroux and 6 years later the compound was synthesized by Löwing, a German chemist working for Bayer. As he had used extracts from plants of the genus Spirea, he called the substance spiric acid, which appears in the brand name Aspirin (acetylsalicylic acid).

Traditional uses
Fever, pain, rheumatic complaints.

Pharmacologic action
Salicin is metabolized to salicylic acid which has antipyretic and analgesic effects.

Conditions frequently treated
Rheumatic diseases, common cold, headache.

Clinical evidence	Few CCTs have been carried out with willow bark preparations. One placebo-controlled RCT in patients with degenerative arthritis has shown positive results after 2 weeks of treatment with willow bark extract (10:1) containing 17.6% of total salicin.[1] A double-blind RCT including 82 patients with chronic arthritic pain over a treatment period of 2 months confirmed these findings.[2] An RCT in 210 patients with lower back pain, using placebo and willow bark dry extracts equivalent to 120 mg of salicin/day and 240 mg of salicin/day respectively, showed significantly positive results. Twenty seven patients in the higher dose group, 15 patients in the lower dose group and four patients in the placebo group were reported to be pain free in the last week of the study.[3]

Dosage   120–240 mg of total salicin daily in divided doses.

Risks

Contraindications
Pregnancy, lactation, patients with salicylate intolerance.

Precautions/warnings
Patients on anticoagulation treatment. Although there are data indicating that willow bark has no effect on coagulation time,[4] patients on this kind of pharmacologic therapy should use willow bark extracts only under careful supervision.

Adverse effects
None known.

Interactions
Anticoagulants.

Quality issues
Preparations standardized to salicin should be used.

Risk–benefit assessment	Although limited, the evidence suggests that willow bark extracts are efficacious in chronic pain. Whether they are as useful as Aspirin (or other NSAIDs) is doubtful. However, the adverse effects profile appears to be more favorable. Therefore willow bark extracts may be worthy of consideration for patients with mild pain who insist on a herbal remedy.

HERBAL AND NON-HERBAL MEDICINE

REFERENCES

1 Schmidt B M. Behandlung von Cox- und Gonarthrosen mit einem Trockenextrakt aus Salix purpurea x daphnoides. Dissertation, University of Tübingen, 1998

2 Mills S Y, Jacoby R K, Chacksfield M, Willoughby M. Effect of a proprietary herbal medicine on the relief of chronic arthritic pain: a double-blind study. Br J Rheumatol 1996; 35:874–878

3 Chrubasik S, Eisenberg E, Balan E, Weinberger T, Luzzati R, Conradt C. Treatment of low back pain exacerbations with willow bark extract: a randomised double-blind study. Am J Med 2000;109:9–14

4 Krivoy N, Pavlotzky F, Eisenberg E, Chrubasik J, Chrubasik S, Brook G. Salix cortex (willow bark dry extract) effect on platelet aggregation. Drug Monit 1999;21:202

YOHIMBE
(Pausinystalia yohimbe K Schumann)

Synonyms	Aphrodien, *Corynanthe yohimbe*, johimbe, Yohimbe (German), yohimbehe, yohimbene, yohimbime, yohimbine.
Examples of trade names	Aphrodyne, Potensan, Prowess, Puamin, Yocon-Glenwood, Yohimbine 'Spiegel', Yohimex.
Source	Bark.
Main constituents	Indole alkaloids of which 10–15% are yohimbine.
Background	Yohimbe is a tall evergreen tree reaching a height of about 30 meters and is native to Central Africa. The ground bark is traditionally used as an aphrodisiac, particularly for male erectile dysfunction. Interestingly, in the US it is also used as an alternative to anabolic steroids for enhancing athletic performance. Yohimbine is the main active constituent of *Pausinystalia yohimbe* and also present in other plants such as the Indian snakeroot (*Rauwolfia serpentina*) and quebracho (*Aspidosperma quebracho-blanco*). Most clinical studies relate to the effects of this isolated constituent of yohimbe bark.
Traditional uses	As an aphrodisiac, skin diseases, pruritus, obesity.
Pharmacologic action	Alpha-2-adrenoceptor blockade. Causes a rise in sympathetic drive by increasing noradrenaline release and firing rate of noradrenergic nuclei in the central nervous system.
Conditions frequently treated	Erectile dysfunction.
Clinical evidence	No evidence from rigorous clinical trials assessing extracts of yohimbe bark was located. A systematic review and meta-analysis of yohimbine for erectile dysfunction assessed seven double-blind RCTs.[1] It concluded that yohimbine is superior to placebo for the treatment of erectile dysfunction of organic or non-organic cause. Other double-blind RCTs indicate no beneficial effects for the treatment of obesity (e.g.[2]) or on gastric emptying rate in obese patients.[3] Another double-blind RCT suggests that yohimbine has no beneficial effects for the treatment of orthostatic hypotension in patients with Parkinson's disease.[4] Single RCTs report positive effects for dry mouth in patients receiving psychotropic drugs[5] and for the treatment of withdrawal symptoms due to drug abuse.[6]

Dosage 16–18 mg of yohimbine hydrochloride daily in divided doses.

Risks

Contraindications
Pregnancy, lactation, children, psychiatric conditions, anxiety, hypertension, cardiac, renal or hepatic diseases.

Precautions/warnings
Individuals with chronic inflammation of the prostate or the reproductive organs.

Adverse effects
Nervous excitation, sleeplessness, anxiety, hypertension, tachycardia, bronchospasm, nausea, vomiting.

Overdose
Doses of 20–30 mg yohimbine hydrochloride daily may cause increased heart rate and raised blood pressure.

Interactions
Increased effects of antidepressants, central nervous system stimulants, phenothiazines and other $alpha_2$-adrenoceptor blocking agents, reduced effects of antihypertensive drugs; interaction with sildenafil is theoretically possible.

Quality issues
Yohimbine hydrochloride preparations may contain other drugs including strychnine and methyltestosterone.

Risk–benefit assessment
There is evidence that yohimbine has beneficial effects in the treatment of erectile dysfunction of various causes. This oral treatment option has obvious advantages over invasive interventions and is relatively safer. Comparative studies with other oral medications such as sildenafil, which has been shown to be effective for this condition, are not available yet comparing the effect sizes derived from systematic reviews, the effectiveness seems to be similar. There is no compelling evidence on yohimbine for the treatment of other conditions.

HERBAL AND NON-HERBAL MEDICINE

REFERENCES

1 Ernst E, Pittler M H. Yohimbine for erectile dysfunction: a systematic review and meta-analysis. J Urol 1998;159:433–436

2 Kucio C, Jonderko K, Piskorska D. Does yohimbine act as a slimming agent? Israel J Med Sci 1991;27:550–556

3 Jonderko K, Kucio C. Effect of anti-obesity drugs promoting energy expenditure, yohimbine and ephedrine, on gastric emptying in obese patients. Aliment Pharmacol Ther 1991;5:413–418

4 Senard J M, Rascol O, Raskol A, Montastruc J L. Lack of yohimbine effect on ambulatory blood pressure recording: a double-blind cross-over trial in Parkinsonians with orthostatic hypotension. Fundament Clin Pharmacol 1993;7:465–470

5 Bagheri H, Schmitt L, Berlan M, Montastruc J L. A comparative study of the effects of yohimbine and anetholtrithioneon salivary secretion in depressed patients treated with psychotropic drugs. Eur J Clin Pharmacol 1997;52:339–342

6 Hameedi F A, Woods S W, Rosen M I, Pearsall H R, Kosten T R. Dose dependent effects of yohimbine on methadone maintained patients. Am J Drug Alcohol Abuse 1997;23:327–333

Table 4.1 **Other medicinal herbs without sufficient evidence of effectiveness**

Name*	Description	Pharmacologic action	Conditions frequently treated	Safety concerns
Andrographis paniculata	Herb native to Asia. Leaves are used medicinally	Antimicrobial	Bacterial dysentery, hepatic and intestinal disorders, common cold	Urticaria
Angelica (Angelica archangelica)	Herb native to Europe and parts of Asia. Root and rhizome are used medicinally	Smooth muscle relaxant	Loss of appetite, abdominal discomfort, flatulence	Photosensitization
Anise (Pimpinella anisum)	Seeds are used medicinally	Expectorant, antispasmodic, antibacterial	Dyspepsia, catarrh	Allergic reactions
Arnica (Arnica montana)	Herb native to Europe and North America. Flowers are used medicinally	Antiinflammatory, antimicrobial	Sprains and bruises (topical)	Oral: should only be taken in homeopathic doses because of toxicity Topical: allergies, dermatitis
Asparagus (Asparagus officinalis),	Cultivated as vegetable. Roots are used medicinally	Diuretic	Urinary tract inflammation, prevention of kidney stones	Allergic reactions
Baizhu (Atractylodis macrocephalus)	Native to China. Rhizomes are used medicinally	Digestive, diuretic	Anorexia, diarrhea	None known
Balloon flower (Platycodon grandiflorum)	Perennial herb native to northern Asia. Roots are used medicinally	Expectorant, antitussive, antiinflammatory	Upper respiratory tract infections	None known
Banxia (Pinellia ternata)	Native to China. Rhizomes are used medicinally	Expectorant, antiemetic	Asthma, cough	Could cause abortion in pregnant women
Beimu (Fritillaria cirrhosa)	Native to China. Bulbs are used medicinally	Antitussive, mucolytic, expectorant	Inflammation of respiratory tract	None known
Bilberry (Vaccinium myrtillus)	Shrub native to northern Europe, Asia and North America; member of Ericaceae family	Antioxidative	Diabetes mellitus, cancer prevention	None known

TABLE 4.1 OTHER MEDICINAL HERBS **167**

Herb	Description	Action	Uses	Side effects/Precautions
Blueberry (*Vaccinium angustifolium*)	Native American fruit; member of the *Ericaceae* family	Antioxidative	Diabetes mellitus, cancer prevention	None known
Borage (*Borage officinalis*)	Annual herb native to Europe and US. Leaves, stems, flowers and seeds are used medicinally	Antiinflammatory	Arthritis	Contains hepatotoxic pyrrolizidine alkaloids
Brucca amarissima	Small tree native to China. Fruits are used medicinally	Antimicrobial	Amebic dysentery, malaria	Anaphylaxis
Butcher's broom (*Ruscus aculeatus*)	Shrub native to the Mediterranean. Rhizome used medicinally	Diuretic, antiinflammatory	Chronic venous insufficiency	Gastrointestinal discomfort, nausea
Calendula (*Calendula officinalis*)	Herb native to the Mediterranean. Flowers are used medicinally	Antiinflammatory, immune stimulating, antimicrobial	Wound healing, gastric ulcers, postmastectomy lymphedema	None known
Caraway (*Carum carvi*)	Fruits are used to produce essential oil	Antispasmodic, antimicrobial	Dyspepsia, flatulence	None known
Cardamom (*Elettaria cardamomum*)	Seeds are used to produce essential oil	Cholagogue, virustatic	Dyspepsia	Precaution: do not use in cases of gallstones
Cascara (*Rhamnus purshiana*)	Tree native to North America. Bark is used medicinally	Increases mobility of colon	Constipation	Fresh bark is toxic and must be stored before use, not for use in inflammatory bowel diseases, gastrointestinal cramps
Chinese goldthread (*Loptis chinensis*)	Perennial herb native to China, Japan and India. Rhizome is used medicinally	Antimicrobial	Diarrhea, conjunctivitis, leishmaniasis, malaria	Gastrointestinal symptoms
Chinese rhubarb (*Rheum officinale*)	Perennial herb resembling the common garden rhubarb cultivated in China and Korea. Rhizomes are used medicinally	Stimulant of colonic activity, increases paracellular permeability	Constipation	Abdominal cramps, diarrhea, fluid loss (overdose)
Cinnamon (*Cinnamonum verum*)	Tree native to southern India. Bark is used medicinally	Carminative, antimicrobial	Loss of appetite, dyspepsia	Allergies

HERBAL AND NON-HERBAL MEDICINE

table continues

HERBAL AND NON-HERBAL MEDICINE

Name*	Description	Pharmacologic action	Conditions frequently treated	Safety concerns
Cloves (Syzygium aromaticum)	Cloves are the dried flower buds used to produce essential oil	Antiseptic, antimicrobial, anesthetic, antispasmodic	Skin or mucosa inflammation and pain (topical)	Skin or mucosa irritation
Comfrey (Symphytum officinale)	Above-ground parts of herb are used medicinally	Antiinflammatory	Bruises and sprains (topical)	Herb contains pyrrolizidine alkaloids which are hepatotoxic, therefore not for internal use
Diahuang (Rehmannia glutinosa)	Native to China. Roots are used medicinally	Antipyretic, antirheumatic, diuretic	Rheumatic pain	None known
Dong quai=Chinese angelica (Angelica sinensis)	Native to China. Volatile oils are extracted from the roots	Vasodilatation, quinidine-like, alters uterine activity	Gynecological disorders, circulation conditions	Bleeding, photosensitivity, interaction with anticoagulants
Eucalyptus (Eucalyptus globulus)	Evergreen tree native to Australia	Expectorant, secretolytic, antiseptic	Inflammation of respiratory tract	Nausea, vomiting, diarrhea
Fennel (Foeniculum vulgare)	Herb native to Mediterranean. Oil obtained from fruit seeds is used medicinally	Antispasmodic, secretolytic	Dyspepsia, flatulence	Allergies
Fenugreek (Trigonella foenum-graecum)	Herbaceous annual plant belonging to Leguminosae family, thought to originate from India or Middle East	Cholagogue, antiinflammatory, galactagogue	Diabetes mellitus, hypercholesterolemia	Minor gastrointestinal symptoms, allergic reactions
Gentian (Gentiana lutea)	Herb native to southern Europe and western Asia. Root is used medicinally	Digestive stimulant	Loss of appetite, flatulence	Headache
Goldenseal (Hydrastis canadensis)	Plant native to North America. Rhizomes are used medicinally	Oxytocic, laxative, antiinflammatory, vasoconstrictive	Wound healing, herpes labialis	Digestive problems, hypertension, hallucinations
Gotu kola (Centella asiatica)	Slender herb native to warmer regions of both hemispheres	Stimulation of collagen synthesis, antiinflammatory	Wound healing (topical), leprosy	Allergic reactions

TABLE 4.1 OTHER MEDICINAL HERBS 169

Herb	Description	Actions	Uses	Adverse effects
Iceland moss (*Cetraria islandica*)	Lichen native to Scandinavia	Antimicrobial, immunostimulant	Loss of appetite, dry cough, irritation of mucous membranes	None known
Ivy (*Hedera helix*)	Climbing plant native to Europe and Asia. Leaves are used medicinally	Expectorant, antispasmodic, antimicrobial, analgesic	Chronic respiratory inflammation	Contact dermatitis
Juniper (*Juniperus communis*)	Shrub native to Europe, Asia and US. Berries are used to produce volatile oil	Diuretic, carminative, antirheumatic	Dyspepsia	Kidney damage (prolonged use or overdose)
Lemon balm (*Melissa officinalis*)	Shrub native to Mediterranean and Asia. Leaves are used medicinally	Sedative, spasmolytic. antimicrobial	Insomnia, herpes labialis (external use)	No serious safety concerns known
Licorice (*Glycyrrhiza glabra*)	Herb native to Mediterranean, Russia and Asia Minor. The genus Glycyrrhiza consists of ~30 species. Licorice is a constituent of many traditional Chinese herbal mixtures. Root is used medicinally	Expectorant, secretolytic. antispasmodic, antiinflammatory, adrenocorticotrophic, aldosterone-like effects	Gastric, ulcers, catarrhs, cancer prevention, detoxification, antiinflammatory, antioxidation	Adverse effects consistent with adrenocorticotrophic actions
Ma huang (*Ephedra*)	Shrub native to Asia	Ephedrine-like effects	Bronchospasm	Abused as a stimulant (e.g. herbal 'ecstasy'), ephedrine-like adverse effects
Marshmallow (*Althaea officinalis*)	Herb native to Europe and Asia. Leaves and roots are used medicinally	Demulcent	Dry cough	None known
Mongolian milk-vetch (*Astragalus mongholicus* or *A. membranaceus*)	Perennial herb native to China, Korea, Mongolia and Siberia. Roots are used medicinally	Immunostimulant, general tonic	Common cold, influenza	None known

table continues

HERBAL AND NON-HERBAL MEDICINE

Name*	Description	Pharmacologic action	Conditions frequently treated	Safety concerns
Myrrh (*Commiphora molmol*)	Oleo-gum resin extruded from stems of the plant	Astringent	Skin or mucosa inflammation	None known
Onion (*Allium cepa*)	Well-known perennial herb used as a food. Probably native to western Asia	Antimicrobial, diuretic, glucose lowering, general tonic	Arteriosclerosis, loss of appetite, wound healing (topical)	Allergic reactions
Pineapple (*Ananas comosus*)	Proteolytic enzyme bromelain, from the fruit, is used medicinally	Platelet inhibition, antiinflammatory, fibrinolytic	Sprains, bruises and posttraumatic edema	Could prolong bleeding time, diarrhea
Poplar = American aspen (*Populus alba*)	The bark of the white poplar is normally used medicinally	Salicylates exert antiinflammatory effects	Rheumatic conditions	Renal dysfunction, GI symptoms, interaction with anticoagulants
Psyllium (*Plantago ovata = Isphagula*)	Leaves, seeds and husks are used medicinally	Bulk-forming laxative	Constipation	Allergic reactions including anaphylaxis
Pumpkin (*Curcurbita pepo*)	Annual vine native to America. Seeds are used medicinally	Antiandrogenic antiinflammatory	Benign prostatic hyperplasia	None known
Qianghuo (*Notopterygium incisum*)	Native to China. Rhizomes are used medicinally	Analgesic	Rheumatic pain, common cold	None known
Sage (*Salvia officinalis*)	Shrub native to the Mediterranean. Leaves are used medicinally	Antimicrobial, antisecretory	Dyspepsia, persistent perspiration	Epileptiform convulsions (prolonged use)
Sarsaparilla (*Smilax*)	Dried roots and rhizomes of various *Smilax* species are used medicinally	Tonic, antiinflammatory, hepatoprotective	Psoriasis, leprosy, appetite stimulant	Renal damage, interaction with hypnotics and digitalis
Shegan (*Belamcanda sinensis*)	Native to China. Rhizomes are used medicinally	Antiphlogistic, expectorant	Asthma, cough, pain	None known
Turmeric (*Curcuma longa*)	Shrub native to southern Asia. Root is used medicinally	Choleritic, antiinflammatory, antioxidant, antimutagenic	Functional gallbladder problems	None known

TABLE 4.1 OTHER MEDICINAL HERBS **171**

White peony (*Paeonia lactiflora*)	Perennial herb native to China, India and Japan. Roots are used medicinally	Antispasmodic, antiinflammatory, analgesic, abortifacient, anticoagulant	Pain (e.g. menstrual)	Could increase action of anticoagulants
Witch hazel (*Hamamelis virginiana*)	Small tree native to North America. Leaves and bark are used medicinally	Astringent, antiinflammatory	Minor skin injuries, hemorrhoids, varicose veins (external use)	None known
Wuweizu (*Schisandra chinensis*)	Native in China. Fruits are used medicinally	Antiinflammatory, antihepatotoxic	Liver protection, asthma	None known
Xixin (*Asarum heterotropoides*)	Native to China. Whole plant is used medicinally	Analgesic, antitussive, sedative	Common cold, headache, other pains	None known
Yarrow (*Achillea millefolium*)	Above-ground parts are used medicinally	Choleretic, antibacterial, astringent, antispasmodic	Loss of appetite, dyspepsia	Allergic reactions
Yuxingcao (*Houttuynia cordata*)	Native to China, Japan, Korea, Vietnam. Aerial parts are used medicinally	Diuretic, antiinflammatory	Inflammation of respiratory tract, acute dysentery, acute urinary tract infections	None known
Zelan (*Lycopus lucidus*)	Native to China. Leaves are used medicinally	Activation of blood circulation, diuretic	Menstrual disorders, postpartum pain	None known

*English or Chinese common name, *Latin name*

HERBAL AND NON-
HERBAL MEDICINE

Table 4.2 Other non-herbal medicines without sufficient evidence of effectiveness

Name	Description	Pharmacologic action	Conditions frequently treated	Safety concerns
Acidophilus	*Lactobacillus acidophilus* is a bacterium which is commercially prepared for oral consumption (probiotic)	Digestive aid, production of B-complex vitamins and a 'healthy' bacterial flora in the gastrointestinal tract	Gastrointestinal problems, prevention of infections, after antibiotic treatments	None known
Agar	Aqueous extract from the cell wall of red marine algae	Promotion of fecal bulk	Constipation	Bowel obstruction, decrease of intestinal absorption of minerals
Bee pollen	Flower pollen and nectar, mixed with digestive enzymes from honeybees	Antioxidative	Allergic conditions including asthma, impotence, prevention of cancer and cardiovascular disease	Allergic reactions including anaphylaxis
Carnitine	Quaternary amine, constituent of muscle cells	Participation in cellular energy production and removal of toxins, cholinergic antagonist, membrane stabilizer	Numerous chronic conditions including cardiovascular disease and Alzheimer's disease	None known
Creatine	Amino acid found in red meat, milk and fish. Also synthesized by the kidneys, liver and pancreas	Maintaining high levels of adenosine triphosphate (main energy source for muscle contraction)	Enhancement of physical performance	Dehydration, gastrointestinal discomfort, muscle cramps
Dehydroepiandrosterone (DHEA)	Precursor of steroid hormones found in some plants (e.g. yam)	Raising levels of androgens and estrogens; assumed antiaging effects	Prevention of cancer, cardiovascular disease, osteoporosis	Hirsutism, insomnia, irritability. Interactions with steroid hormones

TABLE 4.2 OTHER NON-HERBAL MEDICINES **173**

Kelp	Product derived from marine brown algae; used in Japanese folk medicine	Anticarcinogenic	Cancer prevention, obesity, rheumatism	Acne, thrombocytopenia, bleeding, hypotension. Arsenic poisoning. Interactions with anticoagulants possible
Octacosanol	28-carbon long-chain alcohol isolated from vegetable waxes	Enhancement of intramuscular lipolysis	To increase physical endurance	Irritability, orthostatic hypotension
Red yeast rice (*Monascus purpureus*)	Fermentation product of yeast and rice used in traditional Chinese medicine	Reduction of hepatic cholesterol synthesis (contains lorastatin)	Hypercholesterolemia	As lorastatin
Royal jelly	Secretion of worker bees that is fed to the queen bee	Antimicrobial, antitumor	Impotence, baldness, menopause, prevention of cancer and cardiovascular disease	Allergies including anaphylaxis
Thymus extract	Extracts from bovine thymus cells usually for injection	Stimulation of immune system	Cancer, AIDS	Allergic reactions, infection

Table 4.3 **Terminology of medicinal plants**

Common name	Latin name (first describer)	Synonyms
Aloe vera	*Aloe vera* (L)	*Aloe barbadensis* P Miller, Barbados aloe, burn plant, Curacao aloe, elephant's gall, first-aid plant, Hsiang-dan, lily of the desert, Lu-hui, medicine plant, miracle plant, plant of immortality
Artichoke	*Cynara scolymus* (L)	Artischocke (German), bur artichoke, carciofo (Italian), garden artichoke, globe artichoke
Black cohosh	*Cimicifuga racemosa* (L)	*Actaea racemosa* L, black snakeroot, bugbane, rattleroot, rattletop, rattleweed, Traubensilberkerze (German), Wanzenkraut (German)
Butcher's broom	*Ruscus aculeatus* (L)	Box holly, Mäusedorn (German), pungitopo (Italian)
Calendula	*Calendula officinalis* (L)	Gold-bloom, holigold, marigold, marybud, poet's marigold, Ringelbume (German)
Caraway	*Carum carvi* (L)	Cumino (Italian), Kümmel (German)
Cardamom	*Elettaria cardamomum* (L)	*Alpinia cardamomum*, Kardamom (German), Malabar cardamom
Chaste tree	*Vitex agnus castus* (L)	Agneau chaste (French), agnocasto (Italian), agnus castus, chasteberry, gatillier (French), hemp tree, Keuschlamm (German), Mönchspfeffer (German), monk's pepper, vitex
Cloves	*Syzygium aromaticum* (L)	Carophyllum, chiodi di garofano (Italian), *Eugenia carophyllata*, Gewürznelken (German), *Jambosa carophyllus*
Comfrey	*Symphytum officinale* (L)	Beinwell (German), blackwort, bruisewort, slippery root
Cranberry	*Oxycoccus macrocarpus*	Kronsbeere (German), marsh apple, Moosbeere (German), Preisselbeere (German)
Devil's claw	*Harpagophytum procumbens*	Artiglio del diavolo (Italian), grapple plant, Teufelskralle (German), wood spider
Echinacea	*Echinacea angustifolia* (DC), *E. pallida* (Nutt), *E. purpurea* (L)	American cone flower, black sampson hedgehog, Indian head, snakeroot, red sunflower, scurvy root
Elder	*Sambucus nigra* (L)	Black elder, bore tree, bour tree, common elder, hylder, eldrum, sambuco (Italian), Schwarzer Holunder (German)
Evening primrose	*Oenothera biennis* (L)	Fever plant, king's cure-all, Nachtkerze (German), night willow-herb, scabish, sundrop, tree primrose

TABLE 4.3 TERMINOLOGY OF MEDICINAL PLANTS **175**

Common name	Latin name (first describer)	Synonyms
Fennel	*Foeniculum vulgare*	Bitter fennel, garden fennel, Fenchel (German), finocchio (Italian), sweet fennel, wild fennel
Fenugreek	*Trigonella foenum-graecum*	Greek hay, trigonella, Bockshornklee (German), fieno greco (Italian)
Feverfew	*Tanacetum parthenium* (Schultz-Bip)	Altamisa, bachelor's buttons, *Chrysanthemum parthenium* (L), featherfew, motherherb, Mutterkraut (German)
Garlic	*Allium sativum* (L)	Aglio (Italian), ail (French), camphor of the poor, Da-suan, Knoblauch (German), La-juan, poor man's treacle, rustic treacle, stinking rose
German chamomile	*Matricaria recutita* (L)	Camomilla (Italian), *Chamomilla recutita*, fleur de camomile (French), Hungarian chamomile, Kamille (German), pin heads, single chamomile, wild chamomile
Ginger	*Zingiber officinale* (Roscoe)	Ingwer (German), zenzero (Italian), zingiber
Ginkgo	*Ginkgo biloba* (L)	Duck foot tree, icho (Japanese), maidenhair tree, silver apricot
Ginseng, Asian	*Panax ginseng* (C A Meyer)	Allheilkraut (German), Chinese ginseng, Korean ginseng, ninjin (Japanese), true ginseng
Ginseng, Siberian	*Eleutherococcus senticosus* (Maxim)	Devil's shrub, eleuthero ginseng, ninjin (Japanese), Russian ginseng, touch-me-not, wild pepper
Goldenrod	*Solidago vigaurea* (L)	European goldenrod, Goldrute (German)
Goldenseal	*Hydrastis canadensis* (L)	Eye root, hydrastis, idraste (Italian), orange root, yellow root
Gotu kola	*Centella asiatica*	Centella (Italian), Asiatic pennywort, Indian pennywort, Indian water navelwort
Guar gum	*Cyamopsis tetragonolobus* (L)	Cyamopsis gum, gomma guar (Italian), guar (German), guaran, jaguar gum
Grapeseed	*Vitis vinifera*	Grape, semi d'uva (Italian), vitis
Green tea	*Camellia sinensis*	Grüner Tee (German), Matsu-cha
Hawthorn	*Crataegus species*	Biancospino (Italian), maybush, Weißdorn (German), whitethorn
Hop	*Humulus lupulus* (L)	Hopfen (German), houblon (French), humulus, luppolo (Italian), lupulus
Horse chestnut	*Aesculus hippocastanum* (L)	Buckeye, ippocastano (Italian), Rosskastanie (German)

HERBAL AND NON-HERBAL MEDICINE

table continues

Common name	Latin name (first describer)	Synonyms
Horseradish	*Armoriacia rusticana* (P Gaertner)	*Cochlearia armoriacia* L, Meerrettich (German)
Kava kava	*Piper methysticum* (G Forster)	Intoxicating pepper, kava, kawa, kawa pepper, Rauschpfeffer (German), yangona
Lavender	*Lavandula angustifolia* (Miller)	Aspic, English lavender, lavanda (Italian), lavande commun (French), Lavendel (German), true lavender
Licorice	*Glycyrrhiza glabra* (L)	Gancao, glycyrrhiza, Lakritze (German), liquirizia (Italian), sweet root, yasti-madhu
Ma huang	*Ephedra sinica* (Stapf)	Cao mahuang, Chinese ephedra, ephedra, Meerträubchen (German)
Marshmallow	*Althaea officinalis* (L)	Eibisch (German)
Milk thistle	*Silybum marianum* (L)	Cardo mariano (Italian), cardus marianus, holy thistle, lady's thistle, Mariendistel (German), St Mary thistle
Mistletoe	*Viscum album* (L)	All heal, bird lime, devil's fuge, golden bough, Mistel (German), vischio (Italian), viscum
Nettle	*Urtica dioica* (L)	Brennessel (German), common nettle, ortica (Italian), stinging nettle
Passion flower	*Passiflora incarnata* (L)	Apricot vine, fleur de la passion (French), grenadille, maypop passion flower, passiflora (Italian), Passionsblume (German), passion vine, purple passion flower, wild passion flower
Peppermint	*Mentha x piperita* (L)	Brandy mint, Katzenkraut (German), lamb mint, Pfefferminz (German)
Red clover	*Trifolium pratense* (L)	Beebread, cow clover, meadow clover, purple clover, trefoil, trifoglio (Italian), wild clover
Saw palmetto	*Serenoa repens* (Bartram)	American dwarf palm tree, cabbage palm, sabal, *Sabal serrulata*, Sägepalme (German), Zwergsägepalme (German)
Skullcap	*Scutellaria lateriflora* (L)	Helmet flower, hoodwort, quaker bonnet, mad-dog skullcap
Shepherd's purse	*Capsella bursa pastoris* (L)	Hirtentäschel (German), pick-pocket, witches' pouches
St John's wort	*Hypericum perforatum* (L)	Amber touch-and-heal, devil's scourge, goatweed, hypericum, iperico (Italian), Johanniskraut (German), klamath weed, millepertuis (French), rosin rose, Tipton weed, witch's herb
Tea tree	*Melaleuca alternifolia*	Melaleuca, Teebaum (German)

TABLE 4.3 TERMINOLOGY OF MEDICINAL PLANTS **177**

Common name	Latin name (first describer)	Synonyms
Thyme	*Thymus vulgaris* (L)	Common thyme, garden thyme, rubbed thyme, thyme, timo (Italian), *Thymi herba*, Thymian (German)
Turmeric	*Curcuma longa* (L)	*Curcuma domestica* Valeton, *C. aromatica* Salisbury, curcuma, Gelbwurz (German), Indian saffron, Jianghuang (Chinese), kyoo (Japanese)
Uva-ursi	*Arctostaphylus uva-ursi* (L)	Common bearberry, bearberry, beargrape, Bärentraube (German), hogberry, rockberry, sandberry, uva ursina (Italian)
Valerian	*Valeriana officinalis* (L)	All-heal, amantilla. Baldrian (German), fragrant valerian, garden heliotrope, herbe aux chats (French), Indian valerian, Mexican valerian, valeriana (Italian), wild valerian
Willow	*Salix daphnoides* (Villars), *S. purpurea* (L), *S. alba* (L)	White willow, brittle willow, purple willow, salice (Italian), Silberweide (German)
Yarrow	*Achillea millefolium* (L)	Achillea, milfoil, millefolium, Schafgarbe (German)
Yohimbe bark	*Pausinystalia yohimbe* (K Schumann)	Aphrodien, *Corynanthe yohimbe*, johimbe, Yohimbe (German), yohimbehe, yohimbene, yohimbime, yohimbine

HERBAL AND NON-HERBAL MEDICINE

Table 4.4   **Medicinal plants not approved by German Commission E[1] because of safety concerns**

Plant	Possible adverse effect	Responsible constituent
Angelica (seed and herb)	Photosensitivity	Coumarins
Basil	Mutagenicity	Estragole
Bilberry (leaf)	Intoxication	
Bishop's weed (fruit)	Allergic reactions; photosensitivity	Khellin
Bladderwrack	Hyperthyroidism	Iodine
Borage	Liver damage	Pyrrolizidine alkaloids
Bryonia	Numerous risks	Not known
Celery	Allergic skin reactions; phototoxicity	Furanocoumarin
Chamomile (Roman)	Allergic reactions	Not known
Cinnamon (flower)	Allergic reactions	Not known
Cocoa	Allergic reactions, migraine	Not known
Colocynth	Gastrointestinal problems, kidney damage, cystitis	Curcurbitacin
Coltsfoot	Liver damage	Pyrrolizidine alkaloids
Delphinium (flower)	Bradycardia, hypotension, cardiac arrest, central paralyzing and curare-like effects on respiratory system	Alkaloids
Elecampane	Irritation of mucosa, allergic contact dermatitis	Alantolactone
Ergot	Wide spectrum of adverse effects	Alkaloids
Goat's rue	Hypoglycemia	Galegin
Hound's tongue	Liver damage	Pyrrolizidine alkaloids
Kelp	Hyperthyroidism	Iodine
Lemongrass, citronella oil	Toxic alveolitis	Essential oil
Liverwort (herb)	Irritation of skin and mucous membranes	Protoanemonin
Madder (root)	Mutagenic and carcinogenic potential	Lucidin
Male fern	Wide spectrum of adverse effects	Not known
Marjoram	Unclear risks	Arbutin and hydroxyquinone content
Marsh tea	Poisoning, abortions	Not known
Monkshood	Varied spectrum of effects	Cardiotoxic principle
Mugwort	Abortion	Not known
Nutmeg	Psychoactive, abortion	Not known
Nux vomica	Spastic CNS action	Strychnine
Oleander (leaf)	Poisoning, sometimes fatal	Oleandrin

TABLE 4.4 MEDICINAL PLANTS NOT APPROVED **179**

Plant	Possible adverse effect	Responsible constituent
Papain	Bleeding in patients with clotting disorders	Not known
Parsley (seed)	Vascular congestion and contraction of smooth muscles in bladder, intestines, and uterus	Apiol
Pasque (flower)	Severe irritation of skin and mucosa	Protoanemonin
Periwinkle	Suppression immune system	Not known
Petasites (leaf)	Liver damage	Pyrrolizidine alkaloids
Rhododendron, rusty-leaved	Poisoning	Grayanotoxine content
Rue	Phototoxic and mutagenic effects, liver and kidney damage	Furanocoumarins
Saffron	Adverse effects noted in doses over 10 g used for abortion	Not known
Sarsaparilla (root)	Gastric irritation and temporary kidney impairment suspected	Not known
Scotch broom (flower)	Contraindicated in MAOI therapy and hypertension	Not known
Senecio (herb)	Liver damage	Pyrrolizidine alkaloids
Soapwort, red (herb)	Mucous membrane irritation	Saponins
Tansy (flower and herb)	Poisoning due to abuse	Thujone content of oil
Walnut (hull)	Potential mutagenic effect	Juglone
Yohimbe (bark)	Nervousness, tremor, sleeplessness, anxiety, hypertension, and tachycardia, nausea, vomiting associated with therapeutic administration of yohimbine; interaction with psychopharmacological herbs	Sympathomimetic principles

Fetrow & Avila[2] list the following additional plants as 'potentially unsafe'

Common name	Latin name	Possible adverse effects
American yew	*Taxus canadensis*	Cytotoxicity
Autumn crocus	*Colchicum autumnale*	Gastrointestinal toxicity, vomiting, neurologic toxicity, renal failure
Betel palm	*Areca catechu*	Teratogenesis
Bird's foot trefoil	*Lotus corniculatus*	Cyanide poisoning: seizures, paralysis, coma, death
Black locust	*Robinia pseudo-acacia*	Bradycardia, nausea, vomiting, dizziness
Black nightshade	*Solanum americanum*	Cardiac toxicity
Blue flag	*Iris versicolor*	Severe nausea, vomiting, diarrhea

HERBAL AND NON-HERBAL MEDICINE

table continues

Common name	Latin name	Possible adverse effects
Calabar bean	*Physostigma venenosum*	Cholinergic toxicity
Castor oil plant	*Ricinus communis*	Gastrointestinal toxicity or dehydration
Chaparral	*Larrea tridentata*	Fulminant hepatic failure
Comfrey	*Symphytum officinale*	Hepatotoxicity
Cotton	*Gossypium hirsutum*	Hypokalemia, male sterility, heart failure at high doses
Daffodil	*Narcissus pseudonarcissus*	CNS depression, carcinogenicity, coma, death
Foxglove	*Digitalis purpurea*	Bradycardia, heart block, arrhythmias
Germander	*Teucrium scorodonia*	Hepatotoxicity
Goldenseal	*Hydrastis canadensis*	Hyperreflexia, hypertension, seizures, respiratory failure
Hedge mustard	*Sisymbrium officinale*	Cardiac toxicity, heart failure
Hemp dogbane	*Apocynum cannabinum*	Cardiac stimulant, arrhythmias
Henbane	*Hyoscyamus niger*	Anticholinergic toxicity
Indian pink	*Spigelia marilandica*	Death (from overdose)
Indian tobacco	*Lobelia inflata*	Paralysis, hypothermia, cardiovascular collapse, coma, death
Jalap root	*Exagonium purga*	Dramatic purgative, cathartic
Live root	*Senecio longilobus*	Hepatic failure from hepatic venocclusive disease
Marsh marigold	*Caltha palustris*	Inflammation of mucosal tissues and bronchospasm
Mayapple	*Podophyllum peltatum*	Severe gastrointestinal irritation
Moonseed	*Menispermum canadense*	Tachycardia, severe vomiting or diarrhea
Poison hemlock	*Conicum maculatum*	Birth defects
Queen's delight	*Stillingia sylvatica*	Gastrointestinal toxicity, mutagenesis
Wallflower	*Cheiranthus cheiri*	Cardiac toxicity, heart failure, bradycardia
Wild cherry	*Prunus virginiana*	Dyspnea, vertigo, seizures
Wild licorice	*Glycyrrhiza lepidota*	Hypotension, hypertension, hypernatremia, muscle weakness
Wintercress	*Barbarea vulgaris*	Renal damage
Wormseed	*Chenopodium ambrosioides*	Seizures, paralysis
Yellow jessamine	*Gelsemium sempervirens*	Paralysis, death

REFERENCES

1 Blumenthal M (ed). The complete Commission E monographs. Boston: Integrative Medicine Communications, 1998

2 Fetrow C W, Avila J R. Complementary and alternative medicines. Springhouse, PA: Springhouse, 1999

TABLE 4.5 RAW PLANT MATERIAL CAUSING INTOXICATION **181**

Table 4.5 **Raw plant material causing severe intoxication after ingestion of small quantities**

Common names	Latin name	Poisonous plant parts	Symptoms / signs	Treatment
European yew, Eibe (German)	*Taxus baccata* L	All parts except the red coating of the seeds	Nausea, vomiting, intestinal pain, patients become lethargic and comatose, tachycardia, low blood pressure, bradycardia, arrhythmias, cyanosis, pulse rate drops, ECG changes. Fatalities reported	Toxin removal through induced vomiting, gastric lavage, activated charcoal. Treatment of cardiac complications. Specific antidote is not known
Mezereon, Seidelbast (German)	*Daphne mezereum* L	All parts	Inflammation and burning in the mouth, hoarseness, difficulty swallowing, salivation, stomach complaints, bloody stools, diarrhea, neurological symptoms. Fatalities reported.	Toxin removal through induced vomiting, gastric lavage, atropine, symptomatic therapy
Ivy, Efeu (German)	*Hedera helix* L	Stem, leaves, berries	Vomiting, diarrhea, neurological and respiratory symptoms, contact dermatitis. Death from asphyxiation	Toxin removal through induced vomiting, gastric lavage, symptomatic therapy. Assisted ventilation
Boxwood, Immergrüner Buchsbaum (German)	*Buxus sempervirens* L	All parts	Vomiting, severe grayish liquid diarrhea, dizziness. Death by respiratory paralysis has been reported in animals	Toxin removal through induced vomiting, gastric lavage, symptomatic therapy. Specific therapy is not known
Golden chain, Golden rain, Gemeiner Goldregen (German) Laburnum	*Laburnum anagyroides* Medik	All parts	Approximately 30 min after ingestion burning sensation in mouth and throat, salivation, vomiting, delirium, excitation, tonic and clonic convulsions. Death from respiratory paralysis	Toxin removal through induced vomiting, gastric lavage, symptomatic therapy. Assisted ventilation. Specific therapy is not known
Castor, Rizinus (German), Wunderbaum (German), Christuspalme (German)	*Ricinus communis* L	Seeds	Symptoms can occur with a latency of 24 h. Nausea, vomiting, diarrhea, abdominal pain, cold sweats, hypotension, convulsions, cyanosis. Fatalities reported	Toxin removal through induced vomiting, gastric lavage, symptomatic therapy. Control of hydration and electrolytes

table continues

HERBAL AND NON-HERBAL MEDICINE

Common names	Latin name	Poisonous plant parts	Symptoms / signs	Treatment
Deadly nightshade, Tollkirsche (German)	*Atropa belladonna* L	All parts	Dry mouth, mydriasis, tachycardia, restlessness, hallucinations, coma. Death from respiratory paralysis	Toxin removal through gastric lavage. Sedatives. Specific antidote: physostigmine. Assisted ventilation
Datura, Weisser Stechapfel (German)	*Datura stramonium* L	All parts	Dry mouth, mydriasis, sedation, tachycardia, restlessness, hallucinations, coma. Death from respiratory paralysis	Toxin removal through gastric lavage. Sedatives. Specific antidote: physostigmine. Assisted ventilation
Henbane, Schwarzes Bilsenkraut (German)	*Hyoscyamus niger* L	Roots, leaves, seeds	Dry mouth, mydriasis, tachycardia, restlessness, hallucinations, coma. Death from respiratory paralysis	Toxin removal through gastric lavage. Sedatives. Specific antidote: physostigmine-assisted ventilation
Tobacco, Virginischer Tabak (German)	*Nicotiana tabacum* L	All parts except the ripe seeds	Burning sensation in the mouth, nausea, vomiting, ataxia, headaches, hypersalivation, muscle pain and contractions, abdominal pain, visual and auditory perturbations, mental confusion, respiratory difficulties, bradycardia. Death from respiratory paralysis	Toxin removal, activated charcoal, gastric lavage, assisted ventilation, control of blood pressure
Opium poppy, Schlafmohn (German)	*Papaver somniferum* L	All parts except the ripe seeds	Dizziness, vertigo, analgesia, sedation, coma, hypothermia, miosis, cyanosis. Death from respiratory paralysis	Specific antidote: naloxone Gastric lavage, assisted ventilation
Aconite, Eisenhut (German)	*Aconitum napellus* L	All parts	Paresthesia in mouth, face and extremities, pain, anesthesia to nociceptive stimuli, muscle weakness, tetraplegia, vomiting, diarrhea, hypotension, bradycardia, respiratory difficulties. Death from respiratory paralysis	Gastric lavage, activated charcoal, intensive care, correct dehydration and electrolyte imbalance, antiarrhythmics, specific antidote is not known

table continues

TABLE 4.5 RAW PLANT MATERIAL CAUSING INTOXICATION **183**

Common names	Latin name	Poisonous plant parts	Symptoms / signs	Treatment
White hellebore, Weisser Germer (German)	*Veratrum album* L	All parts	Rapid onset of vomiting and nausea, diarrhea, paresthesias, hypersalivation, sneezing, hypotension, bradycardia, neurological signs. Prognosis is poor	Decontamination, activated charcoal, gastric lavage, treat bradycardia with atropine, intensive care
Purple foxglove, Roter Fingerhut (German)	*Digitalis purpurea* L	All parts	Identical to that of drug poisoning. Gastrointestinal symptoms, hallucinations, mental confusion, sleepiness, nausea, visual disturbances such as yellow halos, bradycardia, arrhythmias	Gastric lavage, activated charcoal, atropine, antiarrhythmics, correct electrolyte imbalance, cholestyramine, digoxin antibodies
Lily-of-the-valley, Maiglöckchen (German)	*Convallaria majalis* L	All parts	Gastrointestinal symptoms, nausea, vomiting, diuresis, after massive ingestion symptoms are similar to digitalis poisoning. Fatalities reported	Gastric lavage, activated charcoal, atropine, antiarrhythmics, correct electrolyte imbalance, cholestyramine, digoxin antibodies
Oleander; Oleander (German)	*Nerium oleander* L	All parts	Nausea, vomiting, malaise, weakness, mental confusion, visual disturbances, bradycardia, arrhythmia	Gastric lavage, activated charcoal, atropine, antiarrhythmics, correct electrolyte imbalance, cholestyramine, digoxin antibodies
White bryony, Weisse oder schwarzbeerige Zaunrübe (German)	*Bryonia alba* L	Roots, berries, seeds	Nausea, abdominal pain, diarrhea, vomiting	Toxin removal through induced vomiting, gastric lavage, no specific therapy available
Tutin, Rotbeerige Zaunrübe (German)	*Bryonia dioica* Jacq	Roots, berries, seeds	Nausea, abdominal pain, diarrhea, vomiting	Toxin removal through induced vomiting, gastric lavage, no specific therapy available

table continues

HERBAL AND NON-HERBAL MEDICINE

Common names	Latin name	Poisonous plant parts	Symptoms / signs	Treatment
Jerusalem cherry tree, Korallenbäumchen (German), Korallenstrauch (German), Korallenkirsche (German), Orangenbäumchen (German)	*Solanum pseudocapsicum* L	All parts	Vomiting, nausea, diarrhea, somnolence, abdominal pain, arrhythmia, hyperthermia, Death from cardiac arrest	Toxin removal through induced vomiting, gastric lavage, specific therapy is not known
Water hemlock, Wasserschierling (German)	*Cicuta virosa* L	All parts	Weakness, hypersalivation, burning sensation in the mouth, nausea, tremors, dizziness, abdominal cramps, vomiting, tonic and clonic convulsions. Death from respiratory paralysis	Toxin removal through induced vomiting, gastric lavage, activated charcoal, barbiturates, muscle relaxation, hemodialysis, hemoperfusion, assisted ventilation
Poison hemlock, Gefleckter Schierling (German)	*Conium maculatum* L	All parts	Salivation, nausea, vomiting, pharyngeal irritation, abdominal pain, thirst, swallowing and speaking difficulties, visual and hearing difficulties, convulsive tremors, uncontrolled movements of the limbs, muscle paralysis, respiratory paralysis	Decontamination, assisted ventilation, strychnine as analeptic in small doses
Fool's parsley, Hundspetersilie (German)	*Aethusa cynapium* L	All parts	Salivation, nausea, vomiting, pharyngeal irritation, abdominal pain, thirst, swallowing and speaking difficulties, visual and hearing difficulties, convulsive tremors, uncontrolled movements of the limbs, muscle paralysis, respiratory paralysis	Decontamination, assisted ventilation, strychnine as analeptic in small doses
Autumn crocus, Herbstzeitlose (German)	*Colchicum autumnale* L	All parts	Vomiting, profuse diarrhea, abdominal pain, burning sensation in mouth, difficulties swallowing, convulsions, hyponatremia, oliguria, increased natriuria. Prognosis is very poor	Gastric lavage, activated charcoal, correct electrolyte imbalance, assisted ventilation, analgesics and antispasmodics to relieve intestinal pain

SOURCES

Nowack R. Notfallhandbuch Giftpflanzen. Berlin: Springer, 1998
Bruneton J. Toxic plants. Paris: Lavoisier Publishing, 1999

TABLE 4.6 PRODUCTS REQUIRING THERAPEUTIC MONITORING **185**

Table 4.6
Herbal medicinal products and other food supplements requiring therapeutic monitoring

Name	Recommended test
Aloe	Renal function, electrolytes
Angelica	Coagulation studies
Basil	Blood glucose
Bayberry	Liver function tests
Bearberry	Renal function, electrolytes
Bee pollen	Blood glucose
Betony	Liver function tests
Bistort	Liver function tests
Black haw	Coagulation studies
Blackroot	Liver function tests
Blue cohosh	Blood glucose
Boneset	Liver function tests
Borage	Liver function tests
Buchu	Liver function tests
Cascara	Renal function, electrolytes
Castor bean	Renal function, electrolytes
Cat's claw	Coagulation studies
Chaparral	Liver function tests
Chondroitin	Full blood count, coagulation studies
Condurango	Liver function tests
Cowslip	Liver function tests
Cucumber	Renal function, electrolytes
Dandelion	Blood glucose
Dock, yellow	Renal function, electrolytes
Dong quai	Coagulation studies
Fenugreek	Coagulation studies, blood glucose
Garlic	Full blood count
Ginger	Coagulation studies
Gingko	Coagulation studies
Ginseng	Blood glucose
Gotu kola	Blood glucose
Horse chestnut	Coagulation studies
Jaborandi tree	Liver function tests
Kava	Full blood count
Kelp	Coagulation studies
Kelpware	Renal function, electrolytes, coagulation studies, blood glucose
Khella	Liver function tests
Lovage	Renal function, electrolytes
Lungwort	Coagulation studies
Marshmallow	Blood glucose
Mayapple	Full blood count, liver function tests, renal function, electrolytes
Myrrh	Blood glucose
Myrtle	Blood glucose
Pau d'arco	Coagulation studies
Pennyroyal oil	Liver function tests, renal function, electrolytes
Pomegranate	Liver function tests
Poplar	Liver function tests, coagulation studies
Ragwort	Liver function tests
Red clover	Coagulation studies
Rhatany	Liver function tests

HERBAL AND NON-HERBAL MEDICINE

table continues

Name	Recommended test
Royal jelly	Blood glucose
Sage	Blood glucose
Sarsaparilla	Renal function, electrolytes
Shark cartilage	Liver function tests
Skullcap	Liver function tests
Soapwort	Liver function tests, renal function, electrolytes
Sorrel	Liver function tests, renal function, electrolytes
Squaw vine	Liver function tests
Tonka bean	Liver function tests, coagulation studies
Turmeric	Coagulation studies
Valerian	Liver function tests
Willow	Liver function tests, renal function, electrolytes, coagulation studies
Wintergreen	Coagulation studies
Wormwood	Renal function, electrolytes

SOURCE

Fetrow C W, Avila J R. Complementary and alternative medicine. Springhouse, PA: Springhouse, 1999

TABLE 4.7 INTERACTION WITH HEART MEDICATIONS **187**

Table 4.7 **Herbal medicinal products and other food supplements with the potential to interact with heart medications**

Name	Direction of effect	Concomitant medication
Adonis	⇑	Cardiac glycosides
Agrimony	⇑	Antihypertensives
Aloe vera	⇑	Cardiac glycosides, antiarrhythmic drugs
Arnica	⇓	Antihypertensives
Asafoetida	⇑	Antihypertensives
Avens	⇑	Antihypertensives
Bayberry	⇓	Antihypertensives
Bearberry	⇑	Cardiac glycosides
Betony	⇑	Antihypertensives
Black cohosh	⇑	Antihypertensives
Blue cohosh	⇓	Antihypertensives
Boldo	⇑	Cardiac glycosides
Broom	⇑	Beta-blockers, antihypertensives
Buchu	⇑	Cardiac glycosides
Buckthorn	⇑	Cardiac glycosides
Calamus	⇑	Antiarrhythmics, antihypertensives,
Capsicum	⇓	Antihypertensives
Cascara	⇑	Cardiac glycosides
Cat's claw	⇑	Antihypertensives
Celery	⇑	Antihypertensives
Co-enzyme Q10	⇑	ACE inhibitors and Ca+ channel blockers
Cola	⇓	Antihypertensives
Coltsfoot	⇓	Ca+ channel blockers, antihypertensives
Cornsilk	⇑	Antihypertensives
Cowslip	⇑	Antihypertensives
Dandelion	⇑	Antihypertensives
Devil's claw	⇑	Antihypertensives
Elecampane	⇑	Antihypertensives
Ephedra	⇓	Antihypertensives
Fenugreek	⇑	Antihypertensives
Figwort	⇑	Cardiac glycosides
Fucus	⇑	Antihypertensives
Fumitory	⇑	Antihypertensives, beta-blockers, cardiac glycosides, Ca+ channel blockers
Garlic	⇑	Antihypertensives
Gentian	⇓	Antihypertensives
Ginger	⇓	Antihypertensives
Ginseng, eleutherococcus	⇑	Antihypertensives
Ginseng, panax	⇑	Antihypertensives, cardiac glycosides
Goldenseal	⇑	Antihypertensives
Hawthorn	⇑	Antihypertensives, cardiac glycosides
Horehound, white	⇑	Antihypertensives
Horseradish	⇑	Antihypertensives
Indian snakeroot	⇑	Antihypertensives
Irish moss	⇑	Antihypertensives
Kelp	⇑	Antihypertensives
Khat	⇑	Antihypertensives, antiarrhythmic drugs, beta-blockers
Khella	⇑	Antihypertensives

table continues

Name	Direction of effect	Concomitant medication
Licorice	⇩	Antihypertensives
Lily-of-the-valley	⇧	Cardiac glycosides, beta-blockers, Ca+ channel blockers
Lugwort	⇧	Cardiac glycosides
Maté	⇩	Antihypertensives
Mistletoe	⇧	Antihypertensives
Motherwort	⇧	Cardiac glycosides, antihypertensives
Nettle	⇧	Antihypertensives
Night-blooming cereus	⇧	Cardiac glycosides, ACE inhibitors, antiarrhythmic drugs, Ca+ channel blockers
Oleander	⇧	Cardiac glycosides
Parsley	⇧	Antihypertensives
Pill-bearing spurge	⇧	ACE inhibitors
Plantain	⇧	Antihypertensives
Pokeroot	⇧	Antihypertensives
Prickly ash	⇧	Antihypertensives
Psyllium	⇧	Cardiac glycosides
Queen Anne's lace	⇧	Antihypertensives, cardiac glycosides
Red clover	⇧	Cardiac glycosides
Rhubarb	⇧	Cardiac glycosides
Rue	⇧	Cardiac glycosides, antihypertensives
Sage	⇧	Antihypertensives
Sarsaparilla	⇧	Cardiac glycosides
Senna	⇧	Cardiac glycosides
Shepherd's purse	⇧	Antihypertensives, beta-blockers, cardiac glycosides, Ca+ channel blockers
Squaw vine	⇧	Cardiac glycosides
Squill	⇧	Cardiac glycosides, antihypertensives, antiarrhythmic drugs, Ca+ channel blockers
St John's wort	⇧	Cardiac glycosides, antihypertensives
Strophantus	⇧	Cardiac glycosides
Vervain	⇧	Antihypertensives
Wild carrot	⇧	Antihypertensives
Yarrow	⇧	Antihypertensives
Yohimbine	⇩	Antihypertensives

⇧ increase action
⇩ decrease action

SOURCES

Fetrow C W, Avila J R. Complementary and alternative medicine. Springhouse, PA: Springhouse, 1999

Newall C A, Anderson L A, Phillipson J D. Herbal medicines. A guide for health-care professionals. London: Pharmaceutical Press, 1996

Ernst E. Possible interactions between synthetic and herbal medicinal products. Part 1: a systematic review of the indirect evidence. Perfusion 2000;13:4–15

HERBAL AND NON-HERBAL MEDICINE

TABLE 4.8 INTERACTION WITH ANTICOAGULANTS **189**

Table 4.8
Herbal medicinal products and other food supplements with the potential to interact with anticoagulants

Name	Direction
Agrimony	⇩
Alfalfa	⇧
Angelica	⇧
Aniseed	⇧
Arnica	⇩
Asafoetida	⇧
Bilberry	⇧
Black haw	⇧
Bogbean	⇧
Buchu	⇧
Cat's claw	⇧
Celery	⇧
Chamomile	⇧
Chondroitin	⇧
Cinchona	⇧
Clove	⇧
Co-enzyme Q10	⇧
Cordyceps	⇧
Danshen	⇧
Devil's claw	⇧
Dong quai	⇧
Fenugreek	⇧
Feverfew	⇧
Fucus	⇧
Garlic	⇧
Ginger	⇧
Ginkgo	⇧
Ginseng, panax	⇧
Goldenseal	⇩
Horse chestnut	⇧
Horseradish	⇧
Irish moss	⇧
Kelp	⇧
Khella	⇧
Licorice	⇧
Lovage	⇧
Lugwort	⇧
Meadowsweet	⇧
Mistletoe	⇩
Mugwort	⇧
Pau d'arco	⇧
Pill-bearing spurge	⇧
Pineapple	⇧
Poplar	⇧
Prickly ash	⇧
Quassia	⇧
Red clover	⇧
Reishi	⇧
Senega	⇧
St John's wort	⇩
Sweet clover	⇧

HERBAL AND NON-HERBAL MEDICINE

table continues

Name	Direction
Tonka bean	⇧
Turmeric	⇧
Vervain	⇧
Willow	⇧
Wintergreen	⇧
Woodruff	⇧
Yarrow	⇩

⇧ increasing anticoagulation
⇩ decreasing anticoagulation

SOURCES

Fetrow C W, Avila J R. Complementary and alternative medicine. Springhouse, PA: Springhouse, 1999

Newall C A, Anderson L A, Phillipson J D. Herbal medicines. A guide for health-care professionals. London: Pharmaceutical Press, 1996

Ernst E. Possible interactions between synthetic and herbal medicinal products. Part 1: a systematic review of the indirect evidence. Perfusion 2000;13:4–15

TABLE 4.9 INTERACTION WITH ANTIDIABETIC MEDICATIONS **191**

Table 4.9
Herbal medicinal products and other food supplements with the potential to interact with antidiabetic medications

Name	Direction
Alfalfa	⇧
Aloe vera	⇧
Basil	⇧
Bee pollen	⇩
Burdock	⇧
Celandine	⇧
Celery	⇧
Coriander	⇧
Cornsilk	⇧
Damiana	⇧
Dandelion	⇧
Devil's claw	⇩
Elecampane	⇩
Eucalyptus	⇧
Fenugreek	⇧
Figwort	⇩
Garlic	⇧
Ginseng, eleutherococcus	⇧
Ginseng, panax	⇧
Gotu kola	⇩
Guar gum	⇧
Horehound	⇧
Hydrocotyle	⇩
Juniper	⇧
Licorice	⇩
Marshmallow	⇧
Melatonin	⇧
Myrrh	⇧
Myrtle	⇧
Nettle	⇧
Night-blooming cereus	⇧
Onion	⇧
Sage	⇧
St John's wort	⇩
Tansy	⇧

⇧ increasing antidiabetic effect
⇩ decreasing antidiabetic effect

SOURCES

Fetrow C W, Avila J R. Complementary and alternative medicine. Springhouse, PA: Springhouse, 1999

Newall C A, Anderson L A, Phillipson J D. Herbal medicines. A guide for health-care professionals. London: Pharmaceutical Press, 1996

Ernst E. Possible interactions between synthetic and herbal medicinal products. Part 1: a systematic review of the indirect evidence. Perfusion 2000;13:4–15

HERBAL AND NON-
HERBAL MEDICINE

Table 4.10
Herbal medicinal products with the potential to interact with oral contraceptives

Name	Direction
Chaste tree	⇧
Guar gum	⇩
Herbal laxatives (e.g. aloe vera, senna)	⇩
Hop	⇧
Licorice	⇩
Pokeweed	⇧
Red clover	⇧
Siberian ginseng	⇧
St John's wort	⇩

⇧ increase in plasma levels
⇩ decrease in plasma levels

SOURCES

Fetrow C W, Avila J R. Complementary and alternative medicine. Springhouse, PA: Springhouse, 1999

Newall C A, Anderson L A, Phillipson, J D. Herbal medicines. A guide for health-care professionals. London: Pharmaceutical Press, 1996

Ernst E. Possible interactions between synthetic and herbal medicinal products. Part 1: a systematic review of the indirect evidence. Perfusion 2000;13:4–15

TABLE 4.11 USEFUL WEBSITES **193**

Table 4.11
Some useful websites providing further information on medicines

The following websites contain online information on safety and efficacy of herbal medicinal products and/or dietary supplements. We investigated a large number of sites and selected only those that are searchable, where the information provided is based on research findings and updated frequently, and where the information and any editorial text are balanced, i.e. not limited to positive evidence. The following meet these criteria.

Organization	The Natural Pharmacist
Website	http://www.tnp.com
Access	Partly limited to health professionals (free registration online)
Content	Fully referenced monographs on herbal medicines and dietary supplements detailing safety and efficacy. Further information only available for professionals
Organization	Pharmacist's Letter / Prescriber's Letter
Website	http://www.NaturalDatabase.com
Access	Subscription
Content	Comprehensive, fully referenced monographs on herbal medicines and dietary supplements with extensive information on every aspect (such as interactions with drugs, with other herbs and with foods)
Organization	IBIDS database, run by NIH and US Dept of Agriculture's Food and Nutrition Information Center
Website	http://ods.od.nih.gov/databases/ibids/html
Access	Open
Content	Database of 419 000 journal citations and abstracts (not full texts of articles) with usual database search facilities. Covers herbal medicines and nutritional supplements. Some fact sheets on supplements also available (herbal medicines site under construction, December 2000)

None of the above sites offers to provide information in response to specific enquiries. Urgent information on adverse effects can be obtained from local Poisons Information Centers.

HERBAL AND NON-
HERBAL MEDICINE

Conditions

AIDS/HIV INFECTION

Synonyms   SIDA (French).

Definition   Symptomatic infection with HIV virus associated with immune deficiency.

CAM usage   A systematic review of surveys showed that the prevalence of CAM use in AIDS patients and HIV-positive individuals is high.[1] There was no uniformity as to which treatments were used most. National differences exist and 'flavor of the month' treatments abound. Thus most complementary therapies are relevant in relation to the treatment or palliative/supportive care of AIDS patients.

Clinical evidence It is helpful to differentiate as clearly as possible between alleged CAM 'AIDS cures' (including treatments which are claimed to delay the clinical course of the disease or decrease viral load) and CAM therapies used in palliative or supportive care.

Acupuncture
A rigorous RCT with a complex design tested the effectiveness of acupuncture to treat HIV-related peripheral neuropathic pain.[2] No evidence for effectiveness was found.

Guided imagery
An RCT tested guided imagery or progressive muscle relaxation versus no intervention in 69 HIV-positive individuals.[3] There were no beneficial effects in terms of quality of life but perceived health status was best in the group treated with guided imagery.

Herbal medicine
An RCT tested two different doses of **boxwood** (*Buxus sempervirens*) against placebo in HIV-infected, asymptomatic patients.[4] Results were encouraging but not compelling: 'CD4 counts fell in the low dose group but not in the high-dose group'.

Topical **capsaicin** as a treatment for neuropathic pain was tested against placebo in a recent RCT.[5] After one week's treatment, patients treated with capsaicin cream reported more pain than controls.

A placebo-controlled, double-blind RCT of a complex **Chinese herbal mixture** of eight different herbs yielded promising results:[6] 'life satisfaction' improved in the experimental group but CD4 counts did not. This study was limited by a small sample size and short treatment and follow-up periods. A follow-up study attempted to overcome these problems;[7] 68 HIV-infected adults were randomized to receive either placebo or standardized preparation of 38 Chinese herbs for 6 months. No significant differences in terms of viral load, CD4 cell count, symptoms or psychometric parameters emerged. Thus there is no convincing evidence that Chinese herbal treatments are of benefit to HIV-infected individuals.

St John's wort (*Hypericum perforatum*) has antiretroviral activity in vitro. When 30 HIV-infected individuals were given high-dose intravenous hypericin, no positive effects were seen on virologic markers or CD4 counts.[8] However, a significant degree of phototoxicity was noted.

Many other herbs have antiviral activity and presently feverish research is under way to isolate active compounds and test their therapeutic value. So far, no clinically relevant results have emerged.

Homeopathy

One hundred HIV-positive individuals were randomized to receive either individualized homeopathic remedies or placebo for 15–30 days.[9] There were positive effects on CD4 cell counts only in the homeopathically treated group.

Massage

Twenty-eight neonates born to HIV-positive mothers were randomized to receive either 15-minute massages daily for 10 days or no intervention.[10] The clinical score to evaluate the infants' development showed better outcomes for the neonates treated with massage.

Ozone therapy

A phase I study showed that three out of 10 patients demonstrated improvements with ozone treatment.[11] Thus, an RCT to test ozone therapy was initiated. Regular *ex vivo* ozone treatment of peripheral blood followed by reinjection was carried out for 8 weeks. Compared with placebo treatment, no positive effects on immunological markers were observed.[11]

Spiritual healing

A double-blind RCT of distant healing versus no intervention included 40 patients suffering from advanced AIDS.[12] After 6 months, a blinded review of the medical charts showed significantly better outcomes in the experimental compared with the control group. In another CCT,[13] 20 HIV-infected children were randomized to receive either therapeutic touch or 'mimic therapeutic touch'. The results show that active therapy reduced anxiety while the sham intervention did not.

Stress management

Several forms of stress management may offer useful adjunctive options in caring for AIDS patients. The cumulative evidence

CONDITIONS

Table 5.1 **RCTs of stress management for AIDS/HIV infection**

Reference	Sample size	Interventions [regimen]	Result
Am J Publ Health 1989;79:885–887	64 asymptomatic individuals	A) Stress management training [8 w] B) No intervention	Number of sexual partners decreased, no effect on immune system
Psychol Res 1995;76:451–457	10 asymptomatic individuals	A) Behavioral stress management [10 w] B) No intervention	Positive changes for anxiety, self-esteem and T cell count
Nurs Res 1996;45:246–253	45 AIDS patients and HIV-positive individuals	A) Stress management program [6 w] B) No intervention	Lowering of stress score
J Pediatr Psychol 1996;21:889–897	20 HIV-exposed newborns	A) Daily massage [10 d] B) No intervention	Better results for excitability, stress and other variables
J Consulting Clin Psychol 1997;65:31–43	40 male AIDS patients	A) Cognitive-behavioral stress management [10 w] B) No intervention	Reduction of dysphoria, anxiety and HSV1-2 titre
Psychiat Clin Neurosci 1997; 51:5–8	19 HIV-positive individuals	A) Relaxation therapy [3 mo] B) Psychotherapy C) No intervention	Anger reduced most by relaxation therapy

from these clinical trials is encouraging (Table 5.1), although no study controlled for placebo effects.

Supplements

Advanced stages of AIDS are usually associated with malnutrition which, in turn, impairs immune function. A placebo-controlled RCT of **glutamine** supplementation produced encouraging results.[14] Weight loss was averted in 21 AIDS patients when they were given 40 g of glutamine daily for 12 weeks.

Malnutrition of AIDS patients often results in deficiencies of L-carnitine. **Carnitine** supplementation, in turn, might ameliorate zidovudine-induced myopathies and normalize lymphocyte function.[15] Similarly, vitamin deficiencies of AIDS patients will improve with adequate supplementation. Rigorous clinical trials are warranted.

Other therapies

A CCT[16] evaluated the outcome of a **complex CAM program** including diet, physical activity, smoking cessation, herbal remedies, stress reduction and emotional support in asymptomatic HIV-positive individuals. The results were compared to those in patients who had not received these interventions. After 30 months there were some encouraging differences in terms of

CD4 and CD8 counts. Because of lack of a randomized control group, these findings are not conclusive.

Table 5.2
Summary of clinical evidence for AIDS/HIV infection

Treatment	Weight of evidence	Direction of evidence	Serious safety concerns
Acupuncture (symptomatic)	O	⇩	Yes (see p 29)
Guided imagery (palliative)	O	⇨	No (see p 80)
Herbal medicine			
Boxwood	O	⬀	Yes (see p 5)
Capsaicin cream (symptomatic)	O	⇩	Yes (see p 5)
Chinese herbal mixture	O	⇩	Yes (see p 52)
St John's wort	O	⇩	Yes (see p 156)
Homeopathy	O	⬀	No (see p 55)
Massage (palliative)	O	⇧	No (see p 60)
Ozone therapy	O	⇩	Yes (see p 81)
Spiritual healing (palliative)	O	⬀	No (see p 73)
Stress management (palliative)	OOO	⇧	No
Supplements			
Carnitine	O	⇨	No (see p 172)
Glutamine	O	⇧	Yes (see p 5)

Overall recommendation

None of the numerous 'AIDS cures' which regularly emerge only to vanish months later can be recommended on the basis of reliable data from rigorous clinical trials. CAM interventions used in palliative and supportive care for AIDS patients or HIV-positive individuals may prove to be useful; this applies in particular to stress management programs of various types. At present, it is unclear whether these treatments offer any benefit over and above conventional approaches to caring for AIDS patients and HIV-infected individuals.

REFERENCES

1 Ernst E. Complementary AIDS therapies: the good, the bad and the ugly. Int J STD AIDS 1997;8:281–285

2 Shlay J C, Chaloner K, Max M B et al. Acupuncture and amitriptyline for pain due to HIV-related peripheral neuropathy: a randomized controlled trial. Terry Beirn Community Programs for Clinical Research on AIDS. JAMA 1998;280:1590–1595

3 Eller L S. Effects of cognitive-behavioral interventions on quality of life in persons with HIV. Int J Nurs Stud 1999;36:223–233

4 Durant J, Chantre P, Gonzalez G et al. Efficacy and safety of Buxus sempervirens L. preparations (SPV$_{30}$) in HIV-infected asymptomatic patients: a multicentre, randomized, double-blind, placebo-controlled trial. Phytomedicine 1998;5:1–10

CONDITIONS

5 Paice J A, Ferrams C E V, Lashley F R. Topical capsaicin in the management of HIV-associated peripheral neuropathy. J Pain Sympt Manage 2000;19:45–52

6 Burack J H, Cohen M R, Hahn J A, Abrams D I. Pilot randomized controlled trial of Chinese herbal treatment for HIV-associated symptoms. J Acquir Immun Defic Syndr Hum Retrovirol 1996;12:386–393

7 Weber R, Christen L, Loy M et al. Randomized, placebo-controlled trial of Chinese herb therapy for HIV-1-infected individuals. J AIDS 1999;22:56–64

8 Gulick R M. Phase I studies of hypericin, the active compound in St John's wort, as an antiretroviral agent in HIV-infected adults: AIDS clinical trials group protocols 150 and 258. Ann Intern Med 1999;130:510–514

9 Rastogi D P, Singh V P, Singh V, Dey S K, Rao K. Homeopathy in HIV infection: a trial report of double-blind placebo controlled study. Br Homeopath J 1999;88:49–57

10 Scafidi F, Field T. Massage therapy improves behavior in neonates born to HIV-positive mothers. J Pediatr Psychol 1996;21:889–897

11 Garber G E, Cameron D W, Hawley-Foss N, Greenway D, Shannon M E. The use of ozone-treated blood in the therapy of HIV infection and immune disease: a pilot study of safety and efficacy. AIDS 1991;5:981–984

12 Sicher F, Targ E, Moore D, Smith H S. A randomized double-blind study of the effect of distant healing in a population with advanced AIDS. Report of a small scale study. West J Med 1998;169:356–363

13 Ireland M. Therapeutic touch with HIV-infected children: a pilot study. J Assoc Nurses AIDS Care 1998;9:68–77

14 Wilmore D W. Glutamine-antioxidant supplementation increases body cell mass in AIDS patients with weight loss: a randomized, double-blind controlled trial. Nutrition 1999; 15(11–12):860–864

15 Mintz M. Carnitine in human immunodeficiency virus type 1 infection/acquired immune deficiency syndrome. J Child Neurol 1995;10:2S40–2S44

16 Kaiser J D, Donegan E. Complementary therapies in HIV disease. Alt Ther 1996; 2:42–46

FURTHER READING

Özsoy M, Ernst E. How effective are complementary therapies for HIV and AIDS? A systematic review. Int J STD AIDS 1999;10:629–635
A concise and critical analysis of complementary treatments for AIDS.

ALZHEIMER'S DISEASE

Synonyms/ subcategories	Alzheimer's dementia, presenile dementia, primary neuronal degeneration.
Definition	Progressive mental deterioration that begins in late middle life and usually results in death within 5–10 years, characterized by atrophy of the brain, especially in the frontal, occipital and temporal regions with distortion of the intracellular neurofibrils and the formation of plaques composed of granular filamentous masses with amyloid.
Related conditions	Other forms of (senile) dementia, e.g. vascular dementia, multi-infarct dementia, primary senile dementia.
CAM usage	Herbal treatments and other nutritional supplements are often advocated and used. Several complementary therapies (e.g. massage, reflexology, music therapy), which are aimed at improving

quality of life, are used in palliative care of Alzheimer's patients.

Clinical evidence

In many clinical studies of CAM, the exact diagnosis of the patient groups is unclear; often mixed or ill-defined populations of dementia patients have been studied. Even though this discussion is on Alzheimer's disease (AD), such investigations have been included.

Acupuncture

Several uncontrolled studies from China suggest that acupuncture can be beneficial for dementia patients (e.g. [1]). As these studies lack scientific rigor, conclusions regarding the efficacy of acupuncture for AD cannot be drawn.

Aromatherapy

Several small uncontrolled studies of aromatherapy have been reported (e.g. [2]). Some patients seem to benefit in terms of well-being, but the data are far from compelling.

Herbal medicine

The Kampo mixture **Choto-san** has been tested in an RCT with 139 patients suffering from vascular dementias.[3] Choto-san was superior to placebo in terms of global improvement and several other outcome measures.

Numerous placebo-controlled, double-blind RCTs show that ginkgo (*Ginkgo biloba*) is effective in delaying the deterioration of cognitive function in AD and vascular dementia. Some of these studies are of high methodological quality and include sufficiently large numbers of patients. One narrative systematic review included nine RCTs and arrived at a positive overall conclusion.[4] Similarly, a metaanalysis concluded that ginkgo improved cognitive function (Box 5.1).

Box 5.1
Metaanalysis
Ginkgo for Alzheimer's disease
Arch Neurol 1998;55: 1409–1415

- Inclusion criteria: placebo-controlled, double-blind RCTs, sufficiently characterized patients, use of standardized ginkgo extracts, objective assessment of cognitive function

- Four studies met all the inclusion criteria, including 424 patients

- Their methodological quality was, on average, good

- Overall effect size of 0.40 which translated into a 3% difference in the AD Assessment Scale – cognitive subtest

- Conclusion: there is a small but significant effect of 3–6-month treatment with 120–240 mg of *Ginkgo biloba* extract

Huperzine A, an alkaloid isolated from the Chinese herb *Huperzia serrata*, is a reversible, selective acetylcholinesterase inhibitor. CCTs from China suggest that it improves memory deficiencies in patients with various forms of dementia (e.g. [5]).

Panax ginseng is often advocated for improving mental performance and might therefore have some potential in AD. One Norwegian study with geriatric patients found no benefit in terms of activities of daily living, cognition, somatic symptoms, depression or anxiety.[6] Collectively, the trial data are therefore not fully convincing.

Massage
The evidence from clinical trials suggesting that massage therapy can reduce anxiety or alter behavior in AD patients is encouraging but far from compelling at present.[7]

Music therapy
An RCT including 18 patients implied that exposure to soothing music can reduce aggressive behavior in AD.[8] Other studies confirm positive behavioral changes[7] but the evidence is so far not convincing.

Supplements
Numerous nutritional supplements are being advocated for AD. In most cases the evidence from clinical trials is absent or unconvincing. Some encouraging, albeit preliminary trial evidence exists for the following supplements: **alpha-tocopherol, acetyl-l-carnitine, lecithin, dimethylaminoethanol and**

Table 5.3
Summary of clinical evidence for Alzheimer's disease

Treatment	Weight of evidence	Direction of evidence	Serious safety concerns
Acupuncture	O	⇨	Yes (see p 29)
Aromatherapy	O	⇨	Yes (see p 34)
Herbal medicine			
Choto-san	O	⇧	Yes (see p 5)
Ginkgo	OOO	⇧	Yes (see p 115)
Huperzia serrata	O	⬀	Yes (see p 5)
Ginseng	O	⇩	Yes (see p 88)
Massage	O	⬀	No (see p 60)
Music therapy	O	⬀	No (see p 81)
Supplements			
Acetyl-l-carnitine	O	⬀	No (see p 172)
Alpha-tocopherol	O	⬀	No
Dimethylamino-ethanol	O	⬀	Yes (see p 5)
Lecithin	O	⬀	Yes (see p 5)
Phosphatidylserine	O	⬀	Yes (see p 5)

phosphatidylserine.[9] Unfortunately, the size of the effect is usually small and therefore of questionable clinical relevance.

Overall recommendation

Much of the evidence regarding CAM for AD is too preliminary for strong recommendations. The only exception is *Ginkgo biloba*, which has a modest effect and is reasonably safe. As no comparative trials of ginkgo and conventional drugs for AD exist, its therapeutic value relative to conventional therapies is difficult to assess. One evaluation[10] concluded that cholinesterase inhibitors and ginkgo are equally effective in the treatment of mild to moderate dementia of the Alzheimer type.

REFERENCES

1 Xudong G. The influence of acupuncture modalities on the treatment of senile dementia: a brief review. Am J Acup 1996;24:105–109

2 Brooker D J, Snape M, Johnson E, Ward D, Payne M. Single case evaluation of the effects of aromatherapy and massage on disturbed behavior in severe dementia. Br J Clin Psychol 1997;36:287–296

3 Terasawa K, Shimada Y, Kita T et al. Choto-san in the treatment of vascular dementia: a double-blind, placebo controlled study. Phytomedicine 1997;4:15–22

4 Ernst E, Pittler M H. Ginkgo biloba for dementia. A systematic review of double-blind, placebo-controlled trials. Clin Drug Invest 1999;17:301–308

5 Tang X C, Han Y F. Pharmacological profile of huperzine A, a novel acetylcholinesterase inhibitor from Chinese herb. CNS Drug Rev 1999;5:281–300

6 Thommassen B, Laake K. Ginseng – no identifiable effect in geriatric rehabilitation. Tidsskr Nor Laegeforen 1997;117: 3839–3841

7 Opie J, Rosewarne R, O'Connor D W. The efficacy of psychosocial approaches to behavior disorders in dementia: a systematic literature review. Aust NZ J Psych 1999; 33:789–799

8 Clark M E, Lipe A W, Bilbrey M. Use of music to decrease aggressive behaviors in people with dementia. J Gerontol Nurs 1998;24:10–17

9 Ott B R, Owens N J. Complementary and alternative medicines for Alzheimer's Disease. J Geriatr Psychiatr Neurol 1998;11:163–173

10 Wettstein V A. Cholinesterase inhibitors and Ginkgo extracts: are they comparable in the treatment of dementia? Fortschritte der Medizin 1999;1(suppl 1):11–18

ANXIETY

Synonyms/ subcategories

State anxiety, trait anxiety. ICD-10 categories: Phobic anxiety disorder (agoraphobia, social phobia, specific phobias). Other anxiety disorders (panic disorder, generalized anxiety disorder, mixed anxiety and depression disorder). Obsessive-compulsive disorder. Reaction to severe stress and adjustment disorders (acute stress reaction, posttraumatic stress disorder, adjustment reaction). Dissociative (conversion) disorders. Other neurotic disorders (including neurasthenia and depersonalization or derealization).

Definition

Excessive fearfulness and tensions accompanied by an increased motor tension (restlessness, muscle tension, trembling, fatiguability), autonomic hyperactivity (tachycardia, shortness of breath, dry mouth, cold hands) and increased vigilance and scanning (feeling keyed up, impaired concentration) unattached to a clearly identifiable stimulus.

CAM usage

Forty-three percent of people who suffer from anxiety attacks have used CAM in the previous 12 months, about a quarter of them visiting a practitioner for treatment.[1] The therapies most commonly used include relaxation, exercise, herbs, art/music therapy and megavitamins.[2] In addition, hypnosis, meditation and yoga are widely adopted for the treatment of stress. Many interventions that could be described as CAM may be used in the conventional management of anxiety.

Clinical evidence

Aromatherapy

Aromatherapy is widely promoted for the treatment of 'stress', but a systematic review (Box 5.2) concluded that, although there are clearly significant effects, these are short term and probably too modest to have clinical relevance.

Box 5.2
Systematic review
Aromatherapy for anxiety
Br J Gen Pract 2000;50: 493–496

- Thirteen RCTs, of which six related to treatment of anxiety (452 patients)

- Quality of all studies was poor

- Five showed short-term superiority of aromatherapy

- Conclusion: modest, short-term effect which is unlikely to be clinically relevant

Autogenic training

A systematic review (Box 5.3) found studies of forms of 'autogenic training' that often only included part of the classic technique. Only two studies involved patient groups, but both had positive outcomes for anxiety.

Box 5.3
Systematic review
Autogenic training for anxiety
Compl Ther Med 2000;8:106–110

- Eight CCTs, 245 participants

- Six trials on induced anxiety in volunteers; two on patient groups

- Majority of trials methodologically flawed

- Positive results, in at least some subgroups, in all studies. No significant decrease in panic attacks

- Lack of uniform training procedures and poor methodological quality prevent firm conclusions

Biofeedback

Among 45 individuals with generalized anxiety disorder included in an RCT, eight sessions of EMG and EEG biofeedback were both superior to pseudomeditation control at reducing trait anxiety.[3] Improvements persisted for 6 weeks. Combined alpha-wave EEG and EMG biofeedback training (10 weekly sessions) improved test anxiety in a controlled trial with 163 students with examination phobia, compared with no training (quoted in [4]). Regular EEG biofeedback sessions on 5 days a week for combat-related posttraumatic stress disorder resulted in improvements in several clinical psychology scales compared with standard medication treatments (quoted in[4]). Only three out of 15 biofeedback patients had relapsed at 30 months, compared with all 14 traditionally treated patients. However, there are negative RCTs, such as one involving 66 psychiatric patients where EEG biofeedback showed no difference from placebo biofeedback or untreated controls.[5]

Electrostimulation

A metaanalysis (Box 5.4) found evidence in favor of the effectiveness of electrostimulation although not conclusively so, because of the small size of studies and problems with blinding.

Box 5.4
Metaanalysis
Electrostimulation for anxiety
J Nerv Ment Dis 1995; 183:478–485

- Eight subject-blind RCTs with 249 patients
- Either primary anxiety or alcohol- or drug-related anxiety
- Quality issues limit the findings
- Pooled effect size 0.59 (CI 0.23 to 0.95)
- Cautiously positive conclusion

Exercise

Exercise can reduce anxiety acutely, as shown in an RCT with 85 volunteers randomized to aerobic exercise, relaxation or no treatment control.[6] Both interventions diminished induced anxiety more than the control. In an RCT with 46 patients with panic disorder and agoraphobia, 10 weeks of walking (4 miles three times/week) was less effective than clomipramine, but both were superior to placebo.[7]

Herbal medicine

A systematic review (Box 5.5) concluded that **kava** (*Piper methysticum*) was relatively safe and effective for the treatment of anxiety symptoms.

There is poor-quality evidence for the efficacy of **German chamomile** (*Matricaria recutita* L), **lemon balm** (*Melissa officinalis*), **passion flower** (*Passiflora incarnata*) and **valerian**

CONDITIONS

Box 5.5
Systematic review
Kava for anxiety
J Clin Psychopharmacol
2000;20:84–89

- Seven RCTs involving 377 participants
- Kava extract from 300 to 800 mg/day in divided doses
- Quality was acceptable in six studies
- All studies showed positive effects of kava
- Metaanalysis of three studies showed weighted mean difference of 9.7 (CI 3.5 to 15.8) points on Hamilton Scale
- Conclusion: kava is relatively safe and more efficacious than placebo for the symptomatic treatment of anxiety

(*Valeriana officinalis*) in the treatment of anxiety, which is insufficient to make any recommendations.[8]

Homeopathy

The evidence on the value of homeopathy for this indication is inconsistent. One controlled trial suggested that homeopathy may have an effect in reducing agitation in children after surgery.[9] Another RCT[10] found homeopathy not superior to placebo in 72 adults with anxiety.

Hypnotherapy

Hypnosis is widely offered for dental phobia and in one controlled trial there was no difference between the effect of hypnosis, group therapy and individual desensitization, though all were superior to no treatment.[11] For the management of agoraphobia, hypnosis may be offered as part of desensitization management, at the time of exposure to the anxiety-provoking situation. However, one crossover study in 64 patients found that, although patients preferred it, hypnosis did not make any observable difference to the patients' behavior at the time of the exposure.[12] Anxiety was reduced more effectively by hypnosis when given to children before painful and stressful procedures (bone marrow aspiration, lumbar puncture) than by a non-hypnotic behavioral technique.[13]

Massage

Massage therapy given to depressed pregnant adolescents twice a week for 5 weeks was shown to be superior to relaxation therapy in an RCT involving 26 women. Both groups scored lower anxiety, but the effect in the massage group was accompanied by improvements in mood, sleep and back pain and confirmed by objective measurement of behavior and urinary steroid concentrations.[14] In a further RCT of 21 elderly institutionalized patients, massage was shown to reduce anxiety to a greater extent than no intervention, though it was not significantly different from attention control (conversation).[15] Thus, the specific action of massage itself, as well as its duration of effect, are still not known.

Meditation

There is evidence that meditation can reduce anxiety levels and neuroendocrine responses to stress more effectively than situation control in volunteers placed in stressful conditions[16] and uncontrolled studies have suggested benefits in patients with anxiety. In one RCT, 28 individuals were randomized to receive an 8-week stress reduction program based on mindfulness meditation. Compared with the non-intervention control group, they evidenced greater reductions in overall psychological symptoms, improvements in sense of control and measure of spiritual experiences.[17] A systematic review which included observational studies as well as controlled trials on relaxation techniques for trait anxiety (Box 5.6) found the effect size for meditation to be 0.70 (SD 0.40) compared with progressive muscle relaxation (0.38, SD 0.40). However, there is a shortage of good-quality RCTs to make a convincing case for the effectiveness of meditation for clinical practice.

Music therapy

Music has been used in many health-case settings. Uncontrolled studies of music in coronary care units have had inconsistent results. A rigorous randomized study involving 56 patients admitted to a coronary care unit in Australia compared two or three sessions of either listening to light classical music or following relaxation instructions for 30 minutes. Neither therapy had any effect on anxiety and subjects had no benefit compared with untreated controls.[18] A number of RCTs have failed to show any beneficial effect of music on the anxiety that patients experience during various surgical procedures (e.g. [19]). However, a controlled study found that patients who listened to self-selected music tapes during sigmoidoscopy suffered less anxiety than controls who had no music.[20] The effect of music on clinical anxiety or on phobias has not been tested.

Relaxation

The relaxation response is the diametric opposite of anxiety and there is a host of literature that explores the value of willfully inducing relaxation. Studies in a variety of forms of anxiety were systematically reviewed (Box 5.6). For panic disorder specifically, relaxation was shown to be less effective than cognitive therapy in an RCT of 64 subjects but both were superior to minimal contact control.[21] These results are supported by at least one other good-quality RCT. For management of agoraphobia, relaxation training was as effective as exposure and cognitive treatment and all were more effective than weekly individual therapy sessions in an RCT.[22] There were few differences between the active treatments and the results were maintained at one year.

Relaxation has been used to manage the anxiety associated with major medical conditions. In patients with newly diagnosed cancer,

Box 5.6
Systematic review
**Relaxation
techniques for
anxiety**
J Clin Psychol 1989;45:
957–974

- All observational and controlled trials in which the outcome was trait anxiety

- Relaxation studies involving psychiatric patients were excluded

- Progressive muscle relaxation 22 studies, meditation 70 studies, biofeedback 17 studies (subject numbers not stated)

- Overall effect sizes: progressive muscle relaxation 0.38 (SD 0.40); other forms of relaxation (largely biofeedback) 0.40 (0.35); meditation 0.70 (0.40)

- Effect size related to duration and hours of use of technique

- Conclusion: some grounds for optimism that at least some procedures can reduce trait anxiety

relaxation with or without imagery improved anxiety as well as other aspects of mood.[23] In a similar population, there was a reduction in state anxiety after relaxation compared with untreated controls but there was no significant effect on trait anxiety.[24]

Twenty-six patients with chronic obstructive airways disease were randomized to receive relaxation training or standard management alone.[25] Dyspnea, anxiety and airway obstruction were reduced in the relaxation group while the control group remained the same or became worse.

Relaxation training has been used to reduce the anxiety associated with a variety of medical and surgical procedures and to improve some aspects of healing.[26] For minor surgery there is considerable evidence of patient benefit and one study found relaxation to be superior to attention control in facilitating the ease of general anesthesia in day-case surgery.[27] Audiotapes with relaxation instructions were superior to music tapes or blank tapes at reducing both anxiety and pain (assessed both subjectively and objectively) during femoral angiography.[28] A relaxation procedure before MRI scan reduced the anxiety associated with the scan more than no intervention in an RCT involving 149 subjects.[29] In an RCT of 53 women undergoing radiation therapy for early-stage breast cancer, relaxation with guided imagery was an effective intervention for reducing anxiety and enhancing comfort, compared with no intervention.[30]

Spinal manipulation

Although there are no studies on anxiety as the presenting complaint, in one RCT state anxiety in hypertensives was measured after **chiropractic**, placebo chiropractic or no treatment control in 21 hypertensive patients.[31] There was no difference between the groups though chiropractic was associated with a significant fall in blood pressure.

Spiritual healing

Positive findings for **therapeutic touch** in the treatment of anxiety have been found in RCTs compared with no treatment in 40 healthy professional caregivers/students[32] and compared with sham therapeutic touch in 20 HIV-infected children[33] and 99 hospitalized burn patients[34].

Other treatments

Rolfing (structural integration) was superior to no intervention in reducing state anxiety in an RCT of 48 persons.[35]

A single RCT found **tai chi** to be as effective as moderate walking exercise (and both better than reading control) in alleviating induced anxiety in 96 practitioners of tai chi.[36]

There is surprisingly little research on **yoga** in the treatment of clinical anxiety. In one uncontrolled study, eight obsessive-compulsive patients used yoga for 1 hour daily for a year and attended yoga class for 2 hours each week.[37] The five who persisted with yoga were improved, according to a measure of obsessive-compulsive disorder.

Overall recommendation

For generalized anxiety disorder, drug management is fraught with problems and kava may be a useful short-term alternative when medication is essential. Dependence on kava has not been recorded. Kava can also be recommended for short-term use in

Table 5.4
Summary of clinical evidence for anxiety

Treatment	Weight of evidence	Direction of evidence	Serious safety concerns
Aromatherapy	OO	⬀	Yes (see p 34)
Autogenic training	OO	⬀	Yes (see p 37)
Biofeedback	OO	⇨	No (see p 42)
Electro-stimulation	OO	⬀	Yes (see p 6)
Exercise	O	⇧	Yes (see p 5)
Herbal medicine Kava	OOO	⇧	Yes (see p 129)
Homeopathy	O	⇨	No (see p 55)
Hypnotherapy	O	⬀	Yes (see p 58)
Massage	O	⬀	No (see p 60)
Meditation	OO	⇧	Yes (see p 80)
Music therapy	O	⇨	No (see p 81)
Relaxation	OOO	⇧	No (see p 71)
Spinal manipulation Chiropractic	O	⇩	Yes (see p 47)
Spiritual healing	O	⇧	No (see p 73)

CONDITIONS

acute stress reaction and adjustment reaction. Conventional psychological interventions are as successful as medications for anxiety and often more acceptable. For patients who are willing to undertake a mind–body approach, meditation, and to a lesser extent autogenic training or relaxation, can be encouraged as the evidence is in favor. Electrostimulation may also be recommended, where it is available. Relaxation is also useful for the anxiety associated with particular conditions and medical procedures, although hypnotherapy appears more appropriate for children. Massage is promising in particular clinical situations, e.g. institutionalized patients.

For panic disorder and the various forms of phobia, appropriate medication or conventional psychological management should undoubtedly be used in the first instance, except that hypnotherapy may have specific use in some circumstances (e.g. dental phobia).

REFERENCES

1 Eisenberg D M, Davis R, Ettner S L et al. Trends in alternative medicine use in the United States, 1990–1997. JAMA 1998; 280:1569–1575

2 Astin J A. Why patients use alternative medicine. JAMA 1998;279:1548–1553

3 Rice K M, Blanchard E B, Purcell M. Biofeedback treatments of generalized anxiety disorder: preliminary results. Biofeedback Self Reg 1993;18:93–105

4 Moore N C. A review of EEG biofeedback treatment of anxiety disorders. Clin Electroencephalogr 2000;31:1–6

5 Watson C G, Herder J. Effectiveness of alpha biofeedback therapy: negative results. J Clin Psychol 1980;36:508–513

6 Crocker P R, Grozelle C. Reducing induced state anxiety: effects of acute aerobic exercise and autogenic relaxation. J Sports Med Phys Fitness 1991;31:277–282

7 Broocks A, Bandelow B, Pekrun G et al. Comparison of aerobic exercise, clomipramine and placebo in the treatment of panic disorder. Am J Psychiatr 1998;155:603–609

8 Wong A H C, Smith M, Boon H S. Herbal remedies in psychiatric practice. Arch Gen Psychiatr 1998;55:1033–1044

9 Alibou J P, Jobert J. Aconit en dilution homéopathique et agitation postopératoire de l'enfant. Pédiatrie 1990;45:465–466

10 McCutcheon L E. Treatment of anxiety with a homoeopathy remedy. J Appl Nutr 1996;48:2–6

11 Moore R, Abrahamsen R, Brodsgaard I. Hypnosis compared with group therapy and individual desensitization for dental anxiety. Eur J Oral Sci 1996;104:612–618

12 Van Dyck R, Spinhoven P. Does preference for type of treatment matter? A study of exposure in vivo with or without hypnosis in the treatment of panic disorder with agoraphobia. Behav Modif 1997;21:172–186

13 Zeltzer L, LeBaron S. Hypnosis and nonhypnotic techniques for reduction of pain and anxiety during painful procedures in children and adolescents with cancer. J Pediatr 1982;101:1032–1035

14 Field T, Grizzle N, Scafidi F, Schanberg S. Massage and relaxation therapies' effects on depressed adolescent mothers. Adolescence 1996;31:903–911

15 Fraser J, Kerr J R. Psychophysiological effects of back massage on elderly institutionalized patients. J Adv Nurs 1993;18:238–245

16 MacLean C R K, Walton K G, Wenneberg S R et al. Altered response of cortisol, GH, TSH and testosterone to acute stress after four months' practice of transcendental meditation. Ann NY Acad Sci 1994;746:381–384

17 Astin J A. Stress reduction through mindfulness meditation. Effects on psychological symptomatology, sense of control and spiritual experiences. Psychother Psychosom 1997;66:97–106

18 Elliott D. The effects of music and muscle relaxation on patient anxiety in a coronary care unit. Heart Lung 1994;23:27–35

19 Colt H G, Powers A, Shanks T G. Effect of music on state anxiety scores in patients undergoing fiberoptic bronchoscopy. Chest 1999;116:819–824

20 Pulakanis K C. Effect of music therapy on state anxiety in patients undergoing flexible

sigmoidoscopy. Dis Colon Rectum 1994; 37:478–481

21 Beck J G, Stanley M A, Baldwin L E, Deagle E A 3rd, Averill P M. Comparison of cognitive therapy and relaxation training for panic disorder. J Consult Clin Psychol 1994;62:818–826

22 Ost L G, Westling B E, Hellstrom K. Applied relaxation, exposure in vivo and cognitive methods in the treatment of panic disorder with agoraphobia. Behav Res Ther 1993;31:383–394

23 Bindemann S, Soukop M, Kaye S B. Randomised controlled study of relaxation training. Eur J Cancer 1991;27:170–174

24 Bridge L R, Benson P, Pietroni P C, Priest R G. Relaxation and imagery in the treatment of breast cancer. Br Med J 1988;297:1169–1172

25 Gift A G, Moore T, Soeken K. Relaxation to reduce dyspnea and anxiety in COPD patients. Nurs Res 1992;41:242–246

26 Holden-Lund C. Effects of relaxation with guided imagery on surgical stress and wound healing. Res Nurs Health 1988;11:235–244

27 Markland D, Hardy L. Anxiety, relaxation and anaesthesia for day-case surgery. Br J Clin Psychol 1993;32:493–504

28 Mandle C L, Domar A D, Harrington D P, Leserman J, Bozadjian E M, Friedman R, Benson H. Relaxation response in femoral angiography. Radiology 1990;174:737–739

29 Lukins R, Davan I G, Drummond P D. A cognitive behavioural approach to preventing anxiety during magnetic resonance imaging. J Behav Ther Exp Psychiatr 1997;28:97–104

30 Kolcaba K, Fox C. The effects of guided imagery on comfort of women with early stage breast cancer undergoing radiation therapy. Oncol Nurs Forum 1999;26:67–72

31 Yates R G, Lamping D L, Abram N L, Wright C. Effects of chiropractic treatment on blood pressure and anxiety: a randomized, controlled trial. J Manip Physiol Ther 1998; 11:484–488

32 Olson M, Sneed N. Anxiety and therapeutic touch. Issues Mental Health Nurs 1995;16:97–108

33 Ireland M. Therapeutic touch with HIV-infected children: a pilot study. J Assoc Nurses AIDS Care 1998;9:68–77

34 Turner J G, Clark A J, Gauthier D K, Williams M. The effect of therapeutic touch on pain and anxiety in burn patients. J Adv Nurs 1998;28:10–20

35 Weinberg R S, Hunt V V. Effects of structural integration on state-trait anxiety. J Clin Psychol 1979;35:319–322

36 Jin P. Efficacy of Tai Chi, brisk walking, meditation, and reading in reducing mental and emotional stress. J Psychosom Res 1992; 36:361–370

37 Shannahoff-Khalsa D S, Beckett L R. Clinical case report: efficacy of yogic techniques in the treatment of obsessive compulsive disorders. Int J Neurosci 1996;85:1–17

ASTHMA

Synonyms/ subcategories	Atopic asthma, bronchial asthma, extrinsic asthma, intrinsic asthma, nervous asthma, reflex asthma.
Definition	A condition of the lungs in which there is generalized reversible narrowing of airways due to mucosal edema, spasm of smooth muscle and mucus in bronchi and bronchioles, leading to dyspnea, cough, chest tightness and wheezing.
CAM usage	Surveys of patients with asthma have reported usage in up to 70% of adults in the UK[1] and 55% of children.[2,3] Breathing techniques, relaxation, homeopathy, herbal medicine and yoga are commonly used.
Clinical evidence	*Acupuncture*
	Many studies find positive changes for one outcome among several measured. However, the effects are highly inconsistent

CONDITIONS

and the most rigorous systematic review of RCTs (Box 5.7) concludes that the evidence is insufficient to make recommendations.

Box 5.7
Systematic review
Acupuncture for asthma
Cochrane Library 1998

- Seven placebo-controlled RCTs involving 174 patients
- Quality was moderate overall
- None demonstrated clinically relevant improvements in lung function
- One found improvement in medication use; two found improvement in symptom scores
- Conclusion: 'It is not possible to make any recommendations'

Autogenic training

An RCT comparing autogenic training (AT) with supportive psychotherapy in 24 adults with moderate or severe asthma showed significant and clinically relevant improvement in lung function with AT compared with controls.[4] Two other RCTs were less promising; a study with 38 adults found improvement of anxiety but no changes in lung function[5] and another in 31 adults detected no changes in symptoms or airway resistance, although the use of sympathomimetics decreased.[6]

Biofeedback

The evidence for biofeedback suggests it may have an effect. There were significant improvements in lung function and symptom scores in 33 children given biofeedback over 5 months, whereas those randomized to placebo biofeedback showed improvement in symptom scores only.[7] Another RCT with 20 adolescents showed improvement of symptoms (superior to an untreated control group) but no change in lung function.[8]

Breathing techniques

Breathing techniques have been systematically reviewed (Box 5.8). Although yoga and physiotherapy exercises are promising, there is insufficient evidence to conclude that they are effective.

The **Buteyko breathing technique** (BBT) is based on the concept that people with asthma are under stress and therefore breathe too rapidly and too deeply. The training involves learning to make breathing shallow and slow. There are enthusiastic anecdotal reports of the value of BBT. In the first published RCT (not included in the following systematic review) involving 39 patients with asthma, those who were trained in BBT showed greater reduction in asthma medication use and improvement in quality of life than controls who received asthma education alone.[9] However, there were no significant differences in lung function tests between the groups. There was much longer interaction with the BBT therapist than with the therapist in the control group. In view of flaws such as this, further rigorous trials are awaited with interest.

Box 5.8
Systematic review
Breathing exercises for asthma
Eur Respir J 2000;15: 969–972

- Five RCTs with 150 adults with chronic asthma; one RCT in 38 children with acute asthma

- Interventions included breathing exercises as part of yoga and physiotherapy

- Quality: most studies flawed

- Conclusion: breathing exercises appear promising but insufficient evidence to make firm judgements

Diet

Rigorous tests with randomized, double-blind, placebo-controlled challenge demonstrate that between 2% and 6% of asthmatic patients are hypersensitive to foods.[10] Apart from avoidance of known food allergens, particularly peanuts, in this group of patients, no recommendations can be made for any particular diet on the basis of known evidence. There is some evidence suggesting that reduced dietary intake of vitamins A, C and E as well as selenium and magnesium is associated with brittle asthma in children.[11]

Herbal medicine

A systematic review (Box 5.9) found some promising evidence in single studies with *Picrorrizia kurroa*, *Solanum* spp, *Boswellia serrata*, Saibuko-to, marijuana and dried ivy extract, but insufficient to make firm judgements.

Box 5.9
Systematic review
Herbal medicine for asthma
Thorax 2000;55: 925–929

- Seventeen RCTs included

- Overall quality poor

- Six studies of traditional Chinese herbs (494 patients), eight using traditional Indian herbs (805 patients) and three with Kampo herbs (146 patients)

- Some promising data but no fully convincing evidence for any of the herbal preparations

CONDITIONS

Homeopathy

One derivative version of homeopathy is 'isopathy' which involves high dilutions of a preparation of the allergen(s) to which the individual is sensitive. Isopathic treatment was superior to placebo in improving symptom scores of 28 adults over 21 days in one rigorous study,[12] though the clinical implications of this were far from certain in view of the short duration, small sample and small effect on lung function. The overall evidence from a systematic review (Box 5.10) is insufficient to draw conclusions.

Box 5.10
Systematic review
Homeopathy for asthma
Cochrane Library 1998

- Three placebo-controlled RCTs involving 154 patients

- Quality was variable

- Symptoms alone improved in one study; lung function and medication use improved in the second; no superiority to control group in the third

- Conclusion: not enough evidence to reliably assess the possible role of homeopathy in asthma

Hypnotherapy

The evidence from three published RCTs (Table 5.5) is promising but not convincing. Patients may become less aware of their degree of bronchoconstriction and therefore risk undertreating acute attacks of asthma.

Table 5.5 **RCTs of hypnotherapy for asthma**

Reference	Sample size	Interventions [regimen]	Result	Comment
Br Med J 1962;11: 371–376	62	A) Hypnosis [30 min/d] B) Standard medication	Symptomatic improvement greater with A	No statistical analysis
Br Med J 1968;4:71–76	252	A) Hypnosis [15 min/d] B) Relaxation & breathing exercises	Both groups improved similarly, lung function more with A	Functional changes not clinically relevant
Br Med J 1986;293: 1129–1132	44	A) Hypnosis [6 wkly sessions] B) Attention control (clinic visits)	Benefit in some lung functions in hypnosis-responsive subjects	Stratified by responsiveness

Massage

In one RCT of 32 children, parents either massaged their children each evening or instructed them in relaxation.[13] There were significant improvements in lung function in younger children (aged 6–8 years) after massage for 30 days, compared with relaxation controls, but not in older children aged 9–11. The parents also noted a beneficial effect on themselves.

Meditation

One study attempted to compare transcendental meditation with reading relaxing literature in a crossover study, but was confounded by those who learned to meditate first and then continued to practice after they were crossed over.[14] In the first period, those who meditated experienced a significant decrease in airway resistance.

Relaxation

In view of the association between acute asthma and stress, regular relaxation would seem a promising approach to treatment. Of three RCTs which were performed in the 1970s, two found no clinically relevant improvements with relaxation training[15,16] and one claimed benefit but did not present any data.[17] Three more recent studies are presented (Table 5.6) but have inconsistent inclusion criteria and outcome measures. The overall evidence can be seen to be contradictory.

Table 5.6 **RCTs of relaxation therapy for asthma**

Reference	Sample size	Interventions [regimen]	Result	Comment
J Behav Med 1994;17:1–24	106	A) Relaxation [1 h/d for 8 days] B) Listening to music C) Wait list	No benefit in any group	34 dropped out
Monatsschrift Kinderheilkund 1996;144: 1357–1363	18	A) Relaxation [daily for 3 d] B) Placebo relaxation C) Salbutamol	A and C better than B	Children and adolescents
J Pediatr 1998;132: 854–858	32	A) Massage B) Relaxation [20 min/d for 30 d]	A benefit in under-8s only B no benefit	Children treated by parents

Spinal manipulation

Chiropractic treatment aims to improve the function of the lungs by reducing any restricted movement of the ribs and treating muscle tension in the intercostal muscles. The two most rigorous RCTs (involving 91 children and 31 adults respectively) found no differences in outcomes of chiropractic and sham chiropractic manipulation.[18,19]

Yoga

From 106 subjects included in one controlled trial, those who continued to practice yoga regularly during the follow-up period of 4.5 years showed a significant reduction in asthma medication use and number of asthma attacks and an increase in peak flow rate, compared with the matched controls.[20] However, the drop-out rate was high. Two RCTs failed to find any effect on lung function, although mental improvements were noted.[21,22]

Table 5.7
Summary of clinical evidence for asthma

Treatment	Weight of evidence	Direction of evidence	Serious safety concerns
Acupuncture	OO	⬂	Yes (see p 29)
Autogenic training	O	⇨	Yes (see p 37)
Biofeedback	O	⬈	No (see p 42)
Breathing exercises	OO	⬈	No
Buteyko breathing	O	⬈	No
Diet (allergy avoidance)	O	⇧	No
Herbal medicine Chinese, Indian, Kampo	O	⬈	Yes (see p 52)
Homeopathy	OO	⇨	No (see p 55)
Hypnotherapy	OO	⬈	Yes (see p 58)
Massage	O	⬈	No (see p 60)
Meditation	O	⬈	Yes (see p 80)
Relaxation	OO	⇨	No (see p 71)
Spinal manipulation Chiropractic	OO	⇩	Yes (see p 47)
Yoga	OO	⇨	Yes (see p 77)

Other therapies

An RCT in 30 patients given **reflexology** showed this treatment to have no benefit over an attention control.[23] **Vitamin C** was protective against exercise-induced asthma in a proportion of children.[24] The role of **essential fatty acids** in the diet is probably complex and no recommendation can be made on the present evidence.

Overall recommendation

In comparison with conventional drugs which have reliable effects and known adverse effects, no CAM therapy can be recommended as a sole treatment for asthma. However, some therapies may be useful adjuncts. Hypnotherapy may be helpful for those who are hypnosis responders and yoga for those who are motivated: like any therapy, yoga would need to continue for prolonged periods to maintain any benefit. Autogenic training and Buteyko breathing appear to be the most promising of the other therapies.

REFERENCES

1 Ernst E. Complementary therapies for asthma: what patients use. J Asthma 1998;35:667–671

2 Ernst E. Use of complementary therapies in childhood asthma. Pediatr Asthma Allergy Immunol 1998;21:29–32

CONDITIONS

3 Andrews L, Lokuge S, Sawyer M, Lillywhite L, Kennedy D, Martin J. The use of alternative therapies by children with asthma: a brief report. J Paediatr Child Health 1998;34:131–134

4 Henry M, De Rivera J L G, Gonzalez-Martin I J, Abreu J. Improvement of respiratory function in chronic asthmatic patients with autogenic therapy. J Psychosom Res 1993;17:265–270

5 Speiss K, Sachs G, Buchinger C et al. Zur Auswirkung von Informations- und Entspannungsgruppen auf die Lungenfunktion und psychophysische Befindlichkeit bei Asthmapatienten. Prax Klin Pneumol 1988;42:641–644

6 Deter H C, Allert G. Group therapy for asthma patients: a concept for the psychosomatic treatment of patients in a medical clinic – a controlled study. Psychother Psychosom 1983;40:95–105

7 Kotses H, Harver A, Segreto J, Glaus K D, Creer T L, Young G A. Long-term effects of biofeedback-induced facial relaxation on measures of asthma severity in children. Biofeedback Self Regul 1991;16:1–21

8 Coen B L, Conran P B, McGrady A, Nelson L. Effects of biofeedback-assisted relaxation on asthma severity and immune function. Pediatr Asthma Allergy Immunol 1996;10:71–78

9 Bowler S D, Green A, Mitchell C A. Buteyko breathing techniques in asthma: a blinded randomised controlled trial. Med J Aust 1998;169:575–578

10 Monteleone C A, Sherman A R. Nutrition and asthma. Arch Intern Med 1997;157:23–34

11 Baker J C, Tunnicliffe W S, Duncanson R C, Ayres J G. Reduced dietary intakes of magnesium, selenium and vitamins A, C and E in patients with brittle asthma. Thorax 1995;50 (suppl 2):A75

12 Reilly D, Taylor M, Beattie N G M et al. Is evidence for homoeopathy reproducible? Lancet 1994;344:1601–1606

13 Field T, Henteleff T, Hernandez-Reif M et al. Children with asthma have improved pulmonary functions after massage therapy. J Pediatr 1998;132:854–858

14 Wilson A F, Honsberger R, Chiu J T, Novey H S. Transcendental meditation and asthma. Respiration 1975;32:74–80

15 Alexander A B, Miklich D R, Hershkoff H. The immediate effects of systematic relaxation training on peak expiratory flow rates in asthmatic children. Psychosom Med 1972; 34:388–394

16 Erskine J, Schonell M. Relaxation therapy in bronchial asthma. J Psychosom Res 1979; 23:131–139

17 Hock R A, Bramble J, Kennard D W. A comparison between relaxation and assertive training with asthmatic male children. Bio Psych 1977;12:593–596

18 Balon J, Aker P D, Crowther E R et al. A comparison of active and simulated chiropractic manipulation as adjunctive treatment for childhood asthma. New Engl J Med 1998;339:1013–1020

19 Nielson N H, Bronfort G, Bendix T, Madsen F, Weeke B. Chronic asthma and chiropractic spinal manipulation: a randomised clinical trial. Clin Exp Allergy 1995;25:80–88

20 Nagarathna R, Nagendra H R. Yoga for bronchial asthma: a controlled study. Br Med J 1985;291:1077–1079

21 Fluge T, Richter J, Fabel H, Zysno E, Weller E, Wagner T O. Long-term effects of breathing exercises and yoga in patients with bronchial asthma. Pneumologie 1994;48:484–490

22 Vedanthan P K, Kesavalu L N, Murthy K C et al. Clinical study of yoga techniques in university students with asthma: a controlled study. Allergy Asthma Proc 1998;19:3–9

23 Peterson L N, Faurschou P, Olsen O T, Svendsen U G. Reflexology and bronchial asthma. Ugeskr Laeger 1992;154:2065–2068

24 Cohen H A, Neuman I, Nahum H. Blocking effect of vitamin C in exercise-induced asthma. Arch Pediatr Adolesc Med 1997; 151:367–370

CONDITIONS

ATOPIC ECZEMA

Synonyms/ subcategories   Atopic dermatitis, infantile eczema.

Definition   Inflammatory skin disease characterized by irritation, pruritus, erythema, scaling and thickening of the skin.

CAM usage

A survey of German eczema patients reported homeopathy, acupuncture, dietary therapy, autogenic training and relaxation as the most frequently used forms of CAM.[1]

Clinical evidence

Autogenic training

An RCT (n=113) compared autogenic training (once weekly for 12 weeks) with cognitive-behavioral therapy, a dermatological education program and standard medical care.[2] Results at one year follow-up indicated that autogenic training was as effective as the psychotherapy and superior to the educational program and usual care in terms of skin condition and use of topical steroids.

Diet

Several RCTs[3-6] have investigated egg and cow's milk **exclusion diets**, with two of them showing positive results,[3,6] including one on the effect of maternal antigen avoidance on breast-fed infants.[6] RCTs of prevention of eczema in high-risk infants by maternal antigen avoidance during pregnancy[7] and lactation[8] have been systematically reviewed. Based on only three trials each, it was concluded that the risk of the child developing eczema was likely to be reduced by exclusion diets during lactation, but not during pregnancy.

Table 5.8 Double-blind RCTs of borage oil for atopic eczema

Reference	Sample size	Interventions [dosage]	Result	Comment
Zeitschr Dermatol 1996; 182:131–136	50	A) Borage oil [2×1000 mg/d for 12 w] B) Placebo (palm oil)	A superior to B on severity index	Placebo response of 43%
Br J Dermatol 1999;140: 685–688	160	A) Borage oil [3×500 mg/d for 24 w] B) Placebo (miglyol)	A no different to B on Costa score	Non-compliance seemed likely from plasma lipid measurements

Herbal medicine

Two RCTs of **borage** (*Borago officinalis*) seed oil involving adult patients have produced conflicting results (Table 5.8). A smaller crossover trial in children (n=24) using gamma-linolenic acid from borage seeds reported a strong placebo response and no difference between the interventions.[9]

A systematic review of **Chinese herbs**[10] included only two RCTs from the same researchers who reported positive results for a herbal combination in both adults and children. A subsequent independent crossover RCT of the same preparation found it to be no different to placebo.[11]

A metaanalysis of nine placebo-controlled trials of oil of **evening primrose** (*Oenothera biennis*) demonstrated a significant positive effect.[12] However, the results of subsequent RCTs do not tend to support this result (Table 5.9).

Table 5.9 **Double-blind RCTs of evening primrose oil for atopic eczema**

Reference	Sample size	Interventions [dosage]	Result	Comment
Lancet 1993;341: 1557–1560	123	A) Evening primrose oil [6 g/d for 16 w] B) Evening primrose & fish oil [5 g & 1.3 g] C) Placebo	A or B no different to C on severity scores	Children and adults included but no differential effects
Drugs Exp Clin Res 1994; 20:77–84	51	A) Evening primrose oil [500 mg/kg/d for 8 w] B) Evening Primose oil [250 mg/kg/d] C) Placebo	A superior to C on severity scores; B no different to C	Infants all <8 years; very high doses used; significant difference was borderline
Dermatology 1996;193: 115–120	39	A) Evening primrose oil [600 mg/d for 16 w] B) Placebo	A no different to B on symptom scores	Patients with chronic hand dermatitis
Arch Dis Child 1996; 75:494–497	60	A) Evening primose oil [500 mg/d for 16 w] B) Placebo	A no different to B on symptom scores	Patients aged 1–16 years

A non-randomized trial (n=161) of a topical preparation containing **German chamomile** (*Matricaria recutita*) suggested it may be as useful as hydrocortisone, but no statistical analysis was carried out.[13] A subsequent RCT reported slight superiority over hydrocortisone but little difference with placebo.[14] Again, there was no statistical analysis.

Hypnotherapy
An RCT with children (n=31) compared the effects of hypnotherapy (four sessions over 8 weeks) with biofeedback (skin conductance) and an attention control condition where children discussed their eczema and kept a symptom diary.[15] After 5 months the hypnotherapy and biofeedback groups had

improved significantly more than the control group on severity of eczema, but not area of coverage.

Supplements

A double-blind RCT of supplementation with **selenium** (alone and combined with **vitamin E**) found no difference in severity of eczema compared with placebo.[16]

Zinc has been investigated in a double-blind RCT with children.[17] It was not superior to placebo on any outcome measure.

Table 5.10
Summary of clinical evidence for atopic eczema

Treatment	Weight of evidence	Direction of evidence	Serious safety concerns
Autogenic training	O	⇧	Yes (see p 37)
Biofeedback	O	⬈	No (see p 42)
Diet			
Exclusion in children/adults	OO	⇨	No
Exclusion during pregnancy	O	⇩	No
Exclusion during lactation	O	⬈	No
Herbal medicine			
Borage oil	O	⇝	Yes (see p 167)
Chinese herbs	OO	⇨	Yes (see p 52)
Evening primrose oil	OOO	⇨	Yes (see p 104)
German chamomile	O	⇨	Yes (see p 111)
Hypnotherapy	O	⬈	Yes (see p 58)
Supplements			
Selenium	O	⇩	Yes (see p 5)
Zinc	O	⇩	Yes (see p 5)

Overall recommendation

There is no convincing evidence for the effectiveness of any complementary therapy in treating or preventing eczema and no signs that conventional steroid treatments can be matched. The therapies with the most promising evidence are those with a psychological component: autogenic training, biofeedback and hypnotherapy. These are considered relatively risk free and may be worth considering as an adjunctive treatment in an attempt to minimize use of steroids.

REFERENCES

1 Augustin M, Zschocke I, Buhrke U. Attitudes and prior experience with respect to alternative medicine among dermatological patients: the Freiburg questionnaire on attitudes to naturopathy (FAN). Forsch Komplementärmed 1999;6(suppl 2):26–29

2 Ehlers A, Stangier U, Gieler U. Treatment of atopic dermatitis: a comparison of psychological and dermatological approaches

CONDITIONS

to relapse prevention. J Consult Clin Psychol 1995;63:624–635

3 Lever R, MacDonald C, Waugh P, Aitchison T. Randomised controlled trial of advice on an egg exclusion diet in young children with atopic eczema and sensitivity to eggs. Pediatr Allergy Immunol 1998;9:13–19

4 Atherton D J, Sewall M, Soothill J F, Wells R S, Chilvers C E D. A double-blind controlled cross-over trial of an antigen-avoidance diet in atopic eczema. Lancet 1978;25:401–403

5 Neild V S, Marsden R A, Bailes J A, Bland J M. Egg and milk exclusion diets in atopic eczema. Br J Dermatol 1986;114:117–123

6 Cant A J, Bailes J A, Marsden R A, Hewitt D. Effect of maternal dietary exclusion on breast fed infants with eczema: two controlled studies. Br Med J Clin Res Ed 1986; 293:231–233

7 Kramer M S. Maternal antigen avoidance during pregnancy for preventing atopic disease in infants of women at high risk (Cochrane Review). Cochrane Library. Oxford: Update Software, 1996

8 Kramer M S. Maternal antigen avoidance during lactation for preventing atopic disease in infants of women at high risk. Cochrane Library. Oxford: Update Software, 1996

9 Borreck S, Hildebrandt A, Forster J. Borage seed oil and atopic dermatitis. Klinische Pädiatrie 1997;209:100–104

10 Armstrong N C, Ernst E. The treatment of eczema with Chinese herbs: a systematic review of randomised clinical trials. Br J Clin Pharmacol 1999;48:262–264

11 Fung A Y, Look P C, Chong L Y, But P P, Wong E. A controlled trial of traditional Chinese herbal medicine in Chinese patients with recalcitrant atopic dermatitis. Int J Dermatol 1999;38:387–392

12 Morse P F, Horrobin D F, Manku M S et al. Meta-analysis of placebo-controlled studies of the efficacy of Epogam in the treatment of atopic eczema. Relationship between plasma essential fatty acid changes and clinical response. Br J Dermatol 1989;121:75–90

13 Aertgeerts P, Albring M, Klaschka F, Nasemann T, Patzelt-Wenczler R, Rauhut K, Weigl B. Comparative testing of Kamillosan cream and steroidal (0.25% hydrocortisone, 0.75% fluocortin butyl ester) and non-steroidal (5% bufexamac) dermatologic agents in maintenance therapy of eczematous diseases. Zeitschr für Hautkrankheiten 1985;60(3):270–277

14 Patzelt-Wenczler R, Ponce-Pöschl E. Proof of efficacy of Kamillosan cream in atopic eczema. Eur J Med Res 2000;5:171–175

15 Sokel B, Christie D, Kent A, Lansdown R, Atherton D. A comparison of hypnotherapy and biofeedback in the treatment of childhood atopic eczema. Contemp Hypnosis 1993; 10:145–154

16 Fairris G M, Perkins P J, Lloyd B, Hinks L, Clayton B E. The effect on atopic dermatitis of supplementation with selenium and vitamin E. Acta Derm Venereol 1989;69:359–362

17 Ewing C I, Gibbs A C, Ashcroft C, David T J. Failure of oral zinc supplementation in atopic eczema. Eur J Clin Nutr 1991;45:507–510

BACK PAIN

Synonyms/ subcategories	Mechanical back pain, idiopathic back pain, non-specific back pain, low back pain, back ache, lumbago.
Definition	A common symptom with many (often undefined) causes characterized by pain in and reduced mobility of the back, especially the lumbosacral region.
Related conditions	Back pain with specific causes, i.e. specific back pain (e.g. due to ankylosing spondylitis, vertebral canal stenosis, etc.) can be differentiated from back pain where no cause can be identified. This type is much more common and is often referred to as non-specific, idiopathic or mechanical back pain. Various categories

CONDITIONS

can be differentiated, e.g. acute, subacute and chronic or uncomplicated and complicated (i.e. with neurological signs).

CAM usage

According to most surveys carried out in this area, back pain is the most frequent indication for which patients try CAM (e.g. [1]). The most commonly employed CAM treatments are acupuncture, herbal remedies, massage therapy and spinal manipulation (chiropractic or osteopathy). In our survey of CAM organizations (see p 3) the following treatments were recommended for back pain: Bowen technique, chiropractic, magnet therapy, massage, reflexology and yoga.

Box 5.11
Metaanalysis
Acupuncture for back pain
Arch Intern Med
1998;158:2235–2241

- Twelve RCTs included, nine submitted to metaanalysis

- All types of acupuncture were studied for all types of LBP

- Trial quality was generally adequate

- Odds ratio was 2.30 (CI 1.28 to 4.13) in favor of acupuncture over (various) control treatments

- Odds ratio for all four sham-controlled and evaluator-blinded studies was 1.37 (CI 0.34 to 2.25)

- No clear suggestion emerged as to the optimal type of acupuncture treatment

- Further studies are needed to define with certainty whether acupuncture has specific effects in addition to its non-specific (e.g. placebo) effects

Clinical evidence

Acupuncture
A metaanalysis resulted in a positive verdict for acupuncture (Box 5.11). A non-quantitative systematic Cochrane Review of (almost) the same set of RCTs[2] concluded that the evidence for acupuncture was not fully convincing. A recent comparative RCT of acupuncture versus TENS (transcutaneous electrical nerve stimulation) showed encouraging outcomes for both therapeutic modalities.[3]

Herbal medicine
Several herbal remedies have shown promising results in alleviating musculoskeletal pain.[4] The only one that has been investigated specifically for back pain is **devil's claw** (*Harpagophytum procumbens*). Two independent, uncontrolled studies suggested positive effects. A placebo-controlled, double-blind RCT included 118 patients with acute low back pain (LBP).[5] They received either placebo or devil's claw extract (3×800 mg daily) for 4 weeks. Cumulative Tramalol consumption (the primary endpoint

of the study) did not differ significantly between groups (95 vs 102 mg). The number of patients who were pain free by the end of the trial did, however, show a significant difference in favor of devil's claw.

Massage

This form of therapy is frequently used in Europe for LBP, but has not been extensively studied in controlled clinical trials. A systematic review[6] located four CCTs where massage was used as a control intervention. It concluded that massage therapy seems to have some potential but more research is needed. A recent comparative RCT suggested that the benefit of massage therapy is short-lived.[7]

Box 5.12
Systematic review
Chiropractic spinal manipulation for back pain
J Manipul Physiol Ther 1996;19: 499–507

- Eight RCTs were included

- Various control interventions were used

- All studies had serious methodological flaws

- No convincing evidence for the effectiveness of chiropractic for acute or chronic low back pain

Spinal manipulation

Chiropractic spinal manipulations have been evaluated in several systematic reviews. The most authoritative of these casts considerable doubt on the assumption that its effectiveness has been demonstrated beyond reasonable doubt (Box 5.12). Subsequent studies did not yield results in favor of chiropractic manipulation (Table 5.11). This is an overt contradiction to recent guidelines for treating back pain. A Cochrane Review is in progress and a recent 'best evidence synthesis' suggested that spinal manipulation as a treatment of acute or chronic back pain is supported by moderately conclusive evidence.[8]

Osteopathic spinal manipulation and mobilization has been evaluated less thoroughly than its chiropractic counterpart. A recent RCT compared a complex osteopathic treatment approach, as commonly used by US osteopaths, with standard care in 178 patients with subacute or chronic low back pain.[9] Both groups of patients improved during the 12 weeks' treatment period with no significant difference between them. Thus one might conclude that the osteopathic approach is as effective (or ineffective) as standard medical care. Too few comparative trials exist that examine whether one form of spinal manipulation (e.g. chiropractic) is more effective than another (e.g. osteopathy).

CONDITIONS

Table 5.11 **Recent controlled studies of chiropractic manipulation for back pain**

Reference	Sample size	Interventions	Result	Comment
New Engl J Med 1995;333: 913–917	1555	A) Urban chiropractic B) Rural chiropractic C) Urban primary care physicians D) Rural primary care physicians E) Orthopedic surgeons F) HMO	Functional recovery was similar between groups	Patients were not randomized, mean total outpatient charges were highest for orthopedic surgeons and chiropractors
Pain 1998; 77:201–207	323	A) Chiropractic B) Physiotherapy	No intergroup differences	Treatment was individualized
New Engl J Med 1998;339: 1021–1029	321	A) Chiropractic B) McKenzie physiotherapy C) Minimal intervention (educational booklet)	At 1 month chiropractic was best, but not significant after adjustment for non-normal distribution	Differences were of questionable relevance and essentially all three groups had similar outcomes

Water injections

Sterile water injections have been used for a number of pain syndromes. The theory is that such injections stimulate skin nociceptors and thus close the 'gate' for peripheral pain perception. Two independent placebo-controlled RCTs suggested that they are effective in alleviating back pain of various causes.[7,10] In the most recent of these studies, 34 women suffering from low back pain during labor were randomly assigned to receive intracutaneous sterile water injections, TENS or standard care with massage therapy.[7] The group receiving water injections perceived significantly less pain during 90 minutes following the intervention.

Other therapies

Many if not most forms of CAM have been tried for back pain. For instance, a combination of back school, **relaxation** and **qi gong** yielded promising preliminary results[11] and there are some encouraging data related to **yoga**[12] and **hypnotherapy**.[13] Invariably, however, there are too few clinical trials and a lack of independent replications to allow firm conclusions.

Overall recommendation Based on the evidence available to date, the most promising CAM treatments for back pain are acupuncture (particularly for chronic back pain), spinal manipulation (especially for acute

Table 5.12
Summary of clinical evidence for back pain

Treatment	Weight of evidence	Direction of evidence	Serious safety concerns
Acupuncture	OO	⇗	Yes (see p 29)
Herbal medicine			
Devil's claw	O	⇗	Yes (see p 101)
Massage	O	⇒	No (see p 60)
Spinal manipulation			
(chronic pain)	OO	⇒	Yes (see pp 47, 65)
(acute pain)	OO	⇗	Yes (see pp 47, 65)
Water injections	O	⇗	Yes (see p 81)

back pain) and sterile water injections. None of these therapies is risk free, but serious complications are probably rare. The effect of water injections might be only short-lived and more research is needed. It is difficult to see relevant advantages of herbal over synthetic analgesic medications. The effect sizes of CAM modalities for LBP are invariably small to moderate, yet this also applies to all conventional treatments of back pain available today.[14]

The bottom line therefore is that acupuncture, spinal manipulation and water injections are worth trying, especially in conjunction with standard forms of health care, e.g. (other) analgesics and regular physical exercise. The most important advice to back pain sufferers is to keep up normal activity as much as possible and to realize that having back problems is not a disease but entirely normal.

REFERENCES

1 Eisenberg D M, David R B, Ettner S L et al. Trends in alternative medicine use in the United States, 1990–1997. JAMA 1998; 280:1569–1575

2 Van Tulder M W, Cherkin D C, Berman B, Lao L, Koes B V. Acupuncture for low back pain (Cochrane Review). Cochrane Library. Oxford: Update Software, 1999

3 Grant D J, Bishop-Miller J, Winchester D M, Anderson M, Faulkner S. A randomized comparative trial of acupuncture versus transcutaneous electrical nerve stimulation for chronic back pain in the elderly. Pain 1999; 82:9–13

4 Ernst E, Chrubasik S. Phyto-antiinflammatories. A systematic review of randomized, placebo-controlled, double-blind trials. Rheum Dis Clin North Am 2000;26:13–27

5 Chrubasik S, Zimpfer C, Schütt U, Ziegler R. Effectiveness of *Harpagophytum procumbens* in treatment of acute low back pain. Phytomedicine 1996;3:1–10

6 Ernst E. Massage therapy for low back pain: a systematic review. J Pain Symptom Manage 1999;17:65–69

7 Labrecque M, Nouwen A, Bergeron M, Rancourt J. A randomized controlled trial of non-pharmacologic approaches for relief of low back pain during labor. J Fam Pract 1999;48(4):259–263

8 Bonfort G. Spinal manipulation, current state of research and its indications. Neurol Clin North Am 1999;17(1):91–111

9 Andersson G B J, Lucente T, Davis A M, Kappler R E, Lipton J A, Leurgans S. A comparison of osteopathic spinal manipulation with standard care for patients with low back pain. New Engl J Med 1999;341:1426–1431

CONDITIONS

10 Trolle B, Moller M, Kronborg H, Thomsen S. The effect of sterile water blocks on low back labor pain. Am J Obstet Gynecol 1991; 164:1277–1281

11 Berman B M, Sing B B. Chronic low back pain: an outcome analysis of a mind–body intervention. Compl Ther Med 1997;5:29–35

12 Nespor K. Psychosomatics of back pain and the use of yoga. Int J Psychosom 1989;36:72–78

13 McCauley J D, Thelen M H, Frank R G, Willard R R, Callen K E. Hypnosis compared to relaxation in the outpatient management of chronic low back pain. Arch Phys Med Rehab 1983;64:548–552

14 Van Tulder M W, Koes B W, Bouter L M. Conservative treatment of acute and chronic non-specific low back pain: a systematic review of the most common interventions. Spine 1997;22:2128–2156

FURTHER READING

Ernst E. Back pain. Practical ways to restore health using complementary medicine. London: Godsfield Press, 1998
A practical guide aimed at patients (also available in Spanish and Portuguese).

Frymoyer J W (ed). The adult spine. New York: Raven Press, 1999, vols 1 and 2
An extremely thorough and authoritative text for health-care professionals.

BENIGN PROSTATIC HYPERPLASIA

Synonyms Benign prostatic hypertrophy, nodular hyperplasia of the prostate.

Definition Glandular and stromal hyperplasia occurring very commonly in the middle and lateral lobes of the prostate gland of older men, forming nodules that may increasingly obstruct the urethra.

CAM usage Herbal medicine is the option most commonly used to treat this condition.

Clinical evidence

Herbal medicine

A large double-blind RCT (n=263) was carried out to assess the effects of **African plum** (*Pygeum africanum*) for benign prostatic hyperplasia.[1] African plum extract 100 mg or placebo were administered daily for a treatment period of 60 days. This study and the results of another double-blind RCT (n=120), which administered African plum extract for 6 weeks,[2] suggested significant beneficial effects for nocturia and micturition volume compared with placebo. The results of a small (n=20) double-blind trial, however, do not corroborate these findings.[3]

Several RCTs have assessed the effectiveness of **nettle** (*Urtica dioica*) root extract (Table 5.13). These largely report beneficial effects of nettle root extract compared with placebo. The largest trial on the subject, however, did not report any intergroup differences. Other positive evidence relates to combination preparations including saw palmetto extract[4] or African plum extract.[5]

Table 5.13 **Double-blind RCTs of nettle root extract for benign prostatic hyperplasia**

Reference	Sample size	Interventions [dosage]	Result	Comment
Urologe A 1985;24:49–51	50	A) Nettle [600 mg/d for 9 w] B) Placebo	A superior to B in micturition volume	No difference in subjective complaints
Urologe B 1987; 27:223–226	79	A) Nettle [600 mg/d for 4–6 w] B) Placebo	A Improvement of mean and maximal urinary flow B No improvement	Intergroup differences not reported
Rutishauser G (ed) Benigne Prostata-hyperplasie III. München Zuckerschwerdt, 1992, p 79	40	A) Nettle [1.2 g/d for 6 mo] B) Placebo	A superior to B in symptom score	Long treament period
Urologe B 1996; 36:287–291	41	A) Nettle [6 ml/d for 3 mo] B) Placebo	A superior to B in International Prostate Symptom Score	No difference in micturition volume and maximal urinary flow

A double-blind RCT assessed a combination preparation which contained 80 mg **pumpkin** (*Cucurbita pepo*) seed extract and 80 mg saw palmetto extract.[6] It reports a significant improvement of urinary flow, frequency and time spent urinating after 3 months of treatment with two tablets three times daily, compared with placebo. Beneficial effects as indicated on the International Prostate Symptom Score are suggested by an uncontrolled study.[7] These promising findings require confirmation for a firm judgement on the effectiveness of pumpkin seed extract alone.

The evidence for **saw palmetto** (*Serenoa repens*) extract has been assessed in a metaanalysis (Box 5.13). Some concerns

Box 5.13
Metaanalysis
Saw palmetto for benign prostatic hyperplasia
JAMA 1998;280: 1604–1609

- Eighteen RCTs including 2939 patients; 16 double-blind

- Improvement in self-rating of urinary tract symptoms (risk ratio for improvement 1.72, CI 1.21 to 2.44)

- Improvement in peak urine flow (weighted mean difference 1.93 ml/s, CI 0.72 to 3.14)

- Similar improvements in urinary tract symptom scores and peak urine flow compared with finasteride

- Adverse effects were mild and infrequent

relate to trial quality, but the relatively large body of data provides convincing evidence that saw palmetto improves urinary tract symptoms and peak urine flow. These results are largely corroborated by double-blind RCTs conducted since the metaanalysis (Table 5.14). An involution of prostatic epithelium is reported by a double-blind RCT (n=44), which investigated the effects of a herbal blend containing saw palmetto extract, nettle extract and pumpkin seed oil.[8]

Table 5.14 Double-blind RCTs of saw palmetto for benign prostatic hyperplasia

Reference	Sample size	Interventions [dosage]	Result	Comment
Münch Med Wochenschr 1999;141:62	101	A) Saw palmetto [320 mg/d for 6 mo] B) Placebo	A superior to B in International Prostate Symptom Score and urinary flow measures	No adverse effects
Indian J Urol 1999;16: 26–31	75	A) Saw palmetto [2 × cap/d for 2 mo] B) Placebo	A superior to B in total symptom score and average urinary flow rate	Exact dose of saw palmetto extract not reported
Adv Ther 1999;16: 231–241	100	A) Saw palmetto [1 × 320 mg/d for 3 mo] B) Saw palmetto [2 × 160 mg/d for 3 mo]	Reduction of International Prostate Symptom Score and urinary flow measures from baseline	No differences between regimens

Overall recommendation

The evidence for the short- and medium-term effectiveness of saw palmetto extract is convincing. Saw palmetto seems to improve urinary tract symptom scores and peak urine flow to a similar degree as conventional oral medication. Given the nature and frequency of adverse effects, saw palmetto extract can be recommended as an oral treatment for benign prostatic hyperplasia. However, compelling long-term data are not yet available. For nettle root and African plum extract, the evidence is promising but not compelling.

Table 5.15
Summary of clinical evidence for benign prostatic hyperplasia

Treatment	Weight of evidence	Direction of evidence	Serious safety concerns
Herbal medicine			
African plum	OO	⇗	Yes (see p 5)
Nettle	OO	⇗	Yes (see p 139)
Pumpkin seed	O	⇑	Yes (see p 170)
Saw palmetto	OOO	⇑	Yes (see p 150)

REFERENCES

1 Barlet A, Albrecht J, Aubert A et al. Wirksamkeit eines Extraktes aus Pygeum africanum in der medikamentösen Therapie von Miktionsstörungen infolge einer benignen Prostatahyperplasie: Bewertung objektiver und subjektiver Parameter. Wien Klin Wochenschr 1990;102:667–673

2 Dufour B, Choquenet C, Revol M, Faure G, Jorest R. Controlled study of the effects of Pygeum africanum extract on the functional symptoms of prostatic adenoma. Ann Urol 1984;18:193–195

3 Donkervoort T, Sterling A, Van Ness J, Donker P J. A clinical and urodynamic study of Tadenam in the treatment of benign prostatic hypertrophy. Eur Urol 1977;3:218–225

4 Stepanov V N, Siniakova L A, Sarrazin B, Raynaud J P. Efficacy and tolerability of the lipidosterolic extract of Serenoa repens in benign prostatic hyperplasia. A double-blind comparison of two dosage regimens. Adv Ther 1999;16:231–241

5 Krzeski T, Kazon M, Borkowski A, Witeska A, Kuczera J. Combined extract of Urtica dioica and Pygeum africanum in the treatment of benign prostatic hyperplasia: double-blind comparison of two doses. Clin Therapeut 1993;15:1011–1020

6 Carbin B E, Larsson B, Lindahl O. Treatment of benign prostatic hyperplasia with phytosterols. Br J Urol 1990;66:639–641

7 Schiebel-Schlosser G, Friederich M. Phytotherapy of BPH with pumpkin seeds – a multicentric clinical trial. Zeitschr für Phytotherapie 1998;19:71–76

8 Marks L S, Partin A W, Epstein J I et al. Effects of a saw palmetto blend in men with symptomatic benign prostatic hyperplasia. J Urol 2000;163:1451–1456

CANCER

Synonyms/ subcategories	Malignant tumors or neoplasms.
Definition	General term used to describe any type of malignant neoplasm, most of which invade surrounding tissues, may metastasize and are likely to recur after attempted removal and cause death of the patient unless adequately treated.
Related conditions	Precancerous conditions.
CAM usage	Cancer patients are understandably desperate and would try any treatment that offers hope; therefore, many cancer patients use CAM. A systematic review of surveys on this topic included 26 investigations from 13 countries published between 1977 and 1998.[1] The average prevalence of CAM therapy use was 31%.

Each decade seems to have had its own cancer 'cure' that achieved some prominence, only to fade away as new therapies emerged. Koch antitoxins (1940s), the Hoxie treatment (1950s), Krebiozen (1960s), Laetrile (1970s), metabolic and immunoaugmentative therapy (1980s) are prominent examples. The following treatments are frequently used at present:[1] co-enzyme Q10, diets, herbal remedies, homeopathy, hypnotherapy, meditation, relaxation, reflexology, shark cartilage, spiritual healing/ therapeutic touch, visualization. Some of these therapies are promoted as 'cures', some are used for palliative care and some are promoted for cancer prevention.

CONDITIONS

Clinical evidence

The clinical evidence is divided into three parts: cancer prevention, cancer 'cures' and palliative/supportive care.

Cancer prevention

Diet

Many measures to prevent cancer relate to the dietary intake of plant-derived compounds. Some of those often promoted by proponents of CAM are discussed below.

Several lines of evidence suggest that the regular consumption of **Allium** vegetables, such as onion or garlic, is tumor protective. A systematic review[2] summarized 20 epidemiological studies in this area. With one exception, they all suggest that *Allium* vegetables convey some protection against cancers, particularly those of the gastrointestinal tract. Collectively these data are encouraging but not entirely convincing. Nevertheless, a recommendation for a high regular intake of garlic and onion probably constitutes good advice to individuals who are keen to do something for cancer prevention.

There is a sizable body of evidence to suggest that the polyphenols in **green tea** exhibit protective effects against cancer. Epidemiological studies suggest that the regular consumption of green tea conveys a moderate reduction of cancer risk, particularly cancers of the upper digestive tract. A recent systematic review of the data cautiously concluded that: 'There is some evidence that green tea may prevent the occurrence of some cancers.'[3]

Indirect (e.g. epidemiological) evidence suggests that the regular consumption of **phytoestrogens** lowers the risk of several forms of cancer. For instance, one case-control study showed an inverse association between certain phytoestrogens and prostate cancer risk.[4] These data are not sufficiently compelling to translate into meaningful advice for clinical practice.

Vegetarianism is often claimed to protect against cancer. In a prospective study from the UK, 6000 non-meat eaters and 5000 meat eaters were followed for 12 years.[5] At the end of this period all-cause mortality in the former population was approximately half of that of the control group. The cancer death rate for non-meat eaters was only about 60% of that of omnivores. A metaanalysis of this and four similar studies included a total sample of 76172 men and women. It found no significant difference in mortality between vegetarians and non-vegetarians from stomach, colorectal, lung or breast cancer (yet vegetarians had only 24% the risk of ischemic heart disease of that of omnivores).[6] Strict vegetarianism carries the risk of malnutrition. Sensible advice therefore could be to reduce meat (particularly red meat) consumption without pursuing a strict vegetarian diet.

Herbal medicine

Much basic research implies that **ginseng** (*Panax ginseng*) is tumor protective through its effects on the immune system. An epidemiological study carried out in a ginseng-growing region in Korea[7] included 4634 individuals who were assessed by questionnaire on ginseng intake. During the 5 years of follow-up, 137 cases of cancer occurred. Those individuals who regularly consumed fresh ginseng were associated with a dramatically reduced cancer risk. Even though the data are positive, they are not compelling, and clinical trials are largely lacking.

Table 5.16
Summary of clinical evidence of cancer prevention

Treatment	Weight of evidence	Direction of evidence	Serious safety concerns
Diet			
Allium vegetables	OO	⇧	No (see pp 109, 170)
Green tea	OO	⬈	No (see p 120)
Phytoestrogens	O	⬈	Yes (see p 144)
Vegetarianism	OO	⇨	Yes for vegan diet (see p 6)
Herbal medicine			
Ginseng	O	⇧	Yes (see p 88)

Cancer 'cures'

Treatments which claim to cure cancer, lower the tumor burden or prolong the life of cancer patients are rife within CAM.

Di Bella therapy

The 'Di Bella therapy' consists of melatonin, bromocriptine, either somatostatin or octreotide, and retinoid solution (as well as cyclophosphamide and hydroxyurea in some cases). Eleven independent, multicenter, uncontrolled phase II studies including 386 patients with advanced cancer were initiated in Italy.[8] None of the patients showed complete remission and only three patients had a partial remission. A retrospective matched pair comparison of 314 patients versus matched patients from Italian cancer registers showed a significantly shorter average survival time for Di Bella's patients.[9]

Diet

Proponents of 'alternative' diets claim that their approach can prolong the life of cancer patients. A review of the evidence found no convincing data in support of this hypothesis.[10] In particular, unreplicated data apparently showing a six-fold increase in 5-year survival rates of melanoma patients treated with the **Gerson diet**[11] are unconvincing due to seriously flawed methodology.

Similar claims for a **macrobiotic diet** are also not supported by evidence from rigorous clinical trials. One third of cancer patients on a macrobiotic diet have been shown to experience problems due to weight loss, the restrictive and unpalatable nature of the regimen and the expense and inaccessibility of some ingredients used in this diet.[12]

Herbal medicine

Numerous herbal medicines have been tried for cancer. Fifty patients with advanced solid malignant tumors for whom no effective standard anticancer therapy existed were treated in a CCT, either with melatonin (20 mg/day) or with melatonin and **aloe vera** tincture (1 ml twice daily).[13] No response was seen in the former group while two partial responses were observed in the group treated with aloe vera. This result awaits confirmation in more rigorous trials.

'Destagnation' is a complex mixture of traditional **Chinese herbs**. An RCT with 188 patients suffering from nasopharyngeal carcinomas tested its efficacy against radiation therapy.[14] The 5-year survival rate was 53% in the experimental and 37% in the control group. The difference was statistically significant.

Essiac is a herbal mixture which is popular in North America and consists of *Arctium lappa*, *Rheum palmatum*, *Rumex acetosella* and *Ulmus fulva*. A systematic review did not find a single published clinical trial.[15] Several unpublished investigations were identified and there was some indirect evidence for anticancer activity of several of the constituent herbs. Thus there is insufficient evidence to recommend this herbal mixture.

Mistletoe (*Viscum album*) extracts contain mistletoe lectins and viscotoxins. Both modify intracellular protein synthesis, stimulate cytokine production, inhibit tumor colonization and induce cell necrosis. Two independent systematic reviews on mistletoe[16,17] found only a small number of clinical trials, none of which, due to significant methodological flaws, were conclusive. Kleijnen and colleagues therefore conclude: 'We cannot recommend the use of mistletoe extracts in the treatment of cancer patients with an exception for patients involved in clinical trials'.[17]

The herbal formula **PC-SPES** contains *Chrysanthemum morifolium*, *Gandoderma lucidium*, *Glycyrrhiza glabra*, *Isatis indigotica*, *Panax pseudoginseng*, *Robdosia rubesceus*, *Scutellaria baicalensis* and *Serenoa repens*. The mixture was shown to lower prostate-specific antigen in patients with prostate cancer and to inhibit the growth of prostate cancer cells in vitro.[18] These results are encouraging but require confirmation in clinical trials.

Sho-saiko-to is a Chinese herbal mixture that contains extracts of seven medicinal herbs; 260 patients with hepatocellular carcinoma and cirrhosis were treated with 7.5 g of the mixture daily while the control group received conventional drugs only.[19] The 5-year survival rate showed a (non-significant) trend to be higher in the experimental group compared to the control group.

A hypericin extract from **St John's wort** (*Hypericum perforatum*) was administered intralesionally 3–5 times per week in patients with basal cell carcinoma or squamous cell carcinoma.[20]

The lesions were subsequently irradiated with visible light. The authors claim that hypericin displayed selective tumor targeting. Clinical remissions were observed after 6–8 weeks. These preliminary results require confirmation in a rigorous RCT.

Supplements

A systematic review[21] of all clinical trials of **hydrazine sulfate** included three RCTs from the US. Many studies were methodologically weak. None of the RCTs suggested positive effects. Therefore it was concluded that 'The value of hydrazine sulfate as an antitumor agent – specifically its capacity to stabilize tumor size, cause tumor regression and improve survival – remains uncertain'.[21]

Laetrile has been tested in several rigorous clinical trials (e.g. [22]). No clinically relevant benefit was found, either in terms of cure, survival or stabilization of cancer growth or improvement of symptoms.

Several studies have tested the efficacy of **melatonin** supplementation for slowing tumor progression.[23] One RCT, for instance, suggested that patients with brain metastases treated with melatonin experienced a longer survival time compared with patients who received supportive care only.[24]

The (partly) herbal mixture **714-X** contains camphor, ammonium chloride and nitrate, sodium chloride, ethyl alcohol and water. It is being promoted in North America and Europe, particularly for prostate cancers. A systematic review found several animal studies but no clinical trials that supported its benefit.[25] The conclusion was that 'Side-effects appear to be minimal, but evidence of its effectiveness is limited'.

Shark cartilage is claimed to have antiangiogenesis effects that might inhibit malignant growth. Preclinical investigations supported this hypothesis.[26] Sixty patients with advanced cancers of various types were treated with shark cartilage (1 g/kg/day) as the sole anticancer therapy in an uncontrolled pilot study.[27] No complete or partial responses were noted. The authors concluded that shark cartilage, as a single agent, did not prolong life and had no beneficial effect on quality of life. There is no good evidence to show that shark cartilage is beneficial for cancer patients.

Preclinical studies have demonstrated that bovine **thymus extracts** restore lymphocyte function, improve immunological variables, activate natural killer cells and increase cytotoxic activity as well as mitogen-induced interferon levels in human lymphocytes. Moreover, animal experiments have suggested that thymus extracts inhibit tumor growth. A systematic review of all RCTs did not arrive at positive conclusions (Box 5.14). Injectable thymus preparations can cause severe allergic reactions and have the potential of transmitting serious infections.

Box 5.14
Systematic review
**Thymus extracts
for cancer**
Eur J Cancer 1997;33:
531–535

- Thirteen RCTs were included with a total of 802 patients suffering from various cancers

- Methodological quality was, on average, poor

- Five studies suggested benefits of thymus therapy

- Conclusion: 'no compelling evidence exists for the clinical efficacy of thymus therapy in human cancers'

Support group therapy

There is some, albeit not unequivocal evidence to suggest that psychosocial support groups (usually including therapeutic elements like relaxation or self-hypnosis) prolong survival rates in cancer patients.[23] One much quoted RCT showed that survival was 18 months longer in the experimental compared to the control group.[28]

Other therapies

One hundred and two patients with lung cancer were randomized into one group treated conventionally and one receiving additional individualized treatments accordingly to the principles of traditional **Chinese medicine**.[29] In the latter group, the 2-year survival rate was significantly greater than in the control group (56% vs 16%).

The Bristol Cancer Help Centre Study is a tragic example of the profound confusion that may result from seriously flawed research.[30] The trial apparently demonstrated that the survival rate of those breast cancer patients treated by an adjunctive **package of CAM modalities** was significantly poorer than for controls. Yet the study was not randomized and thus baseline differences are a probable cause for the finding.

A matched-pair comparison was conducted of survival of cancer patients receiving standard care with those receiving a **package of CAM** (autogenous immune-enhancing vaccine, bacille Calmette-Guérin, vegetarian diets and coffee enemas) in addition.[31] There were no differences in survival times but patients in the experimental group reported significantly poorer quality of life.

Eleven patients with inoperable pancreatic adenocarcinomas were treated with a **package of CAM** consisting of large oral doses of pancreatic enzymes, various nutritional supplements, 'detoxification' procedures and an organic diet.[32] The survival rates were 81% at one year and 45% at 2 years. The authors point out that this is far better than expected according to the literature. Thus this pilot study seems to warrant independent replication.

Collectively the evidence for CAM cancer 'cures' is far from compelling. For some therapies, trial results are encouraging but

Table 5.17
Summary of clinical evidence of cancer

Treatment	Weight of evidence	Direction of evidence	Serious safety concerns
Di Bella therapy	OO	⇩	Yes (see p 5)
Diets			
Gerson	O	⇗	Yes (see p 5)
Macrobiotic	O	⇘	Yes (see p 5)
Herbal medicine			
Aloe vera	O	⇗	Yes (see p 84)
Destagnation	O	⇧	Yes (see p 5)
Essiac	O	⇒	Yes (see p 5)
Mistletoe	OO	⇒	Yes (see p 137)
PC-SPES	O	⇗	Yes (see p 5)
Sho-saiko-to	O	⇧	Yes (see p 5)
St John's wort	O	⇧	Yes (see p 156)
Supplements			
Hydrazine sulfate	O	⇒	Yes (see p 5)
Laetrile	OO	⇩	Yes (see p 5)
Melatonin	O	⇗	Yes (see p 133)
'714-X'	O	⇘	Yes (see p 5)
Shark cartilage	O	⇩	Yes (see p 152)
Thymus extracts	OO	⇒	Yes (see p 173)
Support group therapy	O	⇗	No

require independent replication. Most treatments are associated with considerable risks, e.g. direct toxicity, reduction of quality of life or hindering access to conventional treatments.

Palliative/ supportive care

Many CAM modalities have the potential to increase well-being. Thus they are often used in palliative and supportive care for cancer patients.

Acupuncture
A systematic review strongly suggests that acupuncture has a useful role in reducing nausea induced by chemotherapy.[33]

Hypnotherapy
Several (mostly small) RCTs have demonstrated the usefulness of hypnotherapy in palliative cancer care. It has been shown to be effective in controlling pain and nausea/vomiting in various settings.[34] In children, hypnotherapy was more effective than attention control in reducing nausea.[35,36]

Relaxation
The effectiveness of relaxation therapy has been tested repeatedly. In one RCT, for instance, the program consisted of breathing exercises, muscle relaxation and imagery. This regimen was

significantly superior in controlling pain of cancer patients than no intervention.[37] In another RCT, 96 women with advanced breast cancer were randomized to receive either regular relaxation training and imagery or standard care only. The experimental group experienced better quality of life than the control group.[38]

Supplements

Alzoon is a herbal mixture of extracts of *petasites,* juniper, ferns, *brunellias* and dandelions that has been treated with oxygen and UV light. It is promoted (mostly but not exclusively) in Switzerland for the treatment of cancers. An uncontrolled study with 42 cancer patients suggested that 14% of the patients experienced a temporary improvement of quality of life and appetite.[39]

Oral mixtures of proteolytic **enzymes** (Wobe Mucos) are marketed in Germany with the controversial claim of benefiting the well-being of cancer patients. A systematic review included seven prospective clinical studies, including 692 patients in total.[40] The authors concluded: 'Enzyme therapy has generally been found to be a well-tolerated form of treatment for the relief of side-effects caused by other tumor therapies and for improving quality of life'. Due to methodological limitations of the primary data, this hypothesis still requires testing in rigorous RCTs.

Spiritual healing

Several CCTs have tested the effectiveness of **therapeutic touch** to reduce anxiety[41] or increase well-being[42] in cancer patients. Some of these studies have yielded positive results. Due to weaknesses in study design, it is unclear whether the observed effects were due to a specific therapeutic or a non-specific (placebo) effect.

Other therapies

Several CAM treatments might improve the well-being of patients with cancer. These include **mind–body programs** for stress, **acupuncture, acupressure** or **ginger** for nausea, **tai chi** and other gentle exercise techniques for gaining strength, **aromatherapy,** therapeutic **massage** and **relaxation techniques** to reduce stress, **herbal medicines** for depression, anxiety, indigestion and other symptoms, as well as **acupuncture** for pain. The evidence in this area is, however, often anecdotal, inconsistent and collectively unconvincing.[23] More details can be found in the respective chapters of this book.

Collectively, these data suggest that CAM may gain an important role in palliative/supportive cancer care. Unfortunately, the present evidence for most therapies is preliminary at best. This area clearly deserves more research; in particular, we need to know whether treatments are in any way superior to conventional methods of palliative/supportive cancer care. Until more data are available CAM can be cautiously recommended if the risk for harm is minimized through adequate supervision.

Table 5.18
Summary of clinical evidence of palliative care

Treatment	Weight of evidence	Direction of evidence	Serious safety concerns
Acupuncture (nausea)	OO	⇧	Yes (see p 29)
Hypnotherapy	O	⬈	Yes (see p 58)
Relaxation	O	⇧	No (see p 71)
Spiritual healing Therapeutic touch	O	⬈	No (see p 73)
Supplements Alzoon	O	⇨	Yes (see p 5)
Enzymes	O	⬈	No

Overall recommendation

Some dietary regimens aimed at cancer prevention carry little risk and are supported by reasonably good epidemiological evidence; they can thus be recommended provided the principle of a balanced diet is not jeopardized. CAM should be used in conjunction but not instead of mainstream cancer prevention (e.g. smoking cessation). Most CAM cancer 'cures' are burdened with important risks and offer little or no prospect of benefit; they should therefore not be recommended. Those CAM cancer 'cures' for which the evidence is encouraging invariably require further study before sound recommendations can be provided. Some palliative/supportive treatments might eventually gain a place in cancer care, but more research is needed to establish their value relative to conventional palliative care. Meanwhile, they can be cautiously recommended, particularly if cancer patients are strongly in favor of such an approach.

REFERENCES

1 Ernst E, Cassileth B R. The prevalence of complementary/alternative medicine in cancer. A systematic review. Cancer 1998;83:777–782

2 Ernst E. Can allium vegetables prevent cancer? Phytomedicine 1997;4:79–83

3 Kaegi E. Unconventional therapies for cancer: 2 Green tea. Can Med Assoc J 1998; 158:1621–1624

4 Storm S S, Yamamura Y, Duphorne C M. Phytoestrogen intake and prostate cancer: a case control study using a new database. Nutr Cancer 1999;33:20–25

5 Thorogood M, Mann J, Appleby P, McPherson K. Risk of death from cancer and ischaemic heart disease in meat and non meat-eaters. Br Med J 1994;108:1667–1671

6 Key T J, Fraser G E, Thorogood M. Mortality in vegetarians and non-vegetarians: detailed findings from a collaborative analysis of 5 prospective studies. Am J Clin Nutr 1999;70:5165–5245

7 Yun T-K, Choi S-Y. Non-organ specific cancer prevention of ginseng: a prospective study in Korea. Int J Epidemiol 1998;27:359–364

8 Italian Study Group for the Di Bella Multitherapy Trials. Evaluation of an unconventional cancer treatment (the Di Bella

multitherapy): results of phase II trials in Italy. Br Med J 1999;318:224–228

9 Buiatti A, Arniani S, Verdecchia A, Tomatis L and the Italian Cancer Registries. Results from a historical survey of the survival of cancer patients given Di Bella multitherapy. Cancer 1999;86:2143–2149

10 Ernst E, Cassileth B. Cancer diets, fads and facts. Cancer Prevent Int 1996;2:181–187

11 Hildenbrand G. Five-year survival rates of melanoma patients treated by diet therapy after the manner of Gerson: a retrospective review. Alt Ther Health Med 1995;4:29–37

12 Downer S M, Cody M M, McCluskey P et al. Pursuit and practice of complementary therapies by cancer patients receiving conventional treatment. Br Med J 1994; 309:86–89

13 Lissoni P, Giana L, Zerbini S, Trabattoni P, Rovelli F. Biotherapy with the pineal immunomodulating hormone melatonin versus melatonin plus aloe vera in untreatable advanced solid neoplasms. Natural Immunity 1998;16:27–33

14 Xu G Z, Cai W M, Qin D X et al. Chinese herb "destagnation" series I: Combination of radiation with destagnation in the treatment of nasopharyngeal carcinoma (NPC): a prospective randomized trial on 188 cases. Int J Rad Oncol Biol Phys 1989;16:297–300

15 Kaegi E. Unconventional therapies for cancer: 1 Essiac. Can Med Assoc J 1998;158:897–902

16 Kaegi E. Unconventional therapies for cancer: 3 Iscador. Can Med Assoc J 1998; 158:1157–1159

17 Kleijnen J, Knipschild P. Mistletoe treatment for cancer: review of controlled trials in humans. Phytomedicine 1994;1:255–260

18 De La Taille A, Hayek O R, Buttyan R, Bagiella E, Burchardt M, Katz A E. Effects of a phytotherapeutic agent, PC-SPES, on prostate cancer: a preliminary investigation on human cell lines and patients. Br J Urol Int 1999; 84:845–850

19 Oka H, Yamamoto S, Kuroki T et al. Prospective study of chemoprevention of hepatocellular carcinoma with Sho-saiko-to (TJ-9). Cancer 1995;76:743–749

20 Alecu M, Ursaciuc C, Halalau F et al. Photodynamic treatment of basal cell carcinoma and squamous cell carcinoma with hypericin. Anticancer Res 1998;18:4651–4654

21 Kaegi E. Unconventional therapies for cancer: 4 Hydrazine sulfate. Can Med Assoc J 1998; 158:897–902

22 Moertel C G, Fleming T R, Rubin J. A clinical trial of amygdalin (Laetrile) in the treatment of human cancer. New Engl J Med 1982; 306:201–206

23 Jacobson J S, Workman S B, Kronenberg F. Research on complementary/alternative medicine for patients with breast cancer: a review of the biomedical literature. J Clin Oncol 2000;18:668–683

24 Lissoni P. Barni S, Ardizzoa A. A randomized study with pineal hormone melatonin versus supportive care alone in patients with brain metastases due to solid neoplasms. Cancer 1994;73:699–701

25 Kaegi E. Unconventional therapies for cancer: 714-X. Can Med Assoc J 1998;158:1327–1329

26 Ernst E. Antiangiogenic shark cartilage as a treatment for cancer? Perfusion 1998;11:49

27 Miller D R, Anderson G T, Stark J J, Granick J L, Richardson D. Phase I/II trial of the safety and efficacy of shark cartilage in the treatment of advanced cancer. J Clin Oncol 1998; 16:3649–3655

28 Spiegel D, Bloom J R, Kraemer H C. Effect of psychosocial treatment on survival of patients with metastatic breast cancer. Lancet 1989;ii:888–891

29 Li J H. A study on treatment of lung cancer by combined therapy of traditional Chinese medicine and chemotherapy. Chung Kuo Chung Hsi I Chieh Ho Tsa Chih 1996;16:136–138

30 Bagenal F S, Easton D F, Harris E, Chilvers C E D, McElwain T J. Survival of patients with breast cancer attending Bristol Cancer Help Centre. Lancet 1990;336:606–610

31 Cassileth B R, Lusk E J, Guerry D et al. Survival and quality of life among patients receiving unproven as compared with conventional cancer therapy. New Engl J Med 1991;324:1180–1185

32 Gonzalez N J, Isaacs N L. Evaluation of pancreatic proteolytic enzyme treatment of adenocarcinoma of the pancreas, with nutrition and detoxification support. Nutri Cancer 1999;33:115–116

33 Vickers A J. Can acupuncture have specific effects on health – a systematic review of acupuncture trials. J Roy Soc Med 1996; 89:303–311

34 Syrjala K L, Cummings C, Donaldson G W. Hypnosis or cognitive behavioral training for the reduction of pain and nausea during cancer treatment: a controlled clinical trial. Pain 1992;50:237–238

35 Hawkins P J, Liossi C, Ewart W, Hatira P, Kosmidis V H, Varvutsi M. Hypnotherapy for control of anticipatory nausea and vomiting in children with cancer: preliminary findings. Psycho-Oncology 1995;4:101–106

36 Zeltzer L K, Dolgin M J, LeBaron S, LeBaron C. A randomized, controlled study of behavioral intervention for chemotherapy distress in children with cancer. Pediatrics 1991;88:34–42

37 Sloman R, Brown P, Aldana E, Chee E. The use of relaxation for the promotion of comfort and pain relief in persons with advanced cancer. Contemporary Nurse 1994;3:6–12

38 Walker L G, Walker M B, Ogston K et al. Psychological, clinical and pathological effects of relaxation training and guided imagery during primary chemotherapy. Br J Cancer 1999;80(1–2):262–268

39 Hauser S P. Alzoon – anticancer remedy or herbal concoction? Schweizerische Rundschau für Medizin Praxis 1997;86:1113–1115

40 Leipner J, Saller R. Systematic enzyme therapy in oncology. Forsch Komplementärmed Klass Naturheilkd 2000;7:45

41 Samarel N, Fawcett J, Davis M M, Ryan F M. Effects of dialogue and therapeutic touch on preoperative and postoperative experiences of breast cancer surgery: an exploratory study. Oncol Nurs Forum 1998;25:1369–1376

42 Giasson M, Bouchard L. Effect of therapeutic touch on the well-being of persons with terminal cancer. J Holistic Nurs 1998;16:383–398

CHRONIC FATIGUE SYNDROME

Synonyms/ subcategories

Akureyri disease, Iceland disease, myalgic encephalomyelitis, neurasthenia, postviral fatigue syndrome, Royal Free disease, Tapanui flu, yuppie flu.

Definition

A condition of severe disabling fatigue accompanied by a combination of symptoms typically including musculoskeletal pain, sleep disturbances and impairments of concentration and short-term memory.

CAM usage

According to a US survey,[1] massage and exercise were the forms of CAM employed most commonly for chronic fatigue syndrome (CFS). Acupuncture and kinesiology are also used.[2]

Clinical evidence

Exercise

Two RCTs provided evidence that graded exercise can produce improvements on measures of fatigue and functional capacity (Table 5.19). Graded exercise has also been a component of

Table 5.19 **RCTs of graded exercise for chronic fatigue syndrome**

Reference	Sample size	Interventions [regimen]	Result	Comment
Br Med J 1997;314: 1647–1652	66	A) Graded exercise [5×30 min/w for 3 mo] B) Flexibility & relaxation	A superior to B on fatigue & functional capacity	Improvements maintained at 12 mo follow-up
Br J Psychiatr 1998;172: 485–490	136	A) Exercise & 20 mg fluoxetine [3×20 min/w for 6 mo] B) Exercise & placebo C) Fluoxetine & therapist contact D) Therapist contact & placebo	A & B superior to C & D on fatigue & functional capacity	Drop-out rate higher in exercise than non-exercise groups

CONDITIONS

cognitive-behavioral therapy in at least two RCTs that both produced positive results.[3,4] None of these trials found evidence that graded exercise was harmful for CFS patients.

Table 5.20 **Double-blind RCTs of evening primrose oil for chronic fatigue syndrome**

Reference	Sample size	Interventions [dosage]	Result	Comment
Acta Neurol Scand 1990; 82:209–216	63	A) Evening primrose & fish oil [4 g/d for 3 mo] B) Placebo (liquid paraffin)	A superior to B on symptom ratings	Diagnosis was postviral fatigue syndrome not CFS
Acta Neurol Scand 1999; 99:112–116	50	A) Evening primrose & fish oil [4 g/d for 3 mo] B) Placebo (sunflower oil)	A no different to B on symptom ratings	Neither group improved significantly

Herbal medicine

Conflicting results have been reported by two placebo-controlled RCTs of oil of evening primrose (*Oenothera biennis*) combined with fish oil (Table 5.20). There were several key differences between these two trials, i.e. diagnosis, duration of illness and placebo, which may explain the discrepant results, so no conclusion can be drawn on the effectiveness of evening primrose oil for chronic fatigue syndrome. Other herbs have not been clinically investigated despite widespread use by herbalists.[5]

Homeopathy

A double-blind RCT (n=61) of classical homeopathy reported improvements in 33% of the homeopathic group compared with 4% of the placebo group based on self-assessments.[6] No statistical analysis was reported.

Spinal manipulation

A non-randomized trial (n=58) reported superior results with osteopathy (20 sessions over 12 months) than no intervention.[7] It is worth noting that patients had to pay for the osteopathy treatment.

Supplements

In an uncontrolled trial of 3 months of specific amino acid supplementation, 15 of 20 patients reported over 50% improvement in symptoms.[8] Energy and mental function were the areas of greatest improvement.

A small (n=14) double-blind, placebo-controlled, crossover RCT was conducted of an intravenous combination of folic acid, bovine liver extract and vitamin B_{12} given for one week.[9] A substantial placebo response was observed, but no difference between the interventions.

A large double-blind RCT (n=326) of chronic postinfectious fatigue patients investigated the effect of isobutyryl-thiamine disulfide.[10] After 4 weeks of treatment, no improvements were observed with doses of 400 g or 600 g daily compared with placebo.

L-carnitine was compared with amantadine in a crossover RCT (n=30) for 2 months.[11] Clinical improvements were reported for L-carnitine but not amantadine, while tolerability was far superior with L-carnitine.

In a double-blind, placebo-controlled RCT (n=32), intravenous **magnesium** improved energy, pain and emotional symptoms.[12] However, subsequent open studies found no magnesium deficiency in CFS patients and no benefit from magnesium injections.[13,14]

Oral **nicotinamide adenine dinucleotide** (NADH) (10 mg daily for 4 weeks) produced modest improvements in symptoms in a small (n=26) crossover placebo-controlled RCT.[15] No severe adverse events were reported.

Other therapies

Relaxation was used in the control arm of an RCT.[4] It was a successful treatment in 19% of patients, which was significantly less than cognitive-behavior therapy.

Table 5.21
Summary of clinical evidence for chronic fatigue syndrome

Treatment	Weight of evidence	Direction of evidence	Serious safety concerns
Exercise	OO	⇧	Yes (see p 5)
Herbal medicine			
Evening primrose oil	OO	⇨	Yes (see p 104)
Homeopathy	O	⬀	No (see p 55)
Spinal manipulation			
Osteopathy	O	⬀	Yes (see p 65)
Supplements			
Amino acids	O	⬀	No
Folic acid	O	⇩	Yes (see p 5)
Isobutyryl-thiamine disulfide	O	⇩	No
L-carnitine	O	⬀	No (see p 172)
Magnesium	O	⬂	Yes (see p 5)
NADH	O	⬀	No

Overall recommendation

For most complementary therapies there is little positive clinical evidence for chronic fatigue syndrome. This is unsurprising for a condition known to resist most forms of treatment. However, promising evidence is accumulating for graded exercise, although its effectiveness is likely to be enhanced by adjunctive cognitive-behavioral therapy.

CONDITIONS

REFERENCES

1 Astin J A. Why patients use alternative medicine. JAMA 1998;279:1548–1553

2 Az S, Gregg V H, Jones D. Chronic fatigue syndrome: sufferers' evaluation of medical support. J Roy Soc Med 1997;90:250–254

3 Sharpe M C, Hawton K, Simkin S et al. Cognitive behavioural therapy for the chronic fatigue syndrome: a randomised controlled trial. Br Med J 1996;312:22–26

4 Deale A, Chalder T, Marks L, Wessely S. Cognitive behaviour therapy for chronic fatigue syndrome: a randomised controlled trial. Am J Psychiatr 1997;154:408–414

5 Beatty C. Prescriptions used by medical herbalists in the treatment of chronic fatigue syndrome and depression. Eur J Herb Med 1999;4:35–37

6 Awdry R. Homeopathy may help ME. Int J Alt Compl Med 1996;14:12–16

7 Perrin R N, Edwards J, Hartley P. An evaluation of the effectiveness of osteopathic treatment on symptoms associated with myalgic encephalomyelitis. A preliminary report. J Med Engineering Technol 1998;22:1–13

8 Bralley J A, Lord R S. Treatment of chronic fatigue syndrome with specific amino acid supplementation. J Appl Nutr 1994;46:74–78

9 Kaslow J E, Rucker L, Onishi R. Liver extract–folic acid–cyanocobalamin versus placebo for chronic fatigue syndrome. Arch Intern Med 1989;149:2501–2503

10 Tiev K P, Cabane J, Imbert J C. Treatment of chronic postinfectious fatigue: randomised double-blind study of two doses of sulbutiamine (400–600 mg/day) versus placebo. Revue de Médecine Interne 1999;20:912–918

11 Plioplys A V, Plioplys S. Amantadine and L-carnitine treatment of chronic fatigue syndrome. Neuropsychobiology 1997; 35:16–23

12 Cox I M, Campbell M J, Dowson D. Red blood cell magnesium and chronic fatigue syndrome. Lancet 1991;337:757–760

13 Gantz N M. Magnesium and chronic fatigue. Lancet 1991;338:66

14 Clague J E, Edwards R H T, Jackson M J. Intravenous magnesium loading in chronic fatigue syndrome. Lancet 1992;340:124–125

15 Forsyth L M, Preuss H G, MacDowell A L et al. Therapeutic effects of oral NADH on the symptoms of patients with chronic fatigue syndrome. Ann Allergy Asthma Immunol 1999;82:185–191

FURTHER READING

Chaudhuri A, Behan W M H, Behan P O. Chronic fatigue syndrome. Proc Roy Coll Physicians Edinb 1998;28:150–163
Concise but thorough overview of the current state of knowledge of chronic fatigue syndrome.

CHRONIC VENOUS INSUFFICIENCY

Synonyms   Post-thrombotic syndrome; post-thrombophlebitic syndrome.

Definition   Chronic inadequate drainage of venous blood characterized by edema, dermatosclerosis and the feeling of pain, fatigue and tenseness in the lower extremities.

CAM usage   Herbal medicine and hydrotherapy are popular complementary therapies for this condition, particularly in some European countries.

Clinical evidence

Herbal medicine

A double-blind RCT investigated the effects of **buckwheat** (*Fagopyrum esculentum*) tea in 67 patients.[1] One cup of tea, made from one tea bag, was ingested three times daily for 12 weeks. Each bag contained 1.8 g buckwheat herb, amounting to about 270 mg total rutin intake daily. Some beneficial effects were reported for lower leg volume and symptom scores, which were, however, not different from placebo.

The clinical evidence on **butcher's broom** (*Ruscus aculeatus*) is mostly based on RCTs using combination preparations also including hesperidine.[2-4] These studies report some beneficial effects such as edema reduction at the foot and ankle region and a reduction of venous capacity as well as an improvement of symptoms.

One double-blind RCT investigated the effects of a combination preparation containing **ginkgo** (*Ginkgo biloba*) extract, troxerutin and heptaminol.[5] Forty-eight female patients were assessed and received either 625 mg of the preparation or placebo daily for 4 weeks. Clinical symptom scores were not significantly different between treatment and control group. The authors, however, report some beneficial effects on endothelium alterations.

In a placebo-controlled double-blind RCT 87 patients with chronic venous insufficiency (CVI) were given either 30 or 60 mg **gotu kola** (*Centella asiatica*) extract twice daily for 60 days.[6] The results suggest an improvement of microcirculatory parameters such as transcutaneous PO_2 compared with baseline. In a clinical placebo-controlled double-blind RCT 94 outpatients received either 120 mg or 60 mg titrated extract of *Centella asiatica* daily for 2 months.[7] Significant beneficial effects are reported for the symptoms of heaviness in the lower limbs and edema compared with placebo. These findings are corroborated by another double-blind RCT, reporting a significant improvement of night cramps, pruritus and edema after the administration of 60 mg gotu kola extract for 30 days compared with placebo.[8]

A systematic review found compelling evidence for the effectiveness of oral **horse chestnut** (*Aesculus hippocastanum*) seed extract (Box 5.15). The reviewed studies assessed predominantly patients with mild to moderate forms of CVI. Leg edema and symptoms such as pain, tenseness and fatigue were significantly reduced compared with placebo.

Box 5.15
Systematic review
Horse chestnut for chronic venous insufficiency
Arch Dermatol
1998;134:1356–1360

- Thirteen RCTs including 1083 patients
- Trial quality was generally good to excellent
- Seven placebo-controlled trials suggest superiority
- Four trials compared with hydroxyethylrutosides suggest similar effectiveness
- One trial compared with compression therapy suggests similar effectiveness

CONDITIONS

One large double-blind RCT (n=260) compared 360 and 720 mg of **red vine** (*Vitis vinifera*) leaf extract daily with placebo in patients with mild to moderate forms of CVI.[9] This study reports a reduction of lower leg volume and calf circumference compared with placebo and an improvement of CVI symptoms after a treatment period of 12 weeks.

Hydrotherapy

The results of two RCTs which applied cold water stimuli alone or in combination with warm water application suggest beneficial effects for this condition (Table 5.22). The effects of mineral thermal water containing carbon dioxide have been assessed in another RCT.[10] It is reported that venous function was markedly improved after 20 minutes of bathing compared with baseline. Overall, these studies indicate that hydrotherapeutic interventions are of some benefit for patients with CVI.

Table 5.22 **Parallel-armed RCTs of hydrotherapy for chronic venous insufficiency**

Reference	Sample size	Interventions [regimen]	Result	Comment
Vasa 1991; 20:147–152	61	A) Cold water applications [5×w for 24 d] B) No treatment	A superior to B for symptoms of cramps and pain	Beneficial effects also on ankle and calf circumference
Eur J Phys Med Rehabil 1993;3: 123–124	122	A) Cold (12–18°C) and warm (35–38°C) water applications [10 min/d for 24 d] B) No treatment	A superior to B for symptoms of cramps, pain and pruritus	Beneficial effects on foot volume, ankle and calf circumference

Overall recommendation

The evidence for the effectiveness of horse chestnut seed extract is relatively convincing. Given the low frequency of adverse effects and suggestions that it may be as effective as conventional compression therapy, it seems worthy of consideration. Other therapies where the evidence looks promising but not compelling include butcher's broom, gotu kola and hydrotherapy. The current evidence for the effectiveness of other complementary therapies for this condition is weak.

Table 5.23
Summary of clinical evidence for chronic venous insufficiency

Treatment	Weight of evidence	Direction of outcome	Serious safety concerns
Herbal medicine			
Buck wheat	O	⬀	Yes (see p 5)
Butcher's broom	OO	⬀	Yes (see p 167)
Ginkgo	O	⬂	Yes (see p 115)
Gotu kola	OO	⬆	Yes (see p 169)
Horse chestnut	OOO	⬆	Yes (see p 127)
Red vine leaf	O	⬆	Yes (see p 5)
Hydrotherapy	OO	⬆	Yes (see p 5)

REFERENCES

1 Ihme N, Kiesewetter H, Jung F, Hoffmann K H, Birk A, Müller A, Grützner K I. Leg edema protection from a buckwheat herb tea in patients with chronic venous insufficiency: a single blind, randomised, placebo-controlled clinical trial. Eur J Clin Pharmacol 1996; 50:443–447

2 Rudofsky G, Diehm C, Gruß J-D, Hartmann M, Schultz-Ehrenburg H-K, Bisler H. Chronisch venöse Insuffizienz. Münch Med Wochenschr 1990;132:205–210

3 Weindorf N, Schultz-Ehrenburg U. Kontrollierte Studie zur oralen Venentonisierung der primären Varikosis mit Ruscus aculeatus und Trimethylherperidinchalkon. Z Hautkr 1987; 62:28–38

4 Cappelli R, Nicora M, Di Perri T. Use of extract of ruscus aculeatus in venous disease in the lower limbs. Drugs Exp Clin Res 1988; 14:277–283

5 Janssens D, Michiels C, Guillaume G, Cuisinier B, Louagie Y, Remacle J. Increase in circulating endothelial cells in patients with primary chronic venous insufficiency: protective effect of Ginkgor Fort in a randomized double-blind, placebo-controlled clinical trial. J Cardiovasc Pharmacol 1999; 33:7–11

6 Cesarone M R, Laurora G, De Sanctis M T, Incandela L, Grimaldi R, Marelli C, Belcaro G. The microcirculatory activity of Centella asiatica in venous insufficiency.

A double-blind study. Minerva Cardioangiologica 1994;42:299–304

7 Pointel J P, Boccalon H, Cloarec M, Ledevehat C, Joubert M. Titrated extract of Centella asiatica (TECA) in the treatment of venous insufficiency of the lower limbs. Angiology 1987;38:46–50

8 Allegra C, Pollari G, Criscuolo A, Bonifacio M, Tabassi D. L'estratto di Centella asiatica nelle flebopatie degli arti inferiori. Clin Ther 1981; 99:507–513

9 Kiesewetter H, Koscielny J, Kalus U et al. Efficacy of orally administered extract of red vine leaf AS 195 (folia vitis viniferae) in chronic venous insufficiency (stages I–II). A randomized, double-blind, placebo-controlled trial. Arzneimittelforschung 2000;50:109–117

10 Hartmann B, Drews B, Bassenge E. Effects of bathing in CO_2-containing thermal water on the venous hemodynamics of healthy persons with venous diseases. Phys Med Rehabil Kurortmed 1993; 3:153–157

FURTHER READING

London N J M, Nash R. Varicose veins. Br Med J 2000;320:1391–1394
This review article provides reliable information on the symptoms and clinical management of varicose veins.

CONGESTIVE HEART FAILURE

Synonyms/ subcategories   Heart failure, cardiac failure, left ventricular failure, right ventricular failure.

Definition   A state in which circulatory congestion exists as a result of insufficient pumping actions of the heart.

CAM usage   One classic conventional drug for congestive heart failure (CHF) with a plant origin is digitalis. Recently, graded physical exercise has been advocated for this condition. However, neither treatment can be considered to constitute CAM. The CAM treatment modalities that are most frequently recommended for CHF are herbal medicines and various other supplements. A recent survey suggests that garlic, ginger and parsley are most frequently used by CHF patients.[1] For none of these is there any data from rigorous clinical trials to show that it is effective for CHF.

CONDITIONS

Clinical evidence

Acupuncture

One small (n=12) RCT suggested that auriculo-acupuncture might improve left cardiac function in patients with dilating cardiomyopathy and CHF.[2] This study is methodologically weak and requires replication before its results can be accepted as credible.

Herbal medicine

A CCT of **ginseng** (*Panax ginseng*) with three parallel arms included 45 CHF patients.[3] The first group was treated with digoxin, the second with ginseng and the third with a combination of both. Hemodynamic measurements suggested that the results of the two groups treated with ginseng were better than those treated with only digoxin. This trial has several methodological flaws and requires confirmation.

Hawthorn (*Crataegus*) has long been known to possess digitalis-like effects. Moreover, it has vasodilatory and antiarrhythmic properties. An overview of placebo-controlled RCTs showed that it is effective in reducing objective signs and subjective symptoms of CHF in NYHA stage II.[4] Moreover, several comparative clinical trials imply that it is as effective as conventional drugs.[4]

Sunitang is a traditional Chinese remedy used for circulatory disorder. One CCT implied that it might be useful in patients with CHF.[5] Due to methodological shortcomings this study requires confirmation.

The Ayurvedic herb ***Terminalia arjuna*** has been tested in a crossover RCT including 12 patients suffering from CHF NYHA stage IV;[6] 500 mg bark extract was given every 8 hours for 2 weeks in addition to standard therapy. The results show that in the experimental phase of this study there was a significant improvement of all relevant signs and symptoms of CHF. After the trial, all patients received treatment for up to 28 months and the clinical improvement continued, including amelioration in quality of life. These most promising findings require confirmation.

Supplements

Nitric oxide formed by the action of **L-arginine** increases blood flow and could therefore have positive effects in CHF. An RCT tested this hypothesis by treating 15 CHF patients for 6 weeks with 5.6–12.6 g/d oral L-arginine-containing supplements or with placebo following a crossover design.[7] The results show the expected increase in blood flow and significant improvement of functional status was evidenced in an increased 6-minute walking distance (390 ±91 vs 433 ±86 m).

Co-enzyme Q10 is being recommended for, amongst other conditions, hypertension, coronary heart disease and CHF. Several trials, most of which have methodological weaknesses, have suggested that it is effective for CHF.[8] However, two recent rigorous RCTs demonstrated that co-enzyme Q10 supplementation does not improve left ventricular function or quality of life in CHF patients.[9,10]

Other therapies

A small uncontrolled study suggested that a one-hour session of **qi gong** induces beneficial hemodynamic acute effects in CHF patients.[11] This finding requires confirmation in an RCT. A recent uncontrolled pilot study with a small (n=8) sample size showed no relevant benefit of **guided imagery** for patients with congestive heart failure NYHA III.[12]

Overall recommendation

There is conclusive evidence for hawthorn as a symptomatic therapy in mild to moderate CHF. Some tantalizing data exist for *Terminalia arjuna,* but the weight of the evidence is not strong enough for a firm recommendation. The evidence regarding co-enzyme Q10 is ambiguous. These treatments are unlikely to be associated with serious risks when taken under medical supervision. Conventional treatments for CHF are well established and of proven effectiveness. Thus the above herbal medicines should only be prescribed in special cases, e.g. if the patient insists on a 'natural' remedy.

Table 5.24
Summary of clinical evidence for congestive heart failure

Treatment	Weight of evidence	Direction of evidence	Serious safety concerns
Acupuncture	O	⬀	Yes (see p 29)
Herbal medicine			
Ginseng	O	⬀	Yes (see p 88)
Hawthorn	OOO	⬆	Yes (see p 124)
Sunitang	O	⬀	Yes (see p 5)
Terminalia arjuna	O	⬆	Yes (see p 5)
Supplements			
Arginine	O	⬆	No
Co-enzyme Q10	OO	⇨	Yes (see p 97)

REFERENCES

1 Ackman M L, Campbell J B, Buzak K A. Use of nonprescription medications by patients with congestive heart failure. Ann Pharmacother 1999;33:674–679

2 Zhou J R. Effect of auriculo-acupuncture plus needle embedding in heart point on left cardiac, humoral and endocrine function. Chung Kuo Chung Hsi I Chieh Ho Tsa Chih K 1993;13:153–154

3 Ding D Z, Shen T K, Cui Y Z. The effects of red ginseng on the congestive heart failure and its mechanism. Chung Kuo Ching Hsi I Chieh Ho Tsa Chih 1995;15:325–327

4 Weihmayr T, Ernst E. Therapeutic effectiveness of Crataegus. Fortschr Med 1996;114:27–29

5 Chen H C, Hsieh M T. Hemodynamic effects of orally administered Sunitang in humans. Clin Pharmacol Therapeut 1987;41:496–501

6 Bharani A, Ganguly A, Bhargava K D. Salutary effect of Terminalia Arjuna in patients with severe refractory heart failure. Int J Cardiol 1995;49:191–199

7 Rector R S, Bank A J, Mullen K A, Tscumperlin L K, Sih R, Pillai K, Kubo S H. Randomized, double-blind, placebo-controlled study of supplemental oral L-arginine in patients with heart failure. Circulation 1996;93:2135–2141

8 Ernst E. The cardiovascular 'miracle drug' ubiquinone. Herz Kreislauf 1999;31:79–81

9 Watson P S, Scalia G M, Galbraith A, Burstow D J, Bett N. Coenzyme Q did not affect severe heart failure or quality of life. J Am Coll Cardiol 1999;33:1549–1552

10 Khatta M, Alexander B S, Krichten C M, Fisher M L, Freudenberger R, Robinson S W,

Gottlieb S S. The effect of Coenzyme Q10 in patients with congestive heart failure. Ann Intern Med 2000;132:636–640

11 Qian L, Zhou Q, Wang Z, Huang J, Yi F. Effects of Qigong Waiqi on hemodynamics and left ventricular systolic function in patients with congestive heart failure.

Bull Hunan Medical University 1993;18:397–399

12 Klaus L, Beniaminovitz A, Choi L, Greenfield F, Whitworth G L, Oz M C, Mancini D M. Pilot study of guided imagery use in patients with severe heart failure. Am J Cardiol 2000;86:101–104

CONSTIPATION

Synonyms   Obstipation, costiveness.

Definition   A condition characterized by infrequent or incomplete bowel movements.

CAM usage   Herbal medicine is an option frequently used to treat constipation.

Clinical evidence

Acupuncture

Eight patients were assessed during a control period and a treatment period of 3 weeks.[1] Six sessions of acupuncture were administered using needles that were stimulated electrically at 10 Hz. There were no significant differences between control and treatment periods in stool frequency and colonic transit time.

Biofeedback

A number of RCTs have assessed the effectiveness of biofeedback for adult and pediatric patients (Tables 5.25 & 5.26). Collectively these studies imply that biofeedback has beneficial effects for the treatment of constipation. One study suggests that biofeedback is an effective long-term treatment for adult patients,[2] while another reports that long-term recovery rates in children are not increased above those achieved with conventional treatment.[3]

Herbal medicine

A herbal combination preparation containing *Aloe vera*, psyllium and celandin was tested in a double-blind RCT.[4] Thirty-five patients received either up to three capsules (1.5 g) of the herbal preparation or placebo daily for a treatment period of 28 days. There was a significant increase in bowel movements in the treatment group compared with baseline, which was not different from placebo. Overall, significantly more patients in the treatment group considered themselves improved compared with those in the placebo group.

An RCT assessed the effects of a liquid **Ayurvedic** herbal preparation (Misrakasneham) including *Clitoria ternatea*, *Curcuma longa* and *Vitis vinifera* as well as castor oil in the management of opioid-induced constipation.[5] Fifty cancer patients received either the Ayurvedic herbal preparation or up to 360 mg of purified senna extract daily for 14 days. Seventeen of 20 patients

Table 5.25 **RCTs of biofeedback for adult patients for constipation**

Reference	Sample size	Interventions [regimen]	Result	Comment
Am J Gastroenterol 1994;89: 1021–1026	20	A) Electromyographic biofeedback training (EBT) B) Balloon biofeedback [1 session/w for 8 w]	A superior to B in overall improvement	Advised to train at home; small sample size
Gut 1995;37: 95–99	60	A) Muscular training and EBT [1–7 sessions] B) Muscular training [1–4 sessions]	In A 14 of 31 patients improved and in B 12 of 28. Reduction of time spent straining in B compared with baseline	Similar outcome in the two treatment groups
Dis Colon Rectum 1997; 40:889–895	26	A) Anal manometry biofeedback [1–2 session/w for a max. of 10 sessions] B) Sphincter EBT [1–2 session/w for a max. of 10 sessions]	Stool frequency increased in A and B	No significant intergroup difference in terms of efficacy
Dis Colon Rectum 1999; 42:1388–1393	36	A) Intraanal EBT B) EBT plus intrarectal balloon training C) EBT plus home training D) EBT, balloon training and home training	Bowel movements significantly increased in A, B and D compared with baseline	No exact description of treatment regimen

who completed the study in the Ayurveda group had satisfactory bowel movements as compared with 11 of 16 in the senna group. There were no significant intergroup differences.

A double-blind RCT[6] assessed the effectiveness of **psyllium** (*Plantago ovata*) for chronic constipation in 20 patients, of whom 10 had associated irritable bowel syndrome. Patients received either 20 g of psyllium extract or placebo daily for one month. Stools per week and fecal weight increased significantly in the treatment group compared with baseline, while there were no such changes in the placebo group.

Massage

The evidence for abdominal massage has been assessed in a systematic review (Box 5.16). Concerns relate to the heterogeneity of the studies in terms of trial design, patient samples and type of massage used. The review cautiously concludes that abdominal massage could be a promising treatment option for this condition.

Table 5.26 **RCTs of biofeedback for pediatric patients for constipation**

Reference	Sample size	Interventions [regimen]	Result	Comment
J Pediatr 1990;116: 214–222	43	A) EBT [1 session/w for a max. of 6 sessions plus conventional treatment (milk of magnesia, dietary fiber) for 6 mo] B) Conventional treatment	A superior to B for defecation dynamics	Balloon defecation did not improve in those who learned normal defecation dynamics
Lancet 1996; 348: 776–778	192	A) Biofeedback plus conventional treatment (dietary advice, toilet training, laxatives) [5 sessions over 6 w] B) Conventional treatment	A superior to B for defecation dynamics	No intergroup differences after 1 y of follow-up
Ann Behav Med 1998; 20:70–76	87	A) EBT plus toilet training, laxatives and enemas B) Toilet training plus laxatives and enemas C) Conventional treatment (milk of magnesia, senna syrup, enemas)	A and B superior to C in soiling B superior to A and C for laxative use and cost	Patients were assessed for 3 mo following the start of the treatment

Box 5.16
Systematic review
Abdominal massage for constipation
Forsch Komplementärmed 1999;6:149–151

- One RCT and three CCTs including 101 patients

- Trial quality was low

- Two CCTs report an improvement in stool frequency and stool consistency while this is not corroborated by data from an RCT

- Conclusion is limited due to the small number and low quality of available trials

Reflexology

One hundred and thirty postoperative women were randomized to receive one 15-minute session daily for 5 days of either reflexology, leg/foot massage or talking.[7] There were no significant intergroup differences in stool frequency after the treatment period and after 4 days of follow-up.

Other therapies

A CCT investigated the acute effects of **mineral water** containing sulfate (2754 mg/l) on bowel movements and stool consistency.[8] Thirty-four healthy volunteers received either 500 ml mineral water or tap water (29 mg/l sulfate). Significant beneficial effects are reported for the time to bowel movement and stool consistency in favor of mineral water compared with tap water.

Colonic irrigation is often advocated for constipation but no trial data exist and the risk–benefit ratio is uncertain.

Table 5.27
Summary of clinical evidence for constipation

Treatment	Weight of evidence	Direction of evidence	Serious safety concerns
Acupuncture	O	⇩	Yes (see p 29)
Biofeedback	OOO	⇧	No (see p 42)
Herbal medicine			
Aloe vera	O	⬈	Yes (see p 84)
Ayurveda	O	⬈	Yes (see p 52)
Psyllium	O	⬈	Yes (see p 170)
Massage	OO	⬈	No (see p 60)
Reflexology	O	⇩	No (see p 68)

Overall recommendation

The evidence for the short-term effectiveness of biofeedback training is convincing. Given its relative safety and the risks of long-term conventional treatments, it is a reasonable option for constipated patients. In adult patients there is no concrete evidence for its long-term effectiveness, while conventional treatment is also often limited to short-term relief. In pediatric patients the evidence suggests some benefit from adding biofeedback to conventional treatment, but there seems to be little long-term benefit. Encouraging evidence exists for abdominal massage and given its relative safety, it may be beneficial for some patients. For other treatment options the evidence is insufficient for any firm judgement.

REFERENCES

1 Klauser A G, Rubach A, Bertsche O, Müller-Lissner S A. Body acupuncture: effect on colonic function in chronic constipation. Zeitschr für Gastroenterologie 1993; 31:605–608

2 Chiotakakou-Faliakou E, Kamm M A, Roy A J, Storrie J B, Turner I C. Biofeedback provides long term benefit for patients with intractable, slow and normal transit constipation. Gut 1998; 42:517–521

3 Loening-Baucke V. Biofeedback treatment for chronic constipation and encopresis in childhood: long-term outcome. Pediatrics 1995;96:105–110

4 Odes H S, Madar Z. A double-blind trial of a celandin, aloe vera and psyllium laxative preparation in adult patients with constipation. Digestion 1991;49:65–71

5 Ramaesh P R. Kumar K S, Rajagopal M R, Balachandran P, Warrier P K. Managing morphine-induced constipation: a controlled comparison of an Ayurvedic formulation and senna. J Pain Symptom Manage 1998; 16:240–244

6 Tomás-Ridocci M, Añón R, Minguez M, Zaragoza A, Ballester J, y Benages A. Eficacia del Plantago ovaata como regulador del tránsito intestinal. Estudio doble ciego comparativo frente a placebo. Rev Esp Enf Digest 1992;82:17–22

7. Kesselring A, Spichiger E, Müller M. Fussreflexzonenmassage. Pflege 1998; 11:213–218

CONDITIONS

8 Gutenbrunner C, Gundermann G. Kontrollierte Studie über die abführende Wirkung eines Heilwassers. Z Allg Med 1998;74:648–651

FURTHER READING

Moriarty K J, Irving M H. Constipation. Br Med J 1992;304:1237–1240

This review article provides reliable information on the assessment and treatment of constipation.

DEPRESSION

Synonyms/ subcategories

Depressive disorder, depressive illness, dysthymic disorder, neurotic depression, psychotic depression.

Definition

A temporary or chronic mental state characterized by feelings of sadness, loneliness, despair, low self-esteem and self-reproach.

CAM usage

Surveys from the US have identified depression as one of the most common reasons for using CAM. The most popular therapies are exercise, herbal medicine, relaxation and spiritual healing.[1,2]

Clinical evidence

Acupuncture

Three Chinese RCTs indicated similar efficacy between electro-acupuncture and tricyclic antidepressants.[3–5] Three studies using sham or non-specific acupuncture as a control have reported conflicting findings (Table 5.28). It appears that acupuncture treatment is associated with reductions in depressive symptoms, but whether there is a specific effect of needling on depression is unclear.

Autogenic training

An RCT (n=55) was conducted comparing autogenic training (twice weekly for 10 weeks) with no intervention and

Table 5.28 **Sham-controlled RCTs of acupuncture for depression**

Reference	Sample size	Interventions [regimen]	Result	Comment
Psychol Sci 1998;9: 397–401	38	A) Specific acupuncture [1–2 session/w over 8 w] B) Non-specific acupuncture C) Waiting list	A superior to B but no different to C	Therapists were blind to the diagnosis
Fortschr Neurol Psychiatr 2000;68: 137–144	56	A) Acupuncture [10 sessions over 2 w] B) Sham acupuncture	A superior to B	Sample included 43 depressed patients & 13 with anxiety disorder
J Affect Disord 2000; 57:73–81	70	A) Adjunctive acupuncture [3 session/w for 4 w] B) Non-specific adjunctive acupuncture C) No adjunctive intervention	A superior to C but no different to B	All patients treated with mianserin

psychotherapy.[6] Reductions in depression with autogenic training were similar to psychotherapy, but not significantly greater than with no treatment. Subsequently, autogenic training was combined with psychotherapy, which was no more effective than psycho-therapy alone. The authors warned that autogenic training is not generally an appropriate treatment for depression.

Exercise

A large body of unanimously positive evidence exists for the antidepressant effects of exercise. The majority of studies are not of high quality, but over a dozen RCTs collectively provide convincing evidence of efficacy in clinically depressed patients. Two metaanalyses have found significant effects after pooling the data. One included 80 studies of any design with all types of participant.[7] The other was restricted to controlled trials with clinically depressed patients (Box 5.17). The indications are that both aerobic and non-aerobic forms of exercise are effective. Three RCTs have suggested that aerobic exercise may be as effective as psychological or pharmacological treatment (Table 5.29).

Box 5.17
Metaanalysis
Exercise for depression
J Sport Exer Psychol
1998;20:339–357

- Thirty controlled trials including 2158 patients

- Depression as primary disorder or secondary to other psychiatric disorder

- Comparison groups were mainly waiting lists or psycho-therapy

- Trial quality ranged from good to poor

- Significant effect of exercise (mean effect size -0.72; SE 0.10)

- All types of exercise appear to have similar effects

Table 5.29 RCTs of exercise compared with psychiatric treatment for depression

Reference	Sample size	Interventions [regimen]	Result	Comment
Int J Ment Health 1986;13: 148–177	74	A) Running [2×45 min/w for 12w] B) Meditation/relaxation C) Group psychotherapy	A no different to B or C	Improvements maintained at 9 mo
Cog Ther Res 1987;11: 241–251	49	A) Running [3×20 min/w for 10w] B) Cognitive therapy C) Combination of A & B	A no different to B or C	Improvements maintained at 4 mo
Arch Intern Med 1999;159: 2349–2356	156	A) Walking/jogging [3×45 min/w for 16w] B) Sertraline [200 mg/d] C) Combination of A & B	A no different to B or C; less relapse in A after 6 mo	Patients were all ≥50 years

CONDITIONS

Whether the antidepressant effects demonstrated are specific to the exercise itself or are due to associated variables is unclear.

Herbal medicine

There is compelling evidence for the efficacy of St John's wort (*Hypericum perforatum*) versus placebo in mild to moderate depression from metaanalysis (Box 5.18) and systematic reviews including subsequent trials.[8,9] The notion that it is as effective as conventional antidepressants has been strengthened by recent RCTs (Table 5.30). Despite one RCT with severely depressed patients,[10] its value in severe or other forms of depression remains unclear.

Box 5.18
Metaanalysis
St John's wort for depression
Cochrane Library 1998

- Twenty-seven RCTs including 2291 patients

- Mainly mild-moderate depression

- Trial quality generally good

- Fourteen placebo-controlled trials on monopreparations analyzed (pooled rate ratio 2.47; CI 1.69 to 3.61)

- Five compared with other antidepressants (1.01; CI 0.87 to 1.16)

- Adverse events in 26% of St. John's wort groups and 45% of other antidepressants

Table 5.30 **Double-blind RCTs of St John's wort compared with conventional antidepressants**

Reference	Sample size	Interventions [dosage]	Result	Comment
Drug Res 1999;49: 289–296	149	A) St John's wort [800 mg/d for 6 w] B) Fluoxetine [20 mg]	A and B equivalent	ADRs reported for St John's wort similar to fluoxetine
Br Med J 1999;319: 1534–1539	263	A) St John's wort [1050 mg/d for 8 w] B) Imipramine [100 mg] C) Placebo	A and B equivalent; both superior to C	St John's wort dose quite high; impramine dose quite low
Int Clin Psycho- pharmacol 2000;15: 61–68	240	A) St John's wort [500 mg/d for 6 w] B) Fluoxetine [20 mg]	A and B equivalent	Analysis of ADRs favored St John's wort
Br Med J 2000;321: 536–539	324	A) St John's wort [500 mg/d for 6 w] B) Imipramine [150 mg]	A no different to B	Five times as many withdrawals due to ADRs with imipramine than St John's wort

Massage

Massage (once daily for 5 days) was more effective than watching relaxing videos in an RCT (n=72) involving children and adolescent inpatients with depression and adjustment disorder.[11] Improvements were reported in symptoms of depression and anxiety, night time sleep and cortisol levels.

Music therapy

An RCT of depressed elderly patients (n=30) found superior results with a music-based intervention (once weekly for 2 months) than no treatment.[12] The intervention involved various therapeutic modalities (progressive muscle relaxation, massage, exercise, guided imagery, art therapy, visualization) all performed to carefully selected music. As well as music being just one of many parts of the intervention, therapist attention was not controlled for in this study. Other RCTs with depressed adolescent females who listened to rock music while control groups received massage[13] or simply relaxed[14] reported changes to physiological and biochemical parameters but not mood or behavior. The role of music as a therapeutic option remains unclear.

Relaxation

Three small RCTs have suggested that relaxation training is superior to no treatment and potentially similar to cognitive-behavioral therapy (Table 5.31) Clearly, non-specific effects are difficult to control for with this sort of therapy. Nonetheless, the evidence can be considered promising.

Table 5.31 **RCTs of relaxation therapy for depression**

Reference	Sample size	Interventions [regimen]	Result	Comment
J Consult Clin Psychol 1986; 54:653–660	30	A) Relaxation training [10×50 min over 5 w] B) Cognitive-behavioral therapy C) Waiting list	A no different to B; both superior to C	Patients were adolescents; improvements maintained at 5 w follow-up
J Personality Clin Studies 1990;6:83–90	30	A) Progressive muscle relaxation [1×20 min/d for 3 d] B) Yoga & autosuggestion C) Discussion	A no different to B; both superior to C	Patients all on medication
Psychol Rep 1995;77: 403–420	37	A) Relaxation training [1–2×50 min/w for 12 w] B) Cognitive-behavioral therapy C) Desipramine [150–300 mg]	A no different to B; both superior to C	Substantial non-compliance in medication group

Yoga

An RCT with hospitalized melancholic depressives (n=45) compared the effects of Sudarshan Kriya yoga with electroconvulsive therapy and imipramine over 4 weeks.[15] Depression scores improved in all groups to a similar extent. The number of patients in remission at the end of the trial were 93% of the electroconvulsive therapy group, 73% with imipramine and 67% with yoga. No serious adverse events were reported in any group.

Other therapies

In a small non-randomized trial (n=20) with male inpatients, adjunctive **aromatherapy** enabled reductions to be made in the dose of antidepressants compared with patients under usual care.[16]

Single sessions of **dance and movement therapy** produced promising results in two small trials with inpatients when compared with no intervention.[17,18]

Overall recommendation

No complementary treatment is more effective than conventional pharmacological or psychological interventions, but with exercise and in particular St John's wort, there is evidence of therapeutic equivalence and superior tolerability in mild-moderate depression. Other approaches in which research is promising, such as relaxation, yoga and music therapy, are considered relatively risk free and given the sizable placebo response in depression, may benefit some individuals.

Table 5.32
Summary of clinical evidence for depression

Treatment	Weight of evidence	Direction of evidence	Serious safety concerns
Acupuncture	OO	⇨	Yes (see p 29)
Autogenic training	O	⇩	Yes (see p 37)
Exercise	OOO	⇧	Yes (see p 5)
Herbal medicine St John's wort	OOO	⇧	Yes (see p 156)
Massage	O	⇧	No (see p 60)
Music therapy	O	⇗	No (see p 80)
Relaxation	OO	⇧	No (see p 71)
Yoga	O	⇧	Yes (see p 77)

REFERENCES

1 Astin J A. Why patients use alternative medicine. JAMA 1998;279:1548–1553

2 Eisenberg D M, Davis R B, Ettner S L, Appel S, Wilkey S, Rompay M V, Kessler R C. Trends in alternative medicine use in the United States, 1990–1997. JAMA 1998;280:1569–1575

3 Luo H, Jia Y, Zhan L. Electro-acupuncture vs. amitriptyline in the treatment of depressive states. J Trad Chin Med 1985;5:3–8

4 Lou H, Jia Y, Wu X, Dai W. Electro-acupuncture in the treatment of depressive psychosis. Int J Clin Acup 1990;1:7–13

5 Yang X. Clinical observation on needling extrachannel points in treating mental depression. J Trad Chin Med 1994;14:14–18

6 Krampen G. Application of autogenic training before and in addition to integrative psychotherapy of depressive disorders. Z Klin

Psychol Psychiatr Psychother
1997;45:214–232

7 North T C, McCullagh P, Vu Tran Z. Effect of exercise on depression. Ex Sport Sci Rev 1990;18:379–415

8 Stevinson C, Ernst E. Hypericum for depression: an update of the clinical evidence. Eur Neuropsychopharmacol 1999;9:501–505

9 Gaster B, Holroyd J. St. John's wort for depression: a systematic review. Arch Intern Med 2000;160:152–156

10 Vorbach E U, Arnoldt K H, Hübner W D. Efficacy and tolerability of St. John's wort extract LI 160 versus imipramine in patients with severe depressive episodes according to ICD-10. Pharmacopsychiatry 1997;3(suppl):81–85

11 Field T, Morrow C, Valdeon C, Larson S, Kuhn C, Schanberg S. Massage reduces anxiety in child and adolescent psychiatric patients. J Am Acad Child Adolesc Psychiatr 1992; 31:125–131

12 Hanser S B. Thompson L W. Effects of music therapy strategy on depressed older adults. J Gerontol 1994;49:265–269

13 Jones N A, Field T. Massage and music therapies attenuate frontal EEG asymmetry in depressed adolescents. Adolescence 1999; 34:529–534

14 Field T, Martinez A, Nawrocki T, Pickens J, Fox N A, Schanberg S. Music shifts frontal

EEG in depressed adolescents. Adolescence 1998;33:109–116

15 Janakiramaiah N, Gangadhar B N, Naga Venkatesha Murthy P J, Harish M G, Subbakrishna D K, Vedamurthachar A. Antidepressant efficacy of Sudarshan Kriya Yoga in melancholia: a randomized comparison with electroconvulsive therapy and imipramine. J Affect Dis 2000;57:255–259

16 Komori T, Fujiwara R, Tanida M, Nomura J, Yokoyama M M. Effects of citrus fragrance on immune function and depressive states. Neuroimmunomodulation 1995;2:174–180

17 Brooks D, Stark A. The effect of dance/movement therapy on affect: a pilot study. Am J Dance Ther 1989;11:101–112

18 Stewart N J, McMullen L M, Rubin L D. Movement therapy with depressed inpatients: a randomized multiple single-case design. Arch Psychiatr Nurs 1994;8:22–29

FURTHER READING

Ernst E. Depression. New York: Godsfield, 1998
Introduction to ways of treating depression written for a lay population.

Ernst E, Rand J I, Stevinson C. Complementary therapies for depression: an overview. Arch Gen Psychiatr 1998;55:1026–1032
Comprehensive review of clinical trial evidence in this area.

DRUG/ALCOHOL DEPENDENCE

Synonyms
Chemical dependence (dependency), cocaine/opiate dependence, substance abuse, substance misuse.

Definition
Continued or increasing use of a chemical substance, to the extent of having negative consequences upon a person's life, in order to avoid physical or psychological withdrawal symptoms.

CAM usage
Acupuncture and hypnotherapy have been used with the aim of inducing changes in motivation among drug misusers and these therapies as well as others such as reflexology are used in a supportive way with the aim of reducing symptoms and stress during withdrawal. Courses of acupuncture treatment are mandated for this purpose by the state legislature in some areas of the US. Acupuncture and biofeedback are sometimes used as adjuncts in relapse prevention.

CONDITIONS

Clinical evidence

Acupuncture

For alcohol dependence, after some early positive RCTs,[1,2] the balance of evidence (Table 5.33) now suggests that acupuncture has no great value in achieving or maintaining abstinence. However, several of these studies have reported that real acupuncture appears to improve patients' continuing contact with therapy services.

In cocaine and opiate treatment programs, uncontrolled analyses of acupuncture as an adjunct (e.g. [3]) have been promising. However, these results have been contradicted by some rigorous RCTs. For example, in one RCT involving 60 subjects entering a methadone maintenance program, cravings were greater in the group that had real acupuncture compared with those given placebo acupuncture.[4] In another RCT involving 100 subjects with heroin dependence, acupuncture increased the rate of continuation in treatment, although only six subjects remained in the study at 21 days.[5] In cocaine dependence, an RCT of 236 cocaine addicts found no difference in the outcomes after acupuncture compared with placebo acupuncture[6] and the same negative results were achieved using acupuncture as an adjunct to standard cognitive-behavioral therapy in 277 cocaine dependants.[7] A third RCT comparing acupuncture, needle control and relaxation control in 82 patients dependent on cocaine, measured urine drug concentrations and found acupuncture more effective than both controls.[8] The evidence is therefore inconsistent.

Table 5.33 **Sham-controlled RCTs of acupuncture for alcohol dependence**

Reference	Sample size	Interventions [regimen]	Result	Comment
Drug Alcohol Dependence 1992;30: 169–173	56	A) Acupuncture [5 sessions/w initially, total 39] B) Placebo acupuncture	A no different from B	
Am J Acup 1996;24: 19–25	118	A) Acupuncture [12–15 sessions] B) Standard care	A better than B	Subjects already withdrawn from alcohol
Compl Ther Med 1997;5: 19–26	59	A) Acupuncture [weekly for 6] B) Placebo acupuncture C) Standard care	A no different from B or C	
Alcohol Alcoholism 1999;34: 629–635	72	A) Acupuncture [5 sessions/w initially, total 30] B) Placebo acupuncture	A no different from B	

Biofeedback

Biofeedback (BFB) training with relaxation increased the internal locus of control compared with no intervention in an RCT in young alcohol-dependent persons, a change that is associated with improved control over drinking habits.[9] Another RCT found lower relapse rates with EEG biofeedback in chronic alcohol dependency compared with the standard Alcoholic Anonymous 12-step program, as well as reductions in psychopathology.[10] Two RCTs comparing BFB with other treatments and with standard care alone reached inconsistent conclusions (Table 5.34)

Table 5.34 **RCTs comparing biofeedback (BFB) with other active treatments for alcohol dependence**

Reference	Sample size	Interventions [regimen]	Result	Comment
J Subst Abuse Treat 1995; 12:401–413	277	A) EEG BFB [30 days] B) Auricular acupuncture [24–28 sessions over 30 d] C) Bromocriptine [dose as needed up to 7.5 mg 6/d for 9 mo] D) Standard groups & counseling	A, B and C improved retention in project, but not abstinence at 9 mo	Severe alcohol dependence
Alcohol Treat Quart 1994; 11:187–220	250	A) Transcendental meditation [10 h training, 2/d practice] B) EMG BFB [20 1-h sessions] C) Pulsed electro-therapy [15 sessions] D) Standard care [30 d]	A and B more non-drinking days over 18 mo	Severe alcohol dependence

Electrostimulation

Various forms of cranial electrostimulation (using a range of terms including transcranial electrical therapy and neuroelectric therapy) have been applied to patients with drug or alcohol dependency, mainly with the aim of alleviating withdrawal symptoms. The RCTs available in 1990 were reviewed.[11] The variety of electrical parameters (e.g. frequency, intensity, waveform) and treatment regimens used created problems in drawing meaningful conclusions. Several double-blind RCTs had positive results for drug withdrawal but because of methodological problems (principally the large proportion of drop-outs) no firm conclusions could be drawn. Since that time, more rigorous, double-blind RCTs with negative results have been published in cocaine/opiate dependence.[12] However, some authors have argued that they believe the intensity, waveform and frequency of stimulation were not optimal for the drug being withdrawn.[13]

Herbal medicine

Some withdrawal programs in China involve colonic irrigation with **Chinese herbs** as a method of detoxification, but the only RCT located used inappropriate outcome measures and no conclusion can be drawn.[14]

Kudzu (*Pueraria lobata*) is a long-established Chinese herbal remedy which has been used for treatment of alcohol dependence, but a small RCT in 38 persons found no effect on craving or sobriety scores compared with placebo.[15]

Hypnotherapy

For alcohol dependence, a review found that the rigorous evidence about hypnotherapy was restricted to one RCT, the negative outcome of which was weakened by the failure to stratify according to hypnotic susceptibility.[16] There have been no rigorous investigations published since the review.

Relaxation

Relaxation has been used alone as the control method in several controlled trials and found to be of little benefit in drug withdrawal (though it may not have been applied optimally) (e.g. [17]). One small (n=20) RCT found a beneficial effect on sleep patterns in institutionalized chronic alcoholic men, compared with no additional treatment.[18] Relaxation can promote restoration of normal sleep patterns in patients who are withdrawing from long-term hypnotic medication, as compared with no relaxation, but it makes little difference to the temporary disturbance during the actual drug withdrawal, according to an RCT in only 20 subjects.[19]

Other therapies

Regular, aerobic **exercise** was superior at reducing craving in a group of 90 alcohol-dependent patients compared with standard treatment in a controlled trial.[20]

Intercessory **prayer** was found to be of no benefit for alcohol dependency in an RCT of 40 subjects in which it was compared with no additional treatment.[21]

Supplements during withdrawal and recovery may be necessary because appetite and quality of nutritional intake are both often poor in all drug dependence, and metabolic disturbance may also be severe with excessive alcohol use.[22] In addition, **amino acid** supplements have been used with the aim of restoring brain neurotransmitter concentrations: in alcohol dependency, three patients showed improved retention, stress reduction and ease of detoxification compared with 19 controls with standard treatment alone.[23] In another double-blind controlled trial in 23 patients, **gamma-hydroxybutyric acid** reduced symptoms of alcohol withdrawal more effectively than placebo control.[24] These studies are still exploratory and require independent replication.

Yoga was not superior to dynamic group psychotherapy in an RCT of 61 patients undergoing methadone maintenance therapy, as assessed by a range of psychological, sociological and biological measures.[25]

Overall recommendation

For the management of chemical dependence, the major areas of action are in motivating changes in behavior, bringing patients into detoxification and therapy and maintaining abstinence. Acupuncture may have a role in the first two areas, but the evidence is contradictory. Its role in treating the withdrawal symptoms from either alcohol or narcotics appears to be uncertain. Maintenance of abstinence is best attempted with multiple interventions including support and teaching of coping strategies and substitute behaviors. CAM appears to have little to offer in comparison with current methods such as Alcoholics or Narcotics Anonymous or cognitive-behavioral therapy. For dependence on prescribed hypnotic drugs, relaxation may help restore normal sleep patterns.

Table 5.35
Summary of clinical evidence for drug/alcohol dependence

Treatment	Weight of evidence	Direction of evidence	Serious safety concerns
Acupuncture (alcohol)	OO	⬂	Yes (see p 29)
(cocaine & opiates)	OO	⇨	
Biofeedback	O	⇨	No (see p 42)
Electro-stimulation	OO	⇨	Yes (see p 6)
Herbal medicine Chinese herbs (rectally)	O	⬈	Yes (see p 52)
Kudzu	O	⬇	Yes (see p 5)
Hypnotherapy (alcohol)	O	⬇	Yes (see p 58)
Relaxation	O	⇨	No (see p 71)

CONDITIONS

REFERENCES

1 Bullock M L, Umen A J, Culliton P D, Olander R T. Acupuncture treatment of alcohol recidivism: a pilot study. Alcohol Clin Exp Res 1987;11:292–295

2 Bullock M L, Culliton P D, Olander R T. Controlled trial of acupuncture for severe recidivist alcoholism. Lancet 1989; 333:1435–1439

3 Schwartz M, Saitz R, Mulvey K et al. The value of acupuncture detoxification programs in a substance abuse treatment system. J Subst Abuse Treat 1999;17:305–312

4 Wells E A, Jackson R, Dias O R et al. Acupuncture as an adjunct to methadone treatment services. Am J Addict 1995; 4:169–214

5 Washburn A M, Fullilove R E, Fullilove M T et al. Acupuncture heroin detoxification: a single-blind clinical trial. J Subst Abuse Treat 1993;10:345–351

6 Bullock M L, Kiresuk T J, Pheley A M et al. Auricular acupuncture in the treatment of cocaine abuse. J Subst Abuse Treat 1999; 16:31–38

7 Richard A J. Montoya I D, Nelson R, Spence R T. Effectiveness of adjunct therapies in crack cocaine treatment. J Subst Abuse Treat 1995;12:401–413

8 Avants S K, Margolin A, Holford T R, Kosten T R. A randomized controlled trial of auricular acupuncture for cocaine dependence. Arch Intern Med 2000;160:2305–2312

9 Sharp C, Hurford D P, Allison J, Sparks R, Cameron B P. Facilitation of internal locus of control in adolescent alcoholics through a brief biofeedback-assisted autogenic relaxation training procedure. J Subst Abuse Treat 1997;14:55–60

10 Peniston E G, Kulkosky P J. Alpha-theta brainwave training and beta-endorphin levels in alcoholics. Alcohol Clin Exp Res 1989; 13:271–279

11 Alling F A, Johnson B D, Eldoghazy E. Cranial electrostimulation (CES) use in the detoxification of opiate-dependent patients. J Subst Abuse Treat 1990;7:173–180

12 Gariti P. Auriacombe M, Incmikoski R et al. A randomized double-blind study of neuroelectric therapy in opiate and cocaine detoxification. J Subst Abuse 1992;4:299–308

13 Patterson M A, Patterson L, Flood N V et al. Electrostimulation in drug and alcohol detoxification: significance of stimulation criteria in clinical success. Addict Res 1993;1:130–144

14 Sha L J, Zhang Z X, Cheng L X. [Colonic dialysis therapy of Chinese herbal medicine in abstinence of heroin addicts – report of 75 cases] [Chinese]. Chung-Kuo Chung Hsi i Chieh Ho Tsa Chih 1997;17:76–78

15 Shebek J, Rindone J P. A pilot study exploring the effect of kudzu root on the drinking habits of patients with chronic alcoholism. J Alt Compl Med 2000;6:45–48

16 Wadden T A, Penrod J H. Hypnosis in the treatment of alcoholism: a review and appraisal. Am J Clin Hypnosis 1981; 24:41–47

17 Brown R A, Evans D M, Miller I W, Burgess E S, Müller T I. Cognitive-behavioral treatment for depression in alcoholism. J Consult Clin Psychol 1997;65:715–726

18 Greeff A P, Conradie W S. Use of progressive relaxation training for chronic alcoholics with insomnia. Psychol Reports 1998;82:407–412

19 Lichstein K L, Peterson B A, Riedel B W et al. Relaxation to assist sleep medication withdrawal. Behav Modification 1999; 23:379–402

20 Ermalinski R, Hanson P G, Lubin B, Thornby J I, Nahormek P A. Impact of a body-mind treatment component on alcoholic inpatients. J Psychosoc Nurs Ment Health Serv 1997; 35:39–45

21 Walker S R, Tonigan J S, Miller W R, Corner S, Kahlich L. Intercessory prayer in the treatment of alcohol abuse and dependence: a pilot investigation. Alt Ther Health Med 1997; 3:79–86

22 Beckley-Barrett L M, Mutch P B. Position of the American Dietetic Association: nutrition intervention in treatment and recovery from chemical dependence. ADA Reports 1990; 90:1274–1277

23 Blum K, Trachtenberg M C, Ramsay J C. Improvement of inpatient treatment of the alcoholic as a function of neurotransmitter restoration: a pilot study. Int J Addict 1988;23:991–998

24 Gallimberti L, Canton G, Gentile N et al. Gamma-hydroxybutyric acid for treatment of alcohol withdrawal syndrome. Lancet 1989; 334:787–789

25 Shaffer H J, Lasalvia T A. Comparing Hatha yoga with dynamic group psychotherapy for enhancing methadone maintenance treatment: a randomized clinical trial. Alt Ther Health Med 1997;3:57–66

FURTHER READING

Brewington V, Smith M, Lipton D. Acupuncture as a detoxification treatment: an analysis of controlled research. J Subst Abuse Treat 1994;11:289–307

In-depth summary of the available research into acupuncture, broad-based rather than systematic.

ERECTILE DYSFUNCTION

Synonyms   Impotence, male erectile dysfunction.

Definition   Inability of the male to achieve and/or maintain penile erection and thus engage in copulation.

CAM usage   Acupuncture, herbal medicine and hypnotherapy are frequently used.

Clinical evidence

Acupuncture

One RCT evaluated acupuncture as a treatment for patients with non-organic erectile dysfunction.[1] Nine patients were treated at appropriate points and six received placebo acupuncture twice weekly for 6 weeks. Improvements in sexual function were reported in the treatment group, which were not significantly different from the control group. Data from uncontrolled studies indicate some positive effects on the quality of erection and sexual activity in erectile dysfunction due to non-organic[2] and mixed[3] etiologies.

Biofeedback

An RCT (n=30) of biofeedback training assessed patients who received either continuous feedback of erection changes plus excerpts of erotic film delivered contingent on erection increases, contingent film excerpts without continuous feedback or non-contingent film excerpts.[4] There were no intergroup differences in erectile functioning during a 1-month follow-up period. It was concluded that the therapeutic value of erectile feedback remains undemonstrated.

Herbal medicine

An uncontrolled pilot study assessed the effects of ginkgo (*Ginkgo biloba*) extract in antidepressant-induced sexual dysfunction.[5] Sixty-three patients were treated with up to 240 mg daily. Positive effects are reported on all four phases of the sexual response cycle, including penile erection.

Ginseng (*Panax* spp, *Eleutherococcus senticosus*) is widely believed to have aphrodisiac effects for patients with sexual dysfunction. A systematic review of ginseng for any indication, however, found no double-blind RCTs despite extensive searches.[6] One placebo-controlled RCT which was not reported as double blind assessed 90 patients, who were treated with either ginseng or trazodone. Although no intergroup differences were reported for frequency of intercourse, the results suggested superiority of ginseng for penile rigidity, girth, libido and patient satisfaction.[7]

An uncontrolled study assessed the potential of **mustong**, an herbal preparation containing mainly *Mucuna pruriens* and

CONDITIONS

Withania somnifera, as an option for this condition.[8] The report suggests a good to very good improvement of sexual function in 16 of 25 patients.

The effects of **yohimbine**, the main active constituent of yohimbe bark (*Pausinystalia yohimbe*), have been assessed in a metaanalysis (Box 5.19). Its results suggest that yohimbine is effective for this condition. There is no trial that compared yohimbine with sildenafil, but indirect comparison of placebo-controlled trials suggests that yohimbine is less effective, but relatively safer.[9]

Box 5.19
Metaanalysis
Yohimbine for erectile dysfunction
J Urol 1998;159: 433–436

- Seven double-blind RCTs including 419 patients

- Trial quality generally good

- Erectile dysfunction due to organic or non-organic etiologies

- Superior to placebo in response rate (odds ratio 3.85, CI 2.22 to 6.67)

- Adverse effects were reversible and infrequent

Hypnotherapy

Two RCTs assessed the effects of hypnotic suggestions on sexual function.[1,10] Both studies originate from the same research group and included patients with no detectable organic cause. Both studies found improvements in sexual function and report that hypnotic suggestion is significantly more effective than the administration of oral placebo. Independent replication of these findings is warranted.

Pelvic floor exercise

One RCT compared a pelvic floor exercise program with surgery.[11] One hundred and fifty patients with erectile dysfunction and proven vascular leakage were included and 78 randomized to the training program. It was given five times in weekly

Table 5.36
Summary of clinical evidence for erectile dysfunction

Treatment	Weight of evidence	Direction of evidence	Serious safety concerns
Acupuncture	O	⇗	Yes (see p 29)
Biofeedback	O	⇓	No (see p 42)
Herbal medicine			
Ginkgo	O	⇧	Yes (see p 115)
Ginseng	O	⇧	Yes (see p 88)
Mustong	O	⇧	Yes (see p 5)
Yohimbine	OOO	⇧	Yes (see p 165)
Hypnotherapy	O	⇧	Yes (see p 58)
Pelvic floor exercise	O	⇗	No

CONDITIONS

sessions and supervised by a trained physiotherapist. It was concluded that, although in cases of severe venous leakage surgery is superior to a pelvic floor exercise program, in mild forms pelvic floor exercise is an alternative to surgery.

Overall recommendation

There is convincing evidence for the effectiveness of yohimbine for erectile dysfunction from organic or non-organic causes. Its risk–benefit ratio is favorable, which renders it an option worthy of consideration. Comparative studies with conventional oral medication such as sildenafil are not available at present but it has been suggested that yohimbine is less effective but safer. For other therapies such as hypnotherapy, the evidence is not compelling. However, given the possibility of a large placebo response, it may be beneficial for some patients when administered by a responsible therapist.

REFERENCES

1 Aydin S, Ercan M, Çaskurlu T et al. Acupuncture and hypnotic suggestions in the treatment of non-organic male dysfunction. Scand J Urol Nephrol 1997;31:271–274

2 Kho H G, Sweep C G, Chen X, Rabsztyn P R, Meuleman E J. The use of acupuncture in the treatment of erectile dysfunction. Int J Impot Res 1999;11:41–46

3 Yaman L S, Kilic S, Sarica K, Bayar M, Saygin B. The place of acupuncture in the management of psychogenic impotence. Eur Urol 1994;26:52–55

4 Reynolds B S. Biofeedback and facilitation of erection in men with erectile dysfunction. Arch Sexual Behav 1980;9:101–113

5 Cohen A J, Bartlik B. Ginkgo biloba for antidepressant-induced sexual dysfunction. J Sex Marital Ther 1998;24:139–413

6 Vogler B K, Pittler M H, Ernst E. The efficacy of ginseng. A systematic review of randomised clinical trials. Eur J Clin Pharmacol 1999; 55:567–575

7 Choi H K, Seong D H, Rha K H. Clinical efficacy of Korean red ginseng for erectile dysfunction. Int J Impot Res 1995;7:181–186

8 Cjha J K, Roy C K, Bajpai H S. Clinical trial of mustong on secondary sexual impotence in male married diabetics. J Med Assoc Thailand 1987;70:228–230

9 O'Leary M. Erectile dysfunction. In: Godlee F (ed) Clinical evidence. London: BMJ Books, 1999

10 Aydin S, Odabas O, Ercan M, Kara H, Agargun M Y. Efficacy of testosterone, trazodone, and hypnotic suggestion in the treatment of non-organic male sexual dysfunction. Br J Urol 1996;77:256–260

11 Claes H, Baert L. Pelvic floor exercise versus surgery in the treatment of impotence. Br J Urol 1993;71:52–57

FURTHER READING

Lue T F. Erectile dysfunction. New Engl J Med 2000;342:1802–1813

A thorough overview of the physiology of erection and the pathophysiology of erectile dysfunction, followed by a discussion of the drug treatment.

FIBROMYALGIA

Synonyms

Fibromyalgia syndrome, tension myalgia.

Definition

A painful disorder, more common in women, in which diffuse pain, stiffness, fatigue, functional impairment and disrupted sleep are associated with the presence of bilateral tender points.

CAM usage

Sufferers of fibromyalgia commonly use CAM. One survey found that 91% had used CAM, the highest rate for any rheumatic disease.[1] CAM therapies frequently used include massage, dietary therapies, vitamins and herbs, relaxation and imagery, spirituality/prayer, acupressure, acupuncture, biofeedback and meditation.[2]

Clinical evidence

Acupuncture

One good-quality RCT[3] in 70 subjects found that 25% of subjects improved markedly, 50% had satisfactory relief of symptoms and 25% had no benefit. The acupuncture group showed a superior response compared with placebo group in five out of eight measures; 11 subjects withdrew because of reactions to acupuncture treatment. This study was the principal evidence in a systematic review (Box 5.20) which reached a positive overall conclusion.

Box 5.20
Systematic review
Acupuncture for fibromyalgia
J Fam Pract 1999;48: 213–218

- Three RCTs and four cohort studies involving 300 subjects

- Quality of studies highly variable

- A single high-quality RCT suggests that acupuncture is more effective than placebo for relieving pain and morning stiffness

- Other studies are inconclusive, but compatible with this result

- Long-term effects remain unknown

Biofeedback

Although several RCTs have suggested that fibromyalgia patients can benefit from various mind–body therapies, appropriate attention controls have rarely been used. In one controlled study, 12 patients received 15 sessions of either biofeedback or sham biofeedback over 5 weeks.[4] Significant improvements in tender points, pain intensity and morning stiffness were found, which persisted for up to 6 months after the treatment. In an RCT involving 119 subjects, biofeedback with relaxation was compared to exercise, a combination of biofeedback and exercise, and attention control.[5] Biofeedback was associated with improvements in a number of outcomes, but was superior to the control group only in terms of tender points and enhanced self-efficacy of function, i.e. the belief that one can cope with the condition. Biofeedback combined with exercise in the same study produced benefits that persisted over the 2-year follow-up period. The improvements that occur with mind–body interventions appear more likely to be associated with changes in self-efficacy rather than reduction of actual symptoms.[6]

Exercise

Several RCTs of cardiovascular fitness training alone suggest that it can produce benefits in the physical symptoms and quality of life in fibromyalgia (Table 5.37). The benefits are not usually sustained. Some patients find that their disability temporarily increases but improves if the training is pursued for 12 (or sometimes as many as 20) weeks. Other studies, which are of poor quality due to lack of randomization or high drop-out rates, are compatible with the findings of the more rigorous studies.

Table 5.37   **Parallel-arm RCTs of exercise for fibromyalgia**

Reference	Sample size	Interventions [regimen]	Results	Comment
Scand J Rheumatol 1996;25: 77–86	60	A) Aerobics [3 × wkly for 14 w] B) Stress management C) Usual treatment	A and B better than C for pain distribution, pain score, lack of energy, tenderness. A better for work capacity	Only pain changes sustained at 4 y follow-up
Arthritis Care Res 1998;11: 196–209	119	A) Flexibility and strength exercises, walking [6 wkly sessions] B) Biofeedback C) Combination D) Attention control	A, B and C better for tender points, physical activity and self-efficacy than D	C best treatment at 2 y follow-up

Herbal medicine

Forty-five patients were treated with topical **capsaicin** or placebo in a controlled trial. Those receiving capsaicin reported less tenderness and a significant increase in grip strength, but no difference in pain scores.[7]

Homeopathy

In one RCT, 30 patients were selected for inclusion in two stages, first for diagnosis of fibromyalgia and then for matching to the remedy **Rhus Toxicodendron**.[8] The homeopathy group recorded greater reduction in tender points, pain and sleep disturbance, but global assessment was not different.

Massage

Connective tissue massage was compared with no treatment or discussion (attention control) in an RCT involving 52 patients.[9] The treated group experienced greater relief of pain and depression and improvement in quality of life, but were not significantly different in other variables, including activities or sleep.

CONDITIONS

The difference between groups was no longer significant after 3 months.

Other therapies

From one small study (n=39), there is a suggestion that **balneotherapy** with plain fresh-water baths reduces pain and the addition of **valerian** to the bath may improve other outcomes such as well-being and sleep.[10]

A small (n=19) RCT found that, although treatment with **chiropractic** manipulation and soft tissue massage was associated with improvements in many parameters such as spinal pain and mobility, the changes were not significantly superior to no treatment in terms of the physical symptoms.[11] Outcome measures specific to fibromyalgia were not used.

An RCT in which 40 patients with fibromyalgia were randomized to receive either **hypnotherapy** or physical therapy for 12 weeks found improvements in several measures including pain ratings, sleep disturbance and somatic and psychological discomfort scores, though not physicians' global assessments.[12]

Low-dose laser therapy was not found to provide any greater relief of pain than placebo laser in a crossover study involving 60 patients.[13]

A cohort study of **meditation** for 10 weeks in 79 patients with fibromyalgia found improvements in all patients and moderate or great improvement in 51%.[14]

A single trial suggested that **music therapy** was associated with reduced pain and disability in chronic pain patients, including fibromyalgia, compared with untreated controls, but no change in anxiety or depression.[15]

Table 5.38
Summary of clinical evidence for fibromyalgia

Treatment	Weight of evidence	Direction of evidence	Serious safety concerns
Acupuncture	O	⇧	Yes (see p 29)
Biofeedback	O	⇧	No (see p 42)
Exercise	OO	⇗	Yes (see p 5)
Herbal medicine Capsaicin	O	⇗	Yes (see p 5)
Homeopathy	O	⇗	No (see p 55)
Massage	O	⇧	No (see p 60)

Overall recommendation

It is unlikely that any individual complementary therapy can make any greater impact on the progress of fibromyalgia than conventional approaches. However, combinations of therapies are often used for fibromyalgia and CAM may have something to offer in this context. For example, the judicious use of oral medications, such as antidepressants, to deal with pain and insomnia can be usefully combined with biofeedback or (supervised) exercise and perhaps acupuncture. Acupuncture (and aerobic exercise) may exacerbate symptoms but this problem has not been reported with other physical treatments.

REFERENCES

1 Piorro-Boisset M, Esdaile J M, Fitzcharles M-A. Alternative medicine use in fibromyalgia syndrome. Arthritis Care Res 1996;9:13–17

2 Nicassio P M, Schuman C, Kim J et al. Psychosocial factors associated with complementary treatment use in fibromyalgia. J Rheumatol 1997;24:2008–2013

3 Deluze C, Bosia L, Zirbs A, Chantraine A, Vischer T L. Electroacupuncture in fibromyalgia: results of a controlled trial. Br Med J 1992;305:1249–1252

4 Ferraccioli G, Gherilli L, Scita F et al. EMG-biofeedback training in fibromyalgia syndrome. J Rheumatol 1987;14:820–825

5 Buckelew S P, Conway R, Parker J et al. Biofeedback/relaxation training and exercise interventions for fibromyalgia: a prospective trial. Arthritis Care Res 1998;11: 196–209

6 Broderick J E. Mind-body medicine in rheumatologic disease. Rheum Dis Clin North Am 2000;26:161–176

7 McCarty D J, Csuka M, McCarthy G, Trotter D. Treatment of pain due to fibromyalgia with topical capsaicin: a pilot study. Semin Arthritis Rheum 1994;23(suppl 3): 41–47

8 Fisher P, Greenwood A, Huskisson E C, Turner P, Belon P. Effect of homeopathic treatment on fibrositis (primary fibromyalgia). Br Med J 1989;299:365–366

9 Brattberg G. Connective tissue massage in the treatment of fibromyalgia. Eur J Pain 1999; 3:235–245

10 Ammer K, Melnizky P. Medicinal baths for treatment of generalized fibromyalgia [German]. Forsch Komplementärmed 1999;6:80–85

11 Blunt K L, Rajwani M H, Guerriero R C. The effectiveness of chiropractic management of fibromyalgia patients: a pilot study. J Manip Physiol Ther 1997;20:389–399

12 Haanan H C M, Hoenderdos H T W, Romunde L K J et al. Controlled trial of hypnotherapy in the treatment of refractory fibromyalgia. J Rheumatol 1991;18:72–75

13 Waylonis G W, Wilke S, O'Toole D, Waylonis D A, Waylonis D B. Chronic myofascial pain: management by low-output helium-neon laser therapy. Arch Phys Med Rehabil 1998;69:1017–1020

14 Kaplan K H, Goldenberg D L, Galvin-Nadeau M. The impact of a meditation-based stress reduction program on fibromyalgia. Gen Hosp Psychiatr 1993;15:284–289

15 Müller-Busch H C, Hoffmann P. Aktive Musiktherapie bei chronischen Schmerzen. Schmerz 1997;11:91–100

FURTHER READING

Berman B M, Swyers J P. Complementary medicine treatments for fibromyalgia syndrome. Baillière's Best Pract Res Clin Rheumatol 1999;13:487–492
A balanced review of the current state of the evidence.

McCain G A. Treatment of fibromyalgia syndrome. J Musculoskel Pain 1999;7:193–208
A description of all the options available and how they may be integrated for an individual patient.

CONDITIONS

HAY FEVER

Synonyms   Seasonal allergic rhinitis, pollenosis.

Definition   Type I immediate hypersensitivity reaction mediated by specific IgE antibody to a seasonal allergen, leading to mucosal inflammation characterized by sneezing, itching, rhinorrhea, nasal blockage and conjunctivitis.

CAM usage

Allergies are among the most common reasons for using complementary therapies, according to a US survey,[1] with herbal medicine and relaxation used the most. Homeopathy is also popular with hay fever sufferers.

Clinical evidence

Acupuncture

Uncontrolled studies have previously suggested that acupuncture has value in the management of hay fever, but the evidence from RCTs (Table 5.39) suggests that this may be attributable to non-specific factors.

Table 5.39 **RCTs of acupuncture for hay fever**

Reference	Sample size	Interventions [regimen]	Result	Comment
Acup Med 1994;12:84–87	30	A) Acupuncture [1 session/w for 3 w] B) Conventional medication	A superior to B for prevention	Conclusion uncertain due to unclear statistics
Acup Med 1996;14:6–10	102	A) Acupuncture [3–4 sessions over 4 w] B) Sham acupuncture	A no different to B for treatment	Medication use & symptoms decreased in both groups
Wien Med Wochenschr 1998;148:450–453	24	A) Acupuncture [1 session/w for 9 w] B) Sham acupuncture	A no different to B for prevention	Outcome was nasal allergen provocation
Z Allg Med 1998;74:45–46	174	A) Acupuncture [9 sessions over 3 w] B) Laser acupuncture [15 sessions] C) Placebo-laser acupuncture	A & B superior to C for treatment	More therapist time with B & C

Diet

One RCT assessed the effects of an antigen avoidance diet during infancy on later development of atopy.[2] Common allergens such as cow's milk, egg and peanuts were avoided during gestation and first 3 years of life (n=165). Prevalence of hay fever or other allergies was no different from the control group at age 7 years.

Herbal medicine

A double-blind RCT (n=69) of stinging nettle (*Urtica dioica*) taken for one week reported higher global ratings of improvement than for placebo, but no statistical analysis was conducted.[3]

Homeopathy

Seven placebo-controlled RCTs of *Galphimia glauca* from one research group were subjected to metaanalysis by the same researchers (Box 5.21). Collectively the results suggested that the remedy is effective for both ocular and nasal symptoms. The success rate of 79% is comparable to conventional treatments, with minimal adverse events reported.

Box 5.21
Metaanalysis
Homeopathic Galphimia glauca for hay fever
Forsch Komplementärmed 1996;3:230–234

- Seven double-blind placebo-controlled RCTs involving 752 patients

- Quality ratings not performed but methods identical for each trial except only two used intent-to-treat analysis

- Superiority over placebo for ocular symptoms (relative risk: 1.25, CI 1.09 to 1.43) and nasal symptoms (relative risk 1.26, CI 1.05 to 1.50)

Promising results were reported from a small pilot RCT (n=36) of homeopathic grass pollens versus placebo.[4] The same research team conducted a larger (n=144) double-blind placebo-controlled RCT testing homeopathic dilutions of specific antigens identified for each hay fever patient by skin tests.[5] Symptom scores and use of antihistamines were reduced significantly more in the homeopathic group.

A double-blind RCT compared a homeopathic nasal spray with a conventional one (cromolyn sodium) over 42 days in 146 hay fever sufferers.[6] Quality of life assessments indicated therapeutic equivalence of the two treatments.

Supplements

Fish oil supplementation was investigated in a double-blind placebo-controlled RCT (n=37) involving pollen-sensitive individuals with hay fever and asthma.[7] Various outcomes measured over a pollen season revealed no differences between the fish oil and placebo groups.

Other therapies

An RCT (n=47) tested the effects of **hypnotic suggestion** on skin reactions to allergen prick tests in individuals with hay fever and asthma.[8] According to the results, undergoing hypnosis was associated with smaller weals, but specific suggestions had no influence. No clinical trials of hypnotherapy for hay fever symptoms were located, making the potential of this therapy difficult to evaluate.

CONDITIONS

Table 5.40
Summary of clinical evidence for hay fever

Treatment	Weight of evidence	Direction of evidence	Serious safety concerns
Acupuncture			
(prevention)	O	⇨	Yes (see p 29)
(treatment)	OO	⇨	
Diet (prevention)	O	⇩	No
Herbal medicine			
Nettle	O	⬈	Yes (see p 139)
Homeopathy	OO	⇧	No (see p 55)
Supplements			
Fish oil	O	⇩	Yes (see p 5)

Overall recommendation

There is little clinical trial evidence for the effectiveness of most complementary therapies for the prevention or treatment of hay fever. The one exception is homeopathy for which promising evidence exists, particularly for *Galphimia glauca*. There are suggestions that this may be as effective as conventional medication, but this has not been directly investigated. Adverse effects are rare with homeopathic remedies, so for patients dissatisfied with their orthodox medication, homeopathy may be worth considering.

REFERENCES

1 Eisenberg D M, Davis R B, Ettner S L, Appel S, Wilkey S, Rompay M V, Kessler R C. Trends in alternative medicine use in the United States, 1990–1997. JAMA 1998;280:1569–1575

2 Zeiger R S, Heller S. The development and prediction of atopy in high-risk children: follow up at age seven years in a prospective randomized study of combined maternal and infant food allergen avoidance. J Allergy Clin Immunol 1995;95:1179–1190

3 Mittman P. Randomized, double-blind study of freeze-dried *Urtica dioica* in the treatment of allergic rhinitis. Planta Med 1990;56:44–47

4 Reilly D T, Taylor M A. Potent placebo or potency? A proposed study model with initial findings using homoeopathically prepared pollens in hay fever. Br Homoeopath J 1985; 74:65–74

5 Reilly D T, Taylor M A, McSharry C, Aitchison T. Is homoeopathy a placebo response? Controlled trial of homoeopathic potency, with pollen in hay fever as model. Lancet 1986;2:881–886

6 Weiser M, Gegenheimer L H, Klein P. A randomized equivalence trial comparing the efficacy and safety of Luffa comp-Heel nasal spray with cromolyn sodium spray in the treatment of seasonal allergic rhinitis. Forsch Komplementärmed 1999;6: 142–148

7 Thien F C K, Mencia-Huerta J M, Lee T H. Dietary fish oil effects on seasonal hay fever and asthma in pollen-sensitive subjects. Am Rev Respir Dis 1993;147:1138–1143

8 Fry L, Mason A A, Pearson R S. Effect of hypnosis on allergic skin responses in asthma and hay fever. Br Med J 1964;1145–1148

HEADACHE

Synonyms/ subcategories

Tension headache, chronic or episodic tension-type headache, cephalodynia, cephalalgia, cephalea, cerebralgia, encephalalgia, encephalodynia, cervicogenic headache (formerly muscle tension headache).

Definition   Pain in various parts of the head, not confined to the area of distribution of any nerve.

CAM usage   According to Eisenberg's survey,[1] 32% of Americans with headache have used CAM in the previous 12 months, most frequently relaxation and chiropractic. Most other therapies are also used, especially herbal medicine, homeopathy, acupuncture and reflexology.

Clinical
evidence

Acupuncture

Three good-quality studies that yielded analyzable data for tension headache (Table 5.41) were located by a systematic review of acupuncture for all kinds of headache.[2] The review concluded that the current evidence suggests that acupuncture has a role but was not of sufficient quantity or quality to make firm recommendations.

Table 5.41   **RCTs of acupuncture for headache**

Reference	Sample size	Interventions [regimen]	Result	Comment
Cephalalgia 1985;5: 137–142	18	A) Acupuncture [2 session/w for 3 w] B) Sham acupuncture	A superior	Crossover trial
Pain 1992; 48:325–329	30	A) Acupuncture [1 session/w for 8 w] B) Sham acupuncture	Both groups improved, A no different from B	
Headache 1990;30: 593–599	62	A) Acupuncture [4–5 sessions over 2–4 w] B) Physiotherapy [10–12 sessions, intensive]	B superior to A (at 2 and 7 mo)	Sample was all female

Autogenic training

In one study, 146 patients with tension headache were randomized to autogenic training, hypnosis or waiting list control.[3] Autogenic training (but not hypnosis) was significantly better than waiting list immediately after treatment in terms of headache index, but not in terms of headache medication or psychological distress. The improvements were maintained at 6 months, by which time there were no differences in favor of one treatment over the other and both were superior to waiting list. No studies compared autogenic training with an attention control.

CONDITIONS

Biofeedback

A systematic review (Box 5.22) concluded that both relaxation and biofeedback (either on its own or in combination with relaxation) were superior to no treatment and to placebo therapy. However, the review included all prospective studies, whether controlled or not, and aggregated the responses for all groups receiving each therapy or control, which is likely to overestimate the effect size.

Box 5.22
Metaanalysis
Biofeedback and relaxation for headache
Clin J Pain 1994;10: 174–190

- All prospective studies, including uncontrolled studies

- Seventy-eight studies with 175 groups were included in the review, involving 2866 patients

- Mean (SD) effect size from 29 studies of EMG biofeedback was 47% (26%)

- Mean (SD) effect size from 38 studies of relaxation was 36% (20%)

- For comparison, mean (SD) effect size from pharmacological treatment was 39% (23%) and for placebo treatment 20% (38%)

Several subsequent RCTs (Table 5.42) have tested biofeedback in adolescents and adults, mainly in comparison with relaxation. The majority found biofeedback more effective. One study[4] demonstrated that the clinical improvements correlated

Table 5.42 **Parallel-arm RCTs of biofeedback (BFB) for headache**

Reference	Sample size	Interventions [regimen]	Result	Comment
Headache 1995;35: 411–419	26	A) Frontal EMG BFB [12 sessions] B) Trapezius EMG BFB [12 sessions] C) Relaxation [7 sessions]	B better than A or C at 3 mo	
Cephalalgia 1998;18: 463–467	35	A) BFB relaxation [10 sessions in 5 w] B) Relaxation placebo	A better than B at 1 y	Adolescents
Applied Psychophys Biof 1998; 23:143–157	50	A) BFB [12 30-min sessions in 6 w] B) Relaxation [6 1-h sessions in 6 w] C) Untreated control	No difference between A and B. Both better than C for some outcomes	Children. Parental involvement had no influence

with changes in self-efficacy but not in electromyographic or EEG activity. Another study[5] found that patients who have a preference for highly structured practice respond better when they are given explicit guidelines than when they are left to their own devices.

Electrotherapy

Cranial electrotherapy uses a stimulation apparatus to deliver a high-frequency, low-intensity current transcranially. Its role is in treatment of acute headache rather than in prevention. It was found to be significantly more effective than placebo in a multi-center RCT of 100 patients, reducing headache scores by 35% after 20 minutes compared with 18% in the placebo group.[6] However, treatment is detectable so blinding is problematic. The success of blinding was not tested in this study.

Herbal medicine

In an RCT involving 41 adults with a history of tension headache, 164 acute headache attacks were treated with either **peppermint** oil or placebo oil locally and either paracetamol (acetaminophen) or placebo tablet orally.[7] Peppermint oil was superior to placebo and not significantly different from the analgesic drug in reducing headache parameters.

The use of **tiger balm** was supported in one multicenter RCT in which 57 patients were given either tiger balm to apply locally, placebo balm or standard analgesic medication.[8] Tiger balm and medication were both significantly more effective than placebo at reducing the headache intensity, though the success of subject blinding is questionable since tiger balm produces local warmth.

Homeopathy

One rigorous RCT with 98 subjects included patients with tension headache as well as those with migraine and found no benefit from individualized homeopathy compared with placebo.[9]

Hypnotherapy

Like other forms of therapy involving regular relaxation, self-hypnosis appears to be more effective than waiting list control (e.g. [10]). However, it is not clear whether it is superior to other forms of relaxation. Several trials have compared different combinations of therapies including hypnotherapy with various control interventions (e.g. [3,11]). Subjects who are highly hypnotizable tend to show a greater reduction of headaches than those who are less easily hypnotized.[3]

Relaxation

A systematic review of biofeedback and relaxation (Box 5.22) concluded that relaxation is effective, with a mean effect size of 36%. However, the review included all prospective studies, whether controlled or not, and aggregated the responses for all

CONDITIONS

groups receiving each therapy or control, which is likely to overstate the effect size.

In children and adolescents, several RCTs indicate that relaxation has a positive effect on tension headache, though the size of the effect is often modest. Relaxation can be taught efficiently by school nurses; more than two-thirds of the children in one study (n=26) recorded at least 50% improvement at follow-up after 6 months, compared with only a quarter of controls.[12] Follow-up over an average of 4 years found that continuing to practice relaxation maintained the improvements in days free of headache and headache severity, compared with an untreated control group.[13] However, most studies have compared relaxation with no treatment. One exception is a trial among 202 adolescents in which relaxation was compared with placebo relaxation (sitting quietly, thinking of an episode from their life) and no difference was found.[14] It is therefore possible that relaxation techniques are of benefit albeit through non-specific effects.

Spinal manipulation

In a systematic review (Box 5.23) the combined evidence suggested that spinal manipulation has a useful effect on tension, cervicogenic and posttraumatic headaches. In the two studies of patients with tension headache, manipulation was marginally better than amitriptyline in some outcomes of one study and no better than placebo laser in the other. No clear conclusion can be drawn from the latter study since the placebo effect of sham laser is unknown and both groups also received soft tissue massage, the effectiveness of which is also unknown.

Box 5.23
Systematic review
Spinal manipulation for headache
Compl Ther Med 1999; 7:142–155

- Six RCTs for tension, cervicogenic or posttraumatic headache, involving 286 subjects

- Overall moderate quality

- No placebo-controlled studies

- Five studies reported benefit, though no long-term results are available; one reported no additional benefit in addition to deep massage

- No side-effects reported

- Spinal manipulation appears to be as effective as amitriptyline and more effective than ice pack or soft tissue therapy

Other therapies

Guided imagery was used as an adjunct to standard medical treatment in an RCT of 260 adults with chronic tension headache with or without migraine.[15] The intervention group received a guided imagery tape to listen to every day for 1 month and controls received standard medical treatment alone. Guided imagery was superior in global assessment and some quality of life measures.

In one double-dummy RCT involving 32 patients, **reflexology** was compared with flunarizin. Improvements in headache were twice as great with reflexology, but the difference was not statistically significant and methodological flaws prevent any firm conclusions.[16]

Non-contact **therapeutic touch** was significantly more effective than mock therapeutic touch in the treatment of acute headache in an RCT of reasonable quality that involved 90 subjects, though the difference was no longer apparent after 4 hours.[17]

Table 5.43
Summary of clinical evidence for headache

Treatment	Weight of evidence	Direction of evidence	Serious safety concerns
Acupuncture	O	⇨	Yes (see p 29)
Autogenic training	O	⬀	Yes (see p 37)
Biofeedback	OOO	⬀	No (see p 42)
Electrotherapy	O	⬀	Yes (see p 6)
Herbal medicine			
Peppermint (local)	O	⇧	Yes (see p 142)
Tiger balm (local)	O	⬀	Yes (see p 5)
Homeopathy	O	⇩	No (see p 55)
Hypnotherapy	OO	⬀	Yes (see p 58)
Relaxation	OO	⬀	No (see p 71)
Spinal manipulation	OO	⬀	Yes (see pp 47, 65)

Overall recommendation

The evidence is not convincing that any particular CAM therapy is more effective than placebo in preventing tension headaches. However, in the absence of genuinely safe and effective conventional treatment, it is relevant to note that patients may benefit from forms of treatment that involve relaxation. Relaxation in various forms, including straightforward muscular and mental relaxation, hypnotherapy and autogenic training, is simple, relatively safe and beneficial compared with no treatment, though patients should be aware it has not been demonstrated to be superior to placebo. The addition of biofeedback may increase the benefit compared with simple relaxation alone. Therapeutic touch, reflexology and acupuncture may also be worth considering, with the same caveats. Any potential benefit from spinal manipulative therapy is probably outweighed by the risk associated with cervical manipulation. In the treatment of acute headache, there is some evidence to

CONDITIONS

support the use of tiger balm or peppermint locally, and possibly electrotherapy.

REFERENCES

1 Eisenberg D M, Davis R, Ettner S L, Appel S, Wilkey S, Rompay M V. Trends in alternative medicine use in the United States, 1990–1997. JAMA 1998;280:1569–1575

2 Melchart D, Linde K, Fischer P et al. Acupuncture for recurrent headaches: a systematic review of randomized controlled trials. Cephalalgia 1999; 19:779–786

3 Ter Kuile M M, Spinhoven P, Linssen A C G, Zitman F G, Van Dyck R, Rooijmans H G M. Autogenic training and cognitive self-hypnosis for the treatment of recurrent headaches in three different subject groups. Pain 1994;58:331–340

4 Rokicki L A, Holroyd K A, France C R, Lipchik G L, France J L, Kvaal S A. Change mechanisms associated with combined relaxation/EMG biofeedback training for chronic tension headache. Applied Psychophysiol Biofeedback 1997;22:21–41

5 Hart J D. Predicting differential response to EMG biofeedback and relaxation training: the role of cognitive structure. J Clin Psychol 1984;40:453–457

6 Solomon S, Elkind A, Freitag F, Gallagher R M, Moore K, Swerdlow B, Malkin S. Safety and effectiveness of cranial electrotherapy in the treatment of tension headache. Headache 1989;29:445–450

7 Gobel H, Fresenius J, Heinze A, Dworschak M, Soyka D. Effectiveness of Oleum menthae piperitae and paracetamol in therapy of headache of the tension type. Nervenarzt 1996;67:672–681

8 Schattner P, Randerson D. Tiger Balm as a treatment of tension headache. A clinical trial in general practice. Aust Fam Physician 1996;25:216,218,220 passim

9 Walach H, Haeusler W, Lower T et al. Classical homeopathic treatment of chronic headaches. Cephalalgia 1997;17:119–126

10 Melis P M, Rooimans W, Spierings E L, Hoogduin C A. Treatment of chronic tension-type headache with hypnotherapy: a single-blind time controlled study. Headache 1991; 31:686–689

11 Reich B A. Non-invasive treatment of vascular and muscle contraction headache: a comparative longitudinal clinical study. Headache 1989;29:34–41

12 Larsson B, Melin L. Chronic headaches in adolescents: treatment in a school setting with relaxation training as compared with information-contact and self-registration. Pain 1986;25:325–336

13 Engel J M, Rapoff M A, Pressman A R. Long-term follow-up of relaxation training for pediatric headache disorders. Headache 1992;32:152–156

14 Passchier J, Van Den Bree M B, Emmen H H, Osterhaus S O, Orlebeke J F, Verhage F. Relaxation training in school classes does not reduce headache complaints. Headache 1990; 30:660–664

15 Mannix L K, Chandurkar R S, Rybicki L A et al. Effect of guided imagery on quality of life for patients with chronic tension-type headache. Headache 1999;39:326–334

16 Lafuente A, Noguera M, Puy C, Molins A, Titus F, Sanz F. Effekt der Reflexzonenbehandlung am Fuß bezüglich der prophylaktischen Behandlung mit Funarizin bei an Cephalea-Kopfschmerzen leidenden Patienten. Erfahrungsheilkunde 1990; 39:713–715

17 Keller E, Bzdek V M. Effects of therapeutic touch on tension headache pain. Nurs Res 1986;35:101–106

HEPATITIS

Definition Inflammation of the liver usually due to either viral infection or toxic agents.

Related conditions Liver cirrhosis.

CAM usage

Several herbal medicines and some other food supplements are used for various forms of hepatitis.

Clinical evidence

Herbal medicine

CH-100 is a mixture of 19 Chinese herbs. It was tested in a placebo-controlled RCT with 40 patients suffering from chronic hepatitis C.[1] The experimental group had a significant reduction of alanine aminotransferase but no patient cleared the virus.

Compound 861 is a Chinese herbal mixture including *Astralagus membranaceous*, *Salvia militiorrhiza* and *Spatholobus suberectus*. An observational study with 60 patients suffering from chronic hepatitis B has yielded promising results.[2] This was followed by an RCT including 22 patients with the same diagnosis.[3] Liver biopsies showed a significant improvement in histological inflammation and fibrosis in the experimental group and no such changes in the control group.

Jiedu yanggan gao is a Chinese herbal mixture containing 12 medicinal plants. A CCT with 96 patients suffering from chronic hepatitis B showed that 5 months of treatment led to a greater degree of normalization of liver enzymes in the experimental compared with the control group which did not receive the herbal mixture.[4] The authors claim that eight patients in the treatment group were cured.

Kamalahar is an Ayurvedic mixture of six herbs including *Phyllanthus urinaria*. In a placebo-controlled RCT with 52 patients suffering from acute viral hepatitis, 3×500 mg extract were given daily for 15 days.[5] Subsequently the experimental group had improved significantly more than the placebo group in terms of clinical symptoms and liver enzymes.

Licorice (*Glycyrrhiza glabra*) root has immunosuppressive and antiinflammatory effects. (Because of its aldosterone-like properties it should be used cautiously for patients with hypertension, hyperkalemia and ascites.) There are several studies showing beneficial effects for patients with hepatitis. An RCT included 28 patients with chronic hepatitis C who had previously not responded to interferon therapy.[6] Three months' treatment resulted in virus clearance in 33.3% of those patients who had received glycyrrhizin plus interferon while only 13.3% had the same result with interferon alone. A larger (n=84) but retrospective analysis of patients with chronic hepatitis C who had received IV glycyrrhizin 2–7 times weekly for an average of 10 years showed a reduction in risk of hepatocellular carcinomas.[7] Compared to matched patients who had remained untreated for a similar period, the risk was reduced by a factor of 2.5.

LIV 52 is an Ayurvedic herbal mixture which is also marketed in the West. Preliminary data had suggested that the preparation might be effective for hepatitis[8] and liver cirrhosis.[9] However, a 2-year clinical trial including 188 patients with alcoholic liver cirrhosis revealed an increased mortality in the treatment compared with the placebo group (81% vs 40%).[10] This herbal combination should therefore be considered obsolete.

A systematic review included four RCTs of **milk thistle** (*Silybum marianum*) for various forms of viral hepatitis.[11] The results were not uniformly positive, but overall showed an encouraging trend. The safety profile of milk thistle is equally encouraging. Thus the evidence is, on balance, in favor of milk thistle.

Phyllanthus species have been shown to inhibit hepatitis virus DNA polymerase and surface antigen expression. A placebo-controlled trial showed that 59% of all hepatitis B patients treated with *Phyllanthus amarus* lost hepatitis B surface antigen while only 4% in the placebo groups had this result.[12] Unfortunately, these findings could not be confirmed in two subsequent RCTs.[13,14] However, other *Phyllanthus* species seem to yield better results; 123 patients with hepatitis B were randomized to receive either *Phyllanthus amarus*, *P. niruri* or *P. urinaria* or no remedy.[15] Those treated with *P. urinaria* were most likely to lose detectable hepatitis B surface antigen from their serum.

Salvia miltiorrhiza and *Polyporus umbellatus* were tested alone or in combination in a three-armed RCT, including 90 patients with chronic hepatitis B.[16] After 3 months' therapy and at further 3 and 9 months' follow-up there were high rates of liver enzyme normalization and conversion of surface antigen in all these groups. However, results were consistently best for the combination therapy.

Sho-saiko-to is the Japanese name of a Chinese herbal mixture (Xiao-chai-hutang) which is also sometimes called Tj-9. It is composed of skullcap, licorice, bupleurum, ginseng, banxia, jujube and ginger. It has been shown to inhibit lipid peroxidation and hepatocellular membrane damage. A CCT demonstrated that medication with sho-saiko-to normalizes the cytokine production system in patients with hepatitis C.[17] An RCT showed promising clinical results in 222 patients with chronic hepatitis. They received either 54 g sho-saiko-to or placebo daily for 24 weeks.[18] This treatment resulted in significantly more improvement of liver enzymes in the experimental group compared with the control group. The subgroup of patients with hepatitis B also showed a trend towards a decrease of viral antigen and an increase in antibodies. A further RCT including 260 patients with liver cirrhosis showed a trend towards longer survival after 5 years' treatment with sho-saiko-to.[19]

An RCT with 138 hepatitis B patients showed positive results for **Uncaria gambir** compared with placebo.[20] Unfortunately it is burdened with significant toxicity and should therefore be considered obsolete.

Supplements

Epidemiological data from China suggested that **selenium** supplementation protects against hepatitis B infections and subsequent primary liver cancer. This was confirmed in a CCT with 226 hepatitis B surface antigen-positive patients.[21] They were treated either with 200 mcg selenium or placebo daily for 4 years. In the control group, seven patients developed primary liver cancers during this period while in the selenium group no such event was noted.

No evidence for a beneficial effect was found for an extract of bovine **thymus** cells compared with placebo in a rigorous RCT including 38 patients with hepatitis C.[22]

Table 5.44
Summary of clinical evidence for hepatitis

Treatment	Weight of evidence	Direction of evidence	Serious safety concerns
Herbal medicine			
CH-100	O	⬀	Yes (see p 5)
Compound 861	O	⬀	Yes (see p 5)
Jiedu yanggan	O	⬀	Yes (see p 5)
Kamalahar	O	⬀	Yes (see p 5)
Licorice	OO	⇧	Yes (see p 169)
LIV 52	O	⇩	Yes (see p 5)
Milk thistle	OO	⬀	Yes (see p 135)
Phyllanthus spp	OO	⇨	Yes (see p 5)
Salvia miltiorrhiza & Polyporus umbellatus	O	⬀	Yes (see p 5)
Sho-saiko-to	OO	⬀	Yes (see p 5)
Uncaria gambir	O	⇩	Yes (see p 5)
Supplements			
Selenium	OO	⇧	Yes (see p 5)
Thymus extracts	O	⇩	Yes (see p 173)

Overall recommendation

Some forms of hepatitis can be both serious and difficult to treat. Conventional therapy (e.g. interferon) is by no means always successful. Good evidence exists for licorice root and milk thistle as treatments for viral hepatitis and for selenium and licorice root as a means of prevention of liver cancer. The adverse effects of licorice require vigilance. Milk thistle and selenium are associated with markedly fewer safety concerns. These options seem those most worthy of consideration in suitable cases.

CONDITIONS

REFERENCES

1 Batey R G, Bensoussan A, Fan Y Y, Bollipio S, Hossain M A. Preliminary report of a randomized, double-blind placebo-controlled trial of a Chinese herbal medicine preparation CH-100 in the treatment of chronic hepatitis C. J Gastroenterol Hepatol 1998;13:244–247

2 Wang H J, Wang B E. Long term follow-up result of compound 861 in treating hepatofibrosis. Chin J Integr Trad West Med 1995;5:4–5

3 Wang T L, Wang B E, Zhang H H. Pathological study of the therapeutic effect on HBV-related

liver fibrosis with herbal compound 861. Chin J Gastroenterol Hepatol 1998;7:148–153

4   Chen Z. Clinical study of 96 cases with chronic hepatitis B treated with jiedu yanggan gao by a double-blind method. Chin J Modern Develop Trad Med 1990;10:71–74

5   Das D G. A double-blind clinical trial of Kamalahar, an indigenous compound preparation in acute viral hepatitis. Indian J Gastroenterol 1993;12:126–128

6   Abe Y, Ueda T, Kato T, Kohli Y. Effectiveness of interferon, glycyrrhizin combination therapy in patients with chronic hepatitis C. Nippon Rinsho 1994;52:1817–1822

7   Arase Y, Ikeda K, Murashima N et al. The long term efficacy of Glycyrrhizin in chronic hepatitis C patients. Cancer 1997; 79:1494–1500

8   Desai V, Dudhia M, Ghandi V. A clinical study on infective hepatitis treated with LIV 52. Indian Paediatr 1997;3:197

9   Lotterer E, Etzel R. Pilotstudie einer kontrollierten klinischen Prüfung von Liv.52 bei Patienten mit alkoholischer Leberzirrhose. Forsch Komplementärmed 1995;2:12–14

10 Fleig W W, Morgan M Y, Holzer M A. The Ayurvedic drug LIV 52 in patients with alcoholic cirrhosis. Results of a prospective, double-blind, placebo-controlled clinical trial. J Hepatol 1997;26(suppl 1):127

11 Mulrow C, Lawrence V, Jacobs B et al. Report on milk thistle: effects on liver disease and cirrhosis and clinical adverse effects. Evidence Report/Technology Assessment 2000 (unpublished)

12 Thyagarajan S P, Subramanian S, Thirunalasundari T, Venkateswaran P S. Effect of phyllanthus amarus on chronic carriers of hepatitis B virus. Lancet 1988;2:764–766

13 Milne A M, Waldon J, Foo Y. Failure of New Zealand hepatitis B carriers to respond to Phyllanthus amarus. N Z J Med 1994;107:243

14 Leelarasamee A, Trakulosomboon S, Maunwongyathi P. Failure of Phyllanthus amarus to eradicate hepatitis B surface antigen from symptomless carriers. Lancet 1990;335:1600–1601

15 Wang M, Cheng H, Li Y, Meng L, Zhao G, Mai K. Herbs of the genus Phyllanthus in the treatment of chronic hepatitis B: observations with three preparations from different geographic sites. J Lab Clin Med 1995; 126:350–352

16 Xiong L L. Therapeutic effect of combined therapy of Salvia miltiorrhiza and Polyporus umbellatus polysaccharide in the treatment of chronic hepatitis B. Chung Kuo Chung Hsi i Chieh Ho Tsa Chih 1993;13:516–517, 533–535

17 Yamashiki M, Nishimura A, Suzuki H, Sakaguchi S, Kosaka Y. Effects of the Japanese herbal medicine "Sho-Saiko-To" (TJ-9) on in vitro interleukin-10 production by peripheral blood mononuclear cells of patients with chronic hepatitis C. Hepatology 1997;25:1390–1397

18 Hirayama C, Okumura M, Tanikawa K, Yano M, Mizuta M, Ogawa N. A multicenter randomized controlled clinical trial of Shosaiko-to in chronic active hepatitis. Gastroenterologia Japonica 1989; 24:715–719

19 Oha H, Yamamoto S, Kuroki T. Prospective study of chemoprevention of hepatocellular carcinoma with Sho-saiko-to (TJ-9). Cancer 1995;76:743–749

20 Suzuki H, Yamamoto S, Hirayama C. Cianidanol therapy for HBe antigen positive chronic hepatitis. Liver 1986;6:35–44

21 Yu S Y, Zhu Y J, Li W G. Protective role of Selenium against hepatitis B virus and primary liver cancer in Qidong. Biol Trace Element Res 1997;56:117–124

22 Raymond R S, Fallon M B, Abrams G A. Oral thymic extract for chronic hepatitis C in patients previously treated with interferon: a randomized, double-blind, placebo-controlled trial. Ann Intern Med 1998; 129:797–800

HERPES SIMPLEX

Synonyms/ subcategories	Cold sores, herpes labialis, herpes genitalis.
Definition	A variety of infections caused by herpes simplex virus types 1 and 2.

Related conditions	Traumatic herpes, herpes gladiatorum.
CAM usage	Herbal creams are commonly used for the treatment of acute lesions or prevention of recurrences.

Clinical evidence

Herbal medicine

Several studies have suggested that **lemon balm** (*Melissa officinalis*) speeds up the healing of herpes labialis lesions. The most rigorous of these investigations was a placebo-controlled RCT including 66 patients with acute herpes labialis.[1] They applied a commercial cream (Lomaherpan) or placebo cream four times per day for 5 days. The results show significant advantages for the herbal preparation in terms of symptom scores.

A placebo-controlled RCT of **Siberian ginseng** (*Eleuthero-coccus senticosus*) root extract was carried out in 93 individuals with recurrent herpes simplex infections.[2] The aim was to test the effectiveness of this medication in preventing further recurrences. All participants took 4 g extract or placebo for 6 months. In the experimental group, 75% reported improvements in severity duration or frequency of attacks while this figure was 34% in the placebo group.

Supplements

A three-armed RCT tested the effectiveness of Canadian **propolis** against acyclovir or placebo in 30 women with recurrent genital herpes.[3] A tampon with the appropriate ointment was inserted four times per day for 10 days. The average healing time was fastest in the propolis group. Moreover, the incidence of super-infections was reduced in the propolis group.

Table 5.45
Summary of clinical evidence for herpes simplex

Treatment	Weight of evidence	Direction of evidence	Serious safety concerns
Herbal medicine			
Lemon balm (treatment)	OO	⇧	Yes (see p 169)
Siberian ginseng (prevention)	O	⇧	Yes (see p 154)
Supplements			
Propolis (genital herpes)	O	⇧	Yes (see p 147)

Overall recommendation

Herpes simplex infections are difficult to treat with conventional medications and recurrences are even more resistant to therapy. The evidence for CAM is promising but, in most cases, the weight of the evidence is not sufficient for strong recommendations. The exception is topical lemon balm for healing cold sores, which is as effective as conventional therapies and, as far as is known, free of serious adverse effects when applied topically.

CONDITIONS

REFERENCES

1 Koytchev R, Alken R G, Dundarov S. Balm mint extract (Lo-701) for topical treatment of recurring Herpes labialis. Phytomedicine 1999;6:225–230

2 Williams M. Immuno-protection against herpes simplex type II infection by eleutherococcus root extract. Int J Alt Compl Med 1995;13(7):9–12

3 Vynograd N, Vynograd I, Sosnowski Z. A comparative multi-centre study of the efficacy of propolis, acyclovir and placebo in the treatment of genital herpes (HSV). Phytomedicine 2000;7:1–6

HERPES ZOSTER

Synonyms
Shingles.

Definition
An infection caused by the varicella zoster virus, characterized by an eruption of groups of vesicles usually on one side of the body which follow the anatomical course of a nerve or nerve root.

Related conditions
Postherpetic neuralgia.

CAM usage
Various CAM therapies are being advocated for the symptomatic treatment of postherpetic pain. Other treatments are claimed to enhance the healing process of the infection. Acupuncture is used both during infection and to treat neuralgia.

Clinical evidence

Acupuncture
Several CCTs of acupuncture for postherpetic pain have been published. Collectively, they have yielded disappointing results (e.g. [1]). Thus there is no good evidence for its use in this condition.

Enzyme therapy
A commercial enzyme extract (Wobe-Mucos), consisting of trypsin, chymotrypsin, papainase and calf thymus hydrolysate, is promoted in Germany. Two RCTs have suggested that the intramuscular or oral administration of this preparation is equally effective as acyclovir in treating herpes zoster.[2,3] However, this evidence is weak due to methodological shortcomings in both studies.

Herbal medicine
Three placebo-controlled RCTs of topical **capsaicin** for postherpetic pain are available.[4] Collectively they demonstrate that capsaicin cream is superior to placebo for symptomatic pain relief. The effect size, however, is modest.

A topical formulation of ***Clinacanthus nutans*** or placebo was applied five times daily to the affected area for 7–14 days in a CCT with 51 patients suffering from herpes zoster.[5] Compared with placebo, the experimental group exhibited significantly faster healing of the skin lesions. Similarly encouraging results were reported from a subsequent larger RCT.[6]

Table 5.46
**Summary of
clinical evidence
for herpes zoster**

Treatment	Weight of evidence	Direction of evidence	Serious safety concerns
Acupuncture (postherpetic neuralgia)	OO	⇩	Yes (see p 29)
Enzyme therapy (acute herpes)	O	⇗	Yes (see p 80)
Herbal medicine			
Capsaicin (postherpetic neuralgia)	OO	⇧	Yes (see p 5)
Clinacanthus nutans (acute herpes)	O	⇧	Yes (see p 5)

**Overall
recommendation**

Herpes zoster infection and its clinical sequelae are often difficult to control with conventional treatments. The evidence for some forms of CAM is promising but the weight of the evidence is mostly not sufficient for strong recommendations. The exception is topical capsaicin to alleviate postherpetic neuralgia which compares well to conventional therapies in terms of the balance between risk and benefit.

REFERENCES

1 Lewith G T, Field J, Machin D. Acupuncture compared with placebo in post-herpetic pain. Pain 1983;17:361–368
2 Kleine M W, Stauder G M, Beese E W. The intestinal absorption of orally administered hydrolytic enzymes and their effects in the treatment of acute herpes zoster as compared with those of oral acyclovir therapy. Phytomedicine 1995;2:7–15
3 Billigmann V P. Enzymtherapie – eine Alternative bei der Behandlung des Zoster. Fortschr Med 1995;113(4): 39–44

4 Volmink J, Lancaster T, Gray S, Silagy C. Treatments of postherpetic neuralgia – a systematic review of randomized controlled trials. Fam Pract 1996;13:84–91
5 Sangkitporn S, Chaiwat S, Balachandra K, Na-Ayudhaya T D, Bunjob M, Jayavasu C. Treatment of herpes zoster with Clinacanthus nutans (bi yaw yaw) extract. J Med Assoc Thailand 1995;78:624–627
6 Charuwichitratana S, Wongrattanapasson N, Timpatanapong P, Bunjob M. Herpes zoster: treatment with *Clinacanthus nutans* cream. Int J Dermatol 1996;35:665–666

CONDITIONS

HYPERCHOLESTEROLEMIA

Synonyms

Hypercholesteremia, hypercholesterinemia.

Definition

The presence of an abnormally large amount of cholesterol in the plasma of the circulating blood.

**Related
conditions**

Dyslipidemia, hyperlipidemia, hypertriglyceridemia.

CAM usage

Total serum cholesterol can be lowered by reducing fat intake and by increasing regular physical activity. Thus various lifestyle approaches common in CAM can have an effect and are frequently promoted for this purpose. Numerous other modifications of the regular diet are used. These approaches are usually not specific to CAM. Several herbal treatments and other food supplements are used to lower cholesterol levels.

Clinical evidence

Diet

Oat and other fiber products have repeatedly been shown to reduce total and LDL cholesterol. The effect seems to be greater with insoluble fibers.[1] The effect size for oat products seems to be small (Box 5.24).

Box 5.24
Metaanalysis
Oat fiber for hypercholestolemia
JAMA 1992;267: 3317–3325

- Twenty RCTs were included

- Raw data of all trials were obtained and results were recalculated and pooled

- Methodological quality of the trials was, on average, good

- Total cholesterol fell by 0.13 mmol/l

- Stronger effects were noted if initial cholesterol levels were high or dosage of oat fiber was large

- Conclusion: oat fibers cause a modest reduction in total cholesterol

Psyllium (*Plantago ovata*) is a water-soluble fiber product advocated as a bulk laxative. Several RCTs have demonstrated that psyllium can lower total and LDL cholesterol. A metaanalysis of eight RCTs arrived at a positive conclusion (Box 5.25).

Box 5.25
Metaanalysis
Psyllium for hypercholestolemia
Am J Nutr 2000;71: 472–479

- Eight RCTs were included

- In total, 384 patients with mild to moderate hypercholesterolemia received psyllium (10.2 g daily) and 272 received cellulose as placebo

- The quality of these trials was, on average, good

- All subjects were taking a low-fat diet concomitantly

- On average, psyllium lowered total cholesterol by 4% and LDL by 7%

- Psyllium was well tolerated

- Conclusion: psyllium causes a modest reduction of total and LDL cholesterol

Herbal medicine

Dai-saiko-to is a Kampo medicine which was tested in a placebo-controlled RCT including 30 hypertensive patients.[2] Total cholesterol and triglyceride levels did not change significantly but HDL cholesterol increased.

Fenugreek (*Trigonella foenum graecum*) is often advocated for the purpose of normalizing cardiovascular risk factors; 100 g fenugreek seed powder was given daily to a group of patients with insulin-dependent diabetes in an uncontrolled observational study.[3] A fall in fasting blood glucose, total cholesterol, LDL cholesterol and triglycerides was noted.

Garlic (*Allium sativum*) is one of the best clinically investigated herbal remedies. Numerous RCTs have been published, some of high methodological quality. A metaanalysis of 16 RCTs yielded an overall reduction of total cholesterol of 0.77 mmol/l which was a 12% decrease over and above placebo.[4] Since the publication of this article several negative trials have emerged necessitating a reanalysis of this data. The new metaanalysis is cautiously positive (Box 5.26) but the effect size casts doubt on the clinical relevance of the effect.

Box 5.26
Metaanalysis
Garlic for hyper-cholesterolemia
Ann Intern Med
2000;133: 420–429

- Thirteen double-blind, placebo-controlled RCTs were included with 781 patients in total

- The average quality of the studies was good

- On average, there was a significant reduction of 0.41 mmol/l (CI −0.66 to −0.15)

- The six most rigorous, diet-controlled trials showed a non-significant trend only

- Conclusion: garlic is superior to placebo but the effect is small and of debatable clinical relevance

Thirty-six patients with type II diabetes were randomized to receive either 100 mg or 200 mg **ginseng** (*Panax ginseng*) powder or placebo for 8 weeks.[5] Fasting glucose levels decreased but the serum lipid profile did not change significantly.

Guar gum is a dietary fiber product obtained from *Cyamopsis tetragonolobus*. It has been repeatedly shown to lower total cholesterol.[6] In a placebo-controlled, double-blind RCT, 5 g granulated guar gum or placebo was given three times daily for a mean duration of 24 months to patients who had undergone carotid endarterectomy.[7] Both after 12 and 24 months there were statistically significant and clinically relevant reductions of total cholesterol (−1.07 mmol/l) and LDL cholesterol (−1.10 mmol/l).

Saiko-ka-ryukotsu-borei-to is a herbal mixture used in Kampo medicine. An uncontrolled trial with 21 diabetic patients

CONDITIONS

suggested that it lowers total cholesterol and LDL cholesterol levels.[8] This finding, however, was not confirmed by an RCT which compared the effects of two Kampo medicines but did not employ a placebo control group and showed no relevant changes in total cholesterol.[8]

Terminalia arjuna is a herb used in Ayurvedic medicine for various cardiovascular indications. It was used in an uncontrolled trial with patients suffering from coronary heart disease.[9] No relevant changes of total cholesterol or other lipid variables were noted.

A steroid extract from **yam** (*Dioscorea* spp) was tested in an uncontrolled study with elderly individuals.[10] No effect on total cholesterol but an increase in HDL and a decrease in triglycerides were noted.

Supplements

Several studies of dubious quality have implied that **chitosan** is effective. A rigorous, placebo-controlled RCT did not find any effect on blood lipid pattern.[11]

Co-enzyme Q10 (60 mg twice daily) was given orally to 47 patients with slightly elevated levels of lipoprotein (a) and coronary heart disease for 28 days.[12] This regimen did not significantly alter total cholesterol but increased HDL cholesterol and lowered LDL cholesterol and lipoprotein (a).

Phytosterols are plant-derived sterols like sitosterol and campesterol. A review of 16 clinical studies using various methodologies showed that, on average, the supplementation with plant sterols reduced total cholesterol levels by 10% and LDL by 13%.[13]

Red yeast rice is the fermented product of rice on which red yeast (*Monascus purpureus*) has been grown. Traditionally it has been used in China for medicinal purposes and it is now commercially available as a food supplement. Two RCTs are available to show that red yeast rice lowers total cholesterol.[14,15] In the more rigorous recent trial,[15] 83 healthy subjects with hyperlipidemia were given either 2.4 g per day of red yeast rice or placebo for 12 weeks. The total cholesterol level decreased from 6.57 mmol/l to 5.38 mmol/l. Similarly positive effects were also observed for LDL cholesterol and triglycerides.

Other therapies

Ozone therapy was tested in 21 patients with a history of myocardial infarction who were treated with ozone autohemotherapy in an uncontrolled study.[16] A statistically significant decrease in total and LDL cholesterol was observed.

Ninety-three patients with cardiovascular risk factors or coronary heart disease were randomized to either follow a **yoga** lifestyle or continue as usual for 14 weeks.[17] The intervention included yoga and a change in diet. A significant reduction of total cholesterol was noted after 4 weeks and continued for the entire treatment period.

Table 5.47
Summary of clinical evidence for hypercholesterolemia

Treatment	Weight of evidence	Direction of evidence	Serious safety concerns
Diet			
Oat fiber	OOO	⇧	No
Psyllium	OOO	⇧	No
Herbal medicine			
Dai-saiko-to	O	⇧	Yes (see p 5)
Fenugreek	O	⇧	Yes (see p 168)
Garlic	OOO	⇧	Yes (see p 109)
Guar gum	OOO	⇧	Yes (see p 122)
Ginseng	O	⇩	No (see p 88)
Saiko-ka-ryukotsu-borei-to	O	⇨	Yes (see p 5)
Terminalia arjuna	O	⇩	Yes (see p 5)
Yam	O	⇧	Yes (see p 5)
Supplements			
Chitosan	O	⇩	Yes (see p 94)
Co-enzyme Q10	O	⇧	No (see p 97)
Phytosterols	OO	⇧	Yes (see p 5)
Red yeast rice	OO	⇧	Yes (see p 173)

Overall recommendation

CAM offers several options for reducing total cholesterol levels. Fiber supplements are effective but may be seen as conventional dietary treatment. Compelling evidence exists also for garlic. The effect size of all these therapies is modest and considerably less than that of synthetic lipid-lowering drugs. The exception may be red yeast rice, but more data are required for this novel food supplement. The bottom line, therefore, is that some CAM treatments are associated with modest cholesterol-lowering effects which, not least because of their relative safety, warrants their use in cases where diet alone is not sufficiently effective.

CONDITIONS

REFERENCES

1 Glore S R, Van Treeck D, Knehans A W, Guild M. Soluble fiber and serum lipids: a literature review. J Am Dietetic Assoc 1994;94:425–436

2 Saku K, Hirata K, Zhang B et al. Effects of Chinese herbal drugs on serum lipids, lipoproteins and apolipoproteins in mild to moderate essential hypertensive patients. J Hum Hypertens 1992;6:393–395

3 Sharma R D, Raghuram T C, Rao N S. Effect of fenugreek seeds on blood glucose and serum lipids in type I diabetes. Eur J Clin Nutr 1990;44:301–306

4 Silagy C, Neil A. Garlic as a lipid lowering agent – a meta-analysis. J Roy Coll Physicians Lond 1994;28:39–45

5 Sotaneimi E A, Haapakoski E, Rautio A. Ginseng therapy in non-insulin-dependent diabetic patients. Diabetes Care 1995; 18:1373–1375

6 Todd P A, Benfield P, Goa K L. Guar gum: a review of its pharmacological properties, and

use as a dietary adjunct in hyper-cholesterolemia. Drugs 1990;39:917–928

7 Salenius J-P, Harjo E, Jokela H, Reikkinen H, Silvasti M. Long term effects of guar gum on lipid metabolism after carotid endarterectomy. Br Med J 1995;310:95–96

8 Nomura K, Hayashi K, Kuga Y et al. Hypolipidemic effect of Saiko-ka-ryukotsu-borei-to (TJ-12) in patients with type II or type IV hyperlipidemia. Curr Ther Res Clin Exp 1997;58:446–453

9 Dwivedi S, Agarwal M P. Antianginal and cardioprotective effects of *terminalia arjuna*, an indigenous drug, in coronary artery disease. J Assoc Physicians India 1994; 42:287–289

10 Araghiniknam M, Chung S, Nelson-White T, Eskelson C, Watson R R. Antioxidant activity of dioscorea and dehydroepiandrosterone (DHEA) in older humans. Life Sci 1996; 59:PL147–PL157

11 Pittler M H, Abbot N C, Harkness E F, Ernst E. Randomized, double-blind trial of chitosan for body weight reduction. Eur J Clin Nutr 1999; 53:379–381

12 Singh R B. Serum concentration of lipoprotein (a) decreases on treatment with hydrosoluble coenzyme Q10 in patients with coronary

artery disease: discovery of a new role. Int J Cardiol 1999;68:23–29

13 Moghadasian M H, Frohlich J J. Effects of dietary phytosterols on cholesterol metabolism and atherosclerosis: clinical and experimental evidence. Am J Med 1999;107:588–594

14 Wang J, Lu Z, Chi J et al. Multicenter clinical trial of the serum lipid-lowering effects of a *monascus purpureus* (red yeast) rice preparation from traditional Chinese medicine. Curr Ther Res 1997;58:964–978

15 Heber D, Yip I, Ashley J M, Elashoff D A, Elashoff R M, Go V L W. Cholesterol-lowering effects of a proprietary Chinese red-yeast-rice dietary supplement. Am J Clin Nutr 1999; 69:231–236

16 Hernandez F, Menendez F, Wong R. Decrease of blood cholesterol and stimulation of antioxidative response in cardiopathy patients treated with endovenous ozone therapy. Free Radical Biol Med 1995;19:115–119

17 Mahajan A S, Reddy K S, Sachdeva U. Lipid profile of coronary risk subjects following yogic lifestyle intervention. Indian Heart J 1999;51:37–40

INSOMNIA

Synonyms   Sleeplessness, sleep disturbance.

Definition   A persistent condition of unsatisfactory quantity and/or quality of sleep, including difficulty initiating or maintaining sleep.

CAM usage   According to a US survey, insomnia is a common reason for using CAM, with relaxation and herbal medicine being the most popular therapies.[1]

Clinical evidence

Acupuncture

One RCT (n=40) reported greater objective and subjective sleep improvements with acupuncture than sham treatment,[2] while in a trial where patients chose their treatment, sleep improved with both needle and laser acupuncture but also in a waiting list control group.[3] Acupressure produced better results than both sham and no treatment in an RCT (n=84) of elderly insomniacs.[4] Positive effects of acupressure on sleep were also reported in a very small (n=6) sham-controlled crossover RCT with healthy volunteers.[5] Acupuncture/pressure appears to have some promise in promoting sleep, but the evidence is currently limited.

Biofeedback

Several controlled trials have found no or only minimal improvement in sleep with biofeedback compared with other interventions, no treatment or sham feedback.[6-9] However, in two RCTs[8,9] positive results were reported in patients for whom the particular form of feedback was appropriate. For example, EEG feedback benefited those with anxiety-related insomnia and sensorimotor rhythm feedback helped non-anxious insomniacs. The indications are that biofeedback is not helpful for insomnia in general, but may be if tailored for the individual patient.

Exercise

A large body of evidence from healthy volunteers suggests that both acute and chronic exercise can have small to moderate positive effects on sleep duration and quality.[10] An RCT of elderly individuals (n=43) with moderate sleep disturbances improved in several sleep parameters after undertaking a structured exercise program, compared with those on a waiting list.[11]

Box 5.27
Systematic review
**Valerian for
insomnia**
Sleep Med 2000;l:91–99

- Nine double-blind, placebo-controlled RCTs including 390 volunteers

- Volunteers were insomniacs (four trials) or healthy sleepers (five trials)

- Valerian given as single dose (six trials) or for several weeks (three trials)

- Trial quality generally low

- Some positive results but totality of evidence not conclusive

Herbal medicine

Kava (*Piper methysticum*) was shown to improve subjective and objective measures of sleep after acute administration (300 mg) in healthy volunteers (n=12) in a placebo-controlled trial.[12] It has not been investigated in insomniacs.

A systematic review of nine placebo-controlled RCTs of the effects of **valerian** (*Valeriana officinalis*) on sleep reported some positive findings of acute and cumulative effects in patients with insomnia and healthy volunteers (Box 5.27). There was little consistency between studies, though, and the body of evidence is far from compelling. A further RCT (n=75) reported similar results for valerian and oxazepam in improving the sleep quality of insomniacs.[13] A subsequent crossover RCT of valerian compared with placebo (n=16) found no acute effects following a single dose, with improvements after 14 days' administration limited to slow-wave sleep.[14] Positive results also exist from

CONDITIONS

RCTs of preparations combining valerian with other herbs such as hop and lemon balm.[15,16]

Hypnotherapy

Positive results with hypnosis have been reported versus no treatment in a non-randomized trial of 37 female patients[17] and several comparison and placebo interventions in RCTs.[18-20] Taking into account various methodological limitations of these studies, hypnotherapy appears to have some promise in improving sleep.

Relaxation

A large number of clinical trials have suggested that relaxation training can improve sleep, but few are controlled studies and even fewer are randomized. One RCT (n=22) reported that progressive relaxation training (10 sessions over 2 weeks) was superior to no treatment for alcoholic insomniacs,[21] while another (n=53) found it as effective as stimulus control.[22] A further RCT (n=26) reported that compared with no treatment, relaxation and sleep hygiene alone produced better long-term results than when hypnotic drugs were also allowed.[23]

Two metaanalyses of non-pharmacological treatments for insomnia have concluded that relaxation techniques are effective therapies.[24,25] However, they both included uncontrolled studies and categorized various therapies under relaxation (e.g. autogenic training, biofeedback, desensitization, meditation) so do not constitute compelling evidence. Furthermore, the size of improvements was quite small although well maintained over time.

Supplements

The evidence for the efficacy of **melatonin** in treating insomnia consists of a number of small placebo-controlled trials, including at least five that were randomized. Two had negative results,[26,27] while three others reported improvements in several sleep parameters with 2 mg melatonin taken 2 hours before bed (Table 5.48). Positive effects have also been reported with healthy volunteers in controlled studies.[28,29] Although some studies suggest that melatonin supplementation is most effective when natural levels are low, as with the elderly,[30,31] there is contradictory evidence.[32,33] It appears to have good tolerability. The current body of evidence is not conclusive, but suggests that melatonin may have some potential in treating insomnia. The sleep-promoting effects of **vitamin B_{12}** have been investigated in an RCT (n=50) of people with delayed sleep-phase syndrome[34] and a small non-randomized trial (n=10) of shift workers;[35] neither found any superiority over placebo.

Other therapies

An **aromatherapy** study with healthy volunteers under stressful conditions indicated that sleep latency was significantly reduced by the odour of bitter orange essential oil, but not five other oils including lavender and valerian.[36]

Table 5.48 **Double-blind, placebo-controlled, crossover RCTs of melatonin for insomnia**

Reference	Sample size	Interventions [dosage]	Results	Comment
Lancet 1995;346: 541–544	12	A) Melatonin [2 mg 2 h pre-bed for 21 d] B) Placebo	A superior to B on sleep efficiency & time awake after sleep onset, not on sleep latency or total sleep	Elderly chronically ill patients all taking sleep medication
Sleep 1995; 18:598–599	26	A) Melatonin [2 mg fast release 2 h pre-bed for 7 d] B) Melatonin [2 mg slow release] C) Placebo	A superior to C in sleep latency. B superior to C in sleep efficiency & activity	Free-living & institutionalized elderly insomniacs
Arch Gerontol Geriatr 1997; 24:223–231	21	A) Melatonin [2 mg 2 h pre-bed for 21 d] B) Placebo	A superior to B on all sleep parameters	Elderly insomniacs taking benzodiazepines

Table 5.49
Summary of clinical evidence for insomnia

Treatment	Weight of evidence	Direction of evidence	Serious safety concerns
Acupuncture	O	⇧	Yes (see p 29)
Biofeedback	OO	⇩	No (see p 42)
Exercise	O	⇧	Yes (see p 5)
Herbal medicine			
Kava	O	⇧	Yes (see p 129)
Valerian	OO	⇗	Yes (see p 161)
Hypnotherapy	OO	⇧	Yes (see p 58)
Relaxation	OO	⇧	No (see p 71)
Supplements			
Melatonin	OO	⇗	Yes (see p 133)
Vitamin B$_{12}$	O	⇩	No

CONDITIONS

Overall recommendation

There is no compelling evidence for the efficacy of any complementary therapy and little indication that any of them can match conventional hypnotic medications. However, some preliminary, promising evidence exists for valerian and melatonin. Tolerability for both of these medicines appears to be good. Relaxation techniques and regular physical activity appear to convey small to moderate benefits on sleep and, given their harmless nature and other health benefits, are to be encouraged.

REFERENCES

1 Eisenberg D M, Davis R B, Ettner S L, Appel S, Wilkey S, Rompay M V, Kessler R C. Trends in alternative medicine use in the United States, 1990–1997. JAMA 1998;280:1569–1575

2 Montakab H. Acupuncture and insomnia. Forsch Komplementärmed 1999; 1 (suppl):29–31

3 Becker-Carus C, Heyden T, Kelle A. Die Wirksamkeit von Akupunktur und Einstellungs-Entspannungstraining zur Behandlung primärer Schlafstörungen. Z Klin Psychol Psychopathol Psychopath 1985; 33:161–172

4 Chen M L, Lin L C, Wu S C, Lin J G. Effectiveness of acupressure in improving the quality of sleep of institutionalised residents. J Gerontol Med Sci 1999;54A:M389–M394

5 Buguet A, Sartre M, LeKerneau J. Continuous nocturnal automassage of an acupuncture point modifies sleep in healthy subjects. Neurophysiologie Clinique 1995;25:78–83

6 Freedman R, Papsdorf J D. Biofeedback and progressive relaxation treatment of sleep-onset insomnia: a controlled all-night investigation. Biofeedback Self Regulation 1976;1:253–271

7 Nicassio P M, Boylan M B, McCabe T G. Progressive relaxation, EMG biofeedback and biofeedback placebo in the treatment of sleep-onset insomnia. Br J Med Psychol 1982; 55:159–166

8 Hauri P. Treating psychophysiologic insomnia with biofeedback. Arch Gen Psychiatr 1981; 38:752–758

9 Hauri P J, Percy L, Hellekson C, Hartmann E, Russ D. The treatment of psychophysiologic insomnia with biofeedback: a replication study. Biofeedback Self Regulation 1982; 7:223–235

10 Kubitz K A, Landers D M, Petruzzello S J, Han M. The effects of acute and chronic exercise on sleep. Sports Med 1996;21:277–291

11 King A C, Oman R F, Brassington G S, Bliwise D L, Haskell W L. Moderate intensity exercise and self-rated quality of sleep in older adults: a randomized controlled trial. JAMA 1997;277:32–37

12 Emser W, Bartylla K. Verbesserung der Schlafqualität: Zur Wirkung von Kava-Extrakt WS 1490 auf das Schlafmuster bei Gesunden. Neurologie/Psychiatrie 1991;5:636–642

13 Dorn M. Baldrian versus oxazepam: efficacy and tolerability in non-organic and non-psychiatric insomniacs: a randomized,

double-blind, clinical comparative study. Forsch Komplementärmed Klass Naturheilkd 2000;7:79–84

14 Donath R, Quispe S, Diefenbach K, Maurer A, Fietze I, Roots I. Critical evaluation of the effect of valerian extract on sleep structure and sleep quality. Pharmacopsychiatry 2000; 33:47–53

15 Cerny A, Schmid K. Tolerability and efficacy of valerian/lemon balm in healthy volunteers (a double-blind, placebo-controlled, multicentre study). Fitoterapia 1999; 70:221–228

16 Gerhard U, Linnenbrink N, Georghiadou C, Hob V. Effects of two plant-based sleep remedies on vigilance. 1996;85:473–481

17 Borkovec T D, Fowles D C. Controlled investigation of the effects of progressive and hypnotic relaxation on insomnia. J Abnormal Psychol 1973; 82:153–158

18 Anderson J A, Dalton E R, Basker M A. Insomnia and hypnotherapy. J Roy Soc Med 1979;72:734–739

19 Barabasz A F. Treatment of insomnia in depressed patients by hypnosis and cerebral electrotherapy. Am J Clin Hypnos 1976; 19:120–122

20 Stanton H E. Hypnotic relaxation and the reduction of sleep onset insomnia. Int J Psychosom 1989;36:64–68

21 Greeff A P, Conradie W S. Use of progressive relaxation training for chronic alcoholics with insomnia. Psychol Reps 1998; 82:407–412

22 Engle Friedman M, Bootzin R R, Hazlewood L, Tsao C. An evaluation of behavioural treatments for insomnia in the older adult. J Clin Psychol 1992;48:77–90

23 Hauri P J. Can we mix behavioural therapy with hypnotics when treating insomniacs? Sleep 1997;20:1111–1118

24 Morin C M, Culbert J P, Schwartz S M. Nonpharmacological interventions for insomnia: a meta-analysis of treatment efficacy. Am J Psychiatr 1994;151:1172–1180

25 Murtagh D R, Greenwood K M. Identifying effective psychological treatments for insomnia: a meta-analysis. J Consult Clin Psychol 1995;63:79–89

26 Dawson D, Rogers N L, Van Den Heuvel C, Kennaway D J, Lushington K. Effect of sustained nocturnal transbuccal melatonin administration on sleep and temperature in elderly insomniacs. J Biol Rhythms 1998; 13:532–538

27 Ellis C M, Lemmens G, Parkes J D. Melatonin and insomnia. J Sleep Res 1996;5:61–65

28 Waldhauser F, Saletu B, Trinchard-Lugan I. Sleep laboratory investigations on hypnotic properties of melatonin. Psychopharmacology 1990;100:222–226

29 Dollins A B, Zhdanova I V, Wurtman R J, Lynch H J, Deng M H. Effect of inducing nocturnal serum melatonin concentrations in daytime on sleep, mood, body temperature and performance. Proc Natl Acad Sci 1994; 91:1824–1828

30 Nave R, Peled R, Lavie P. Melatonin improves evening napping. Eur J Pharmacol 1995; 275:213–216

31 Haimov I, Laudon M, Zisapel N et al. Sleep disorders and melatonin rhythms in elderly people. Br Med J 1994;309:167

32 Lushington K, Pollard K, Lack L, Kennaway D J, Dawson D. Daytime melatonin administration in elderly good & poor sleepers: effects on core body temperature and sleep latency. Sleep 1997;20:1135–1144

33 Hughes R J, Sack R L, Lewy A J. The role of melatonin and circadian phase in age-related sleep maintenance insomnia: assessment in a clinical trial of melatonin replacement. Sleep 1997;21:52–68

34 Okawa M, Takahashi K, Egashira K et al. Vitamin B12 treatment for delayed sleep phase syndrome: a multi-centre double-blind study. Psychiatr Clin Neurosci 1997;51:275–279

35 Bohr K C. Effect of vitamin B12 on sleep quality and performance of shift workers. Wien Medizin Wochenschr 1996;146:289–291

36 Miyake Y, Nakagawa M, Asakura Y. Effects of odors on humans (I). Effects on sleep latency. Chemical Senses 1991;16:183

FURTHER READING

Ernst E. Insomnia. New York: Godsfield, 1998
Introduction to ways of treating insomnia written for a lay population.

Morin C M, Mimeault V, Gagné A. Nonpharmacological treatment of late-life insomnia. J Psychosom Res 1999;46:103–116
Overview of the evidence for psychological and behavioral techniques in treating insomnia in elderly people.

INTERMITTENT CLAUDICATION

Synonyms

Charcot's syndrome, myasthenia angiosclerotica, peripheral arterial occlusive disease, peripheral vascular disease stage II.

Definition

A condition usually caused by atherosclerotic stenoses of peripheral arteries characterized by ischemia of the muscles, predominantly the calf muscles, causing attacks of pain and lameness brought on by walking.

CAM usage

Hydrotherapy, chelation therapy, herbal medicine and lifestyle changes are interventions frequently used for the treatment of this condition.

Clinical evidence

Chelation therapy

A systematic review reported that none of the available double-blind RCTs found beneficial effects for pain-free and maximal walking distances compared with placebo (Box 5.28). It is associated with severe adverse events[1,2] and the review concluded that chelation therapy should be regarded as obsolete for intermittent claudication.

CONDITIONS

Box 5.28
Systematic review
Chelation therapy for intermittent claudication
Circulation 1997;96: 1031–1033

- Four double-blind, placebo-controlled RCTs including 225 patients

- Three were of good quality

- Largest trial assessed 153 patients for 6 mo

- All trials report no intergroup differences for walking distances

- Adverse events included kidney damage and hypocalcemia

Herbal medicine

A double-blind RCT (n=64) found positive results for **garlic** (*Allium sativum*) extract.[3] It reports that garlic powder given in a daily dose of 800 mg for 12 weeks increases pain-free walking distance significantly more than placebo. All patients included in this trial also received physical therapy twice weekly.

The evidence from rigorous studies of **ginkgo** (*Ginkgo biloba*) for this condition has been assessed in a metaanalysis (Box 5.29). According to these data and other evidence from comparative trials (e.g. [4]) ginkgo extract is effective for patients with intermittent claudication. It increased pain-free and maximal walking distances to a similar degree compared with other conventional oral treatments. The overall effect, however, is modest.

Box 5.29
Metaanalysis
Ginkgo for intermittent claudication
Am J Med 2000;108: 276–281

- Eight double-blind, placebo-controlled RCTs including 415 patients

- Trial quality was good to excellent

- Pain-free walking distance: weighted mean difference 34 m, (CI 26 to 43).

- Six trials report significant differences in favor of ginkgo for maximal walking distance

Several double-blind RCTs exist for **Padma 28**, a Tibetan mixture including 22 different, mainly herbal ingredients (Table 5.50). These studies reported a modest increase in pain-free and maximal walking distance. Overall the available data suggest that this herbal mixture is an effective option for intermittent claudication.

Hydrotherapy

Two RCTs investigated the effects of water containing carbon dioxide (CO_2) on microcirculatory parameters in patients with intermittent claudication.[5,6] These studies report an increase in

Table 5.50 **Double-blind, placebo-controlled RCTs of Padma 28 for intermittent claudication**

Reference	Sample size	Interventions [dosage]	Result	Comment
Schweiz Med Wschr 1985;115: 752–756	43	A) Padma 28 [2.28 g/d for 4 mo] B) Placebo	A superior to B for maximal walking distance	No concomitant relevant interventions allowed
Herb Pol 1987;33:29–41	100	A) Padma 28 [1.52 g/d for 4 mo] B) Placebo	A superior to B for maximal walking distance	Rigorous trial
Angiology 1993;44: 836–867	36	A) Padma 28 [1.36 g/d for 4 mo] B) Placebo	A superior to baseline for pain-free and maximal walking distances	Intergroup difference not stated
Forsch Komplementärmed 1994;1:18–26	93	A) Padma 28 [1.52 g/d for 4 mo] B) Placebo	A superior to B for maximal walking distance	Rigorous trial

skin blood flow at the dorsum of the foot. A small clinical RCT (n=24) assessing the effects of water containing CO_2 reports an increase in pain-free walking distance after immersion of the lower extremities for 30 min five times weekly for 4 weeks compared with fresh water.[7]

Table 5.51
Summary of clinical evidence for intermittent claudication

Treatment	Weight of evidence	Direction of evidence	Serious safety concerns
Chelation therapy	OO	⇩	Yes (see p 44)
Herbal medicine			
Garlic	O	⇧	Yes (see p 109)
Ginkgo	OOO	⇧	Yes (see p 115)
Padma 28	OO	⇧	Yes (see p 5)
Hydrotherapy	O	⇗	Yes (see p 5)

Overall recommendation

No therapy is as effective as conventional regular physical exercise. It can be recommended as a beneficial lifestyle change in addition to smoking cessation. Convincing evidence exists for the effectiveness of ginkgo extract, which seems to be as effective as other conventional oral interventions. Although the overall effect seems modest, given the nature and frequency of adverse events, it can be recommended as an oral treatment.

CONDITIONS

Padma 28 seems to be of some benefit, while for other interventions such as hydrotherapy, the evidence looks promising but insufficient for firm recommendations.

REFERENCES

1 Nissel H. Arteriosklerose und Chelattherapie. Wien Med Wochenschr 1986;136:586–588
2 Wirebaugh S R, Geraets D R. Apparent failure of coronary arteriosclerosis. DICP Ann Pharmacother 1990;24:22–25
3 Kiesewetter H, Jung F, Jung E M et al. Effects of garlic coated tablets in peripheral arterial occlusive disease. Clin Invest 1993;71:383–386
4 Böhmer D, Kalinski S, Michaelis P, Szögy A. Behandlung der PAVK mit Ginkgo-biloba-extrakt (GBE) oder Pentoxifyllin. Herz Kreislauf 1988;20:5–8
5 Hartmann B R, Bassenge E, Pittler M H. Effect of carbon dioxide-enriched water and fresh water on the cutaneous microcirculation and oxygen tension in the skin of the foot. Angiology 1997;48:337–343
6 Hartmann B, Drews B, Bassenge E. Carbon dioxide-induced increase in foot blood flow and oxygen partial pressure in peripheral arterial occlusive disease. Dtsch Med Wochenschr 1991;116:1617–1621
7 Hartmann B R, Bassenge E, Hartmann M. Effects of serial percutaneous application of carbon dioxide in intermittent claudication: results of a controlled trial. Angiology 1997;48:957–963

FURTHER READING

London N J M, Nash R. Ulcerated lower limb. Br Med J 2000;320:1589–1591
This review article provides reliable information on the symptoms and clinical management of arterial and venous ulcers.

Tooke J E, Lowe G D O. A textbook of vascular medicine. London: Arnold, 1996
A comprehensive account of vascular medicine.

IRRITABLE BOWEL SYNDROME

Synonyms   Irritable colon, mucous colitis, spastic colitis, spastic colon.

Definition   Non-specific term used to describe symptoms such as abdominal pain, flatulence and alternating diarrhea with constipation, thought to reflect increased muscular tone of the colon.

CAM usage   According to surveys from North America herbal medicine, relaxation and homeopathy are most frequently used for irritable bowel syndrome.[1,2]

Clinical evidence

Acupuncture
There are few data from rigorous trials of acupuncture for this condition. One RCT reported beneficial effects compared with sham acupuncture[3] but important details are missing, preventing full appraisal of the report. In an uncontrolled study seven patients received acupuncture once weekly for 4 weeks.[4] The results suggested an improvement in general well-being and in symptoms of bloating.

Biofeedback
Forty patients were entered in an uncontrolled study assessing computer-aided thermal biofeedback training.[5] Patients achieved

progressively deeper levels of relaxation after four 30-minute sessions. The results suggested a reduction of global and bowel symptom scores. Two controlled studies including 122 patients altogether assessed a multi-component treatment consisting of thermal biofeedback, relaxation and cognitive therapy and found no advantage over attention control for overall symptom scores.[6]

Herbal medicine

A combination preparation (**Appital**) containing various herbal extracts, e.g. caraway oil, was tested in a double-blind RCT, which included 59 patients who were diagnosed according to the Manning criteria.[7] At the end of an 8-week treatment period, there were no differences in symptom scores in the treatment group compared with placebo.

A double-blind placebo-controlled RCT assessed the effects of **Asa foetida** (0.1% alcoholic dilution) and asa foetida in a combination preparation also containing **Nux vomica** (0.01% alcoholic dilution).[8] The results indicate some beneficial effect in the global improvement of symptoms in the active groups, but this did not reach significance when compared with placebo.

In a placebo-controlled, double-blind RCT 169 patients were treated for 6 weeks with either standard therapy consisting of clidinium bromide, chlordiazepoxide and isphagula or an **Ayurvedic** preparation containing *Aegle marmelos correa* and *Bacopa monniere.*[9] Long-term results show that neither form of therapy was better than placebo.

A double-blind RCT compared individualized with standard **Chinese herbal** formulations and placebo in 103 patients, who were diagnosed according to accepted criteria.[10] After 16 weeks global improvements in symptoms were reported in both treatment groups compared with placebo. Individualized treatment was no better than standard Chinese herbal formulation.

A double-blind RCT tested a combination of extracts from bitter candytuft, matricaria flower, peppermint leaves, caraway fruit, licorice root and melissa balm (**Iberogast**) in 103 patients.[11] After 4 weeks of treatment the authors report a significant improvement in the global IBS symptom score compared with placebo.

Three RCTs have assessed preparations containing **isphagula** (*Plantago ovata*) (Table 5.52). Two trials report beneficial effects, while one study found no significant global improvement of symptoms compared with placebo. Overall, the evidence is encouraging, but the heterogeneity of the available data in terms of medication used, dosage and treatment period prevents a firm judgement.

A metaanalysis assessed the available evidence for **peppermint** oil.[12] Of eight RCTs of peppermint oil monopreparations, seven trials included patients who were not diagnosed according

Table 5.52 **Double-blind RCTs of isphagula for irritable bowel syndrome**

Reference	Sample size	Interventions [dosage]	Result	Comment
Br Med J 1979;1: 376–378	96	A) Isphagula husk [2×1 sachet/d for 3 mo] B) Hyoscine butylbromide (Buscopan) [4×10 mg/d] C) Lorazepam [2×1 mg/d] D) Placebo	A superior to D for global improvement	Only in the group treated with isphagula was the difference between real and placebo preparations statistically significant
J Assoc Phys India 1982;30: 353–355	26	A) Isphagula husk [2.5 g/d for 3 w] B) Placebo	A superior to B for global improvement	Patients with additional psychiatric symptoms had the least improvement
Ir Med J 1983; 76:253	80	A) Isphagula poloxamer [2 sachets/d for 4 w] B) Placebo	No significant intergroup differences including global improvement	All patients received 30 g dietary fiber

to accepted criteria. Although the metaanalysis suggested beneficial effects, it was concluded that the effectiveness of peppermint oil for the symptomatic treatment of IBS is not established beyond reasonable doubt (Box 5.30). A double-blind RCT, which became available after the metaanalysis, reports beneficial effects for abdominal pain, distension and stool frequency, but also failed to diagnose patients according to the accepted Rome or Manning criteria.[13]

Box 5.30
Metaanalysis
Peppermint oil for irritable bowel syndrome
Am J Gastroenterol 1998;93:1131–1135

- Eight RCTs (seven double-blind) including 295 patients
- The only study that diagnosed patients according to accepted criteria (Manning) was negative
- Dosage was 3×0.2–0.4 ml/d for 2–4 w
- Significant effect for global improvement of symptoms ($n=5$) (odds ratio 0.20; CI 0.04 to 0.89)
- Two of three studies not subjected to metaanalysis were positive
- Adverse effects included heartburn, perianal burning, blurred vision, nausea and vomiting

A double-blind RCT compared two different preparations of a fixed combination of **peppermint and caraway oil;**[14] 223 patients with non-ulcer dyspepsia in combination with IBS received either enteric-coated capsules containing 90 mg peppermint oil and 50 mg caraway oil or an enteric-soluble formulation containing 36 mg peppermint oil and 20 mg caraway oil. The results indicate a reduction in pain intensity compared with baseline and equivalent effectiveness of the preparations.

Hypnotherapy

Three RCTs investigated whether hypnotherapy is effective for the treatment of IBS (Table 5.53). These studies and a further follow-up study[15] report symptomatic relief after hypnotherapy compared with various control interventions. These encouraging results indicate that hypnotherapy is a promising option, but the heterogeneity of the available studies in terms of trial design and the small sample size prevent a firm judgement.

Table 5.53 **RCTs of hypnotherapy for irritable bowel syndrome**

Reference	Sample size	Interventions [regimen]	Result	Comment
Lancet 1984; 2:1232–1234	30	A) Hypnotherapy [7 sessions over 3 mo] B) Oral placebo plus psychotherapy	A superior to B for abdominal pain, bowel habit, abdominal distension and well-being	Patients were encouraged to use autohypnosis daily; considerable placebo response
Lancet 1989; 1:424–425	33	A) Group hypnotherapy [4 sessions over 7 w] B) Individual hypnotherapy	No intergroup differences; 20 patients improved in symptom scores	Patients were encouraged to use autohypnosis daily
Appl Psycho-physiol Biofeedback 1998;23: 219–232	12	A) Hypnotherapy [12 sessions over 6 w] B) Wait list control	A superior to B for global improvement of symptoms	Small sample size

Supplements

A multicenter RCT investigated the effectiveness of a supplement (**Florelax**) containing yeast, vitamin B, nicotinamide, folic acid and herbal extracts of camomile, angelica, valerian and peppermint;[16] 380 patients received either a high-fiber diet plus two tablets of supplement daily or diet alone for 6 weeks. The results indicate a reduction of the intensity, frequency and duration of the symptoms in the treatment group compared with diet alone.

Table 5.54
Summary of clinical evidence for irritable bowel syndrome

Treatment	Weight of evidence	Direction of evidence	Serious safety concerns
Acupuncture	O	⇧	Yes (see p 29)
Biofeedback	O	⇩	No (see p 42)
Herbal medicine			
Appital	O	⇩	Yes (see p 5)
Asa foetida	O	⇩	Yes (see p 5)
Ayurveda	O	⇩	Yes (see p 52)
Chinese herbs	O	⇧	Yes (see p 52)
Isphagula	OO	⇗	Yes (see p 170)
Peppermint	OOO	⇗	Yes (see p 142)
Hypnotherapy	OO	⇧	Yes (see p 58)
Supplements			
Florelax	O	⇧	Yes (see p 5)

Overall recommendation

The evidence is not compelling for any complementary treatment. Many conventional therapies are similarly unsatisfactory for this condition although when abdominal pain is the predominant symptom, smooth muscle relaxants have shown to be beneficial. The data for peppermint oil are encouraging but are still not sufficiently reliable to allow firm recommendations. However, given the few treatment options available and its favorable safety profile, peppermint oil might be worth considering. The evidence for hypnotherapy looks promising, making it a possible option for some patients when administered by a responsible therapist. Other treatments which have shown some beneficial effects but are less convincing include Chinese herbal formulations and isphagula extract.

REFERENCES

1 Smart H L, Mayberry J F, Atkinson M. Alternative medicine consultations and remedies in patients with the irritable bowel syndrome. Gut 1986;27:826–828

2 Eisenberg D M, Davis R B, Ettner S L, Appel S, Wilkey S, Rompay M V, Kessler R C. Trends in alternative medicine use in the United States, 1990–1997. JAMA 1998;280:1569–1575

3 Kunze M, Seidel H-J, Stübe G. Vergleichende Untersuchung zur Effektivität der kleinen Psychotherapie, der Akupunktur und der Papaverintherapie bei Patienten mit Colon irritabile. Z Gesamte Inn Med 1990; 45:625–627

4 Chan J, Carr I, Mayberry J F. The role of acupuncture in the treatment of irritable bowel syndrome: a pilot study. Hepato-Gastroenterol 1997;44:1328–1330

5 Leahy A, Clayman C, Mason I, Lloyd G, Epstein O. Computerised biofeedback games: a new method for teaching stress management and its use in irritable bowel syndrome. J Roy Soc Phys Lond 1998;32:552–556

6 Blanchard E B, Schwartz S P, Suls J M et al. Two controlled evaluations of multicomponent psychological treatment of irritable bowel syndrome. Behav Res Ther 1992;30:175–189

7 Pedersen B S, Helø O H, Jørgensen F B, Kromann-Andersen H. Behandling af colon irritabile med kosttilskuddet Appital. Ugeskr Læger 1998;160:7259–7262

8 Rahlfs V W, Mössinger P. Zur Behandlung des Colon irritabile. Arzneim-Forsch Drug Res 1976;26:2230–2234

9 Yadav S K, Jain A K, Tripathi S N, Gupta J P. Irritable bowel syndrome: therapeutic

evaluation of indigenous drugs. Ind J Med Res 1989;90:496–503

10 Bensousson A, Talley N J, Hing M, Menzies R, Guo A, Ngu M. Treatment of irritable bowel syndrome with Chinese herbal medicine. A randomized controlled trial. JAMA 1998; 280:1585–1589

11 Madisch A, Plein K, Mayr G, Buchert D, Hotz J. Benefit of a herbal preparation in patients with irritable bowel syndrome: results of a double-blind, randomized placebo-controlled, multicenter trial. Dig Dis Week (in press)

12 Pittler M H, Ernst E. Peppermint oil for irritable bowel syndrome: a critical review and meta-analysis. Am J Gastroenterol 1998;93:1131–1135

13 Liu J-H, Chen G-H, Yeh H-Z, Huang C-K, Poon S-K. Enteric-coated peppermint-oil capsules in the treatment of irritable bowel syndrome: a prospective, randomized trial. J Gastroenterol 1997;32:765–768

14 Freise J, Köhler S. Pfefferminzöl/Kümmelöl-Fixkombination bei nicht-säurebedingter Dyspepsie – Vergleich der Wirksamkeit und Verträglichkeit zweier galenischer Zubereitungen. Pharmazie 1999;54:210–215

15 Whorwell P J, Prior A, Colgan S M. Hypnotherapy in severe irritable bowel syndrome: further experience. Gut 1987;28:423–425

16 Grattagliano A, Anti M, Luchetti R, Marino P, Gasbarrini G. Studie clinico randomizzato sull'efficacia di un integratore biologico nei pazienti affetti da sindrome dell'intestino irritabile. Minerva Gastroenterol Dietol 1998;44:51–55

FURTHER READING

Harris M S. Irritable bowel syndrome: a cost-effective approach for primary care physicians. Postgrad Med 1997;101:3–15

Jailwala J, Imperiale T F, Kroenke K. Pharmacological treatment of the irritable bowel syndrome: a systematic review of randomized, controlled trials. Ann Intern Med 2000;133:136–147

MENOPAUSE

Synonyms	Climacteric.
Definition	The physiologic cessation of menstruation characterized by symptoms such as hot flushes, night sweats, dizziness, palpitations, low energy, decreased sexual interest and depression.
CAM usage	The CAM modalities most popular with menopausal women have been identified as dietary or nutritional supplements, spiritual approaches, exercise, herbal medicine and homeopathy.[1]

Clinical evidence

Acupuncture

In an RCT of electroacupuncture and superficial needling, both techniques reduced hot flushes, but with electroacupuncture the effect lasted for up to 3 months and there were also beneficial effects on other menopausal symptoms.[2] In a small sham-controlled RCT (n=10) Chinese acupuncture provided relief of menopausal symptoms lasting less than two months.[3] These studies suggest that small, transitory improvements may be possible with acupuncture, but meaningful changes are unlikely.

Herbal medicine

In addition to several uncontrolled trials (e.g.[4]) at least three RCTs from Germany have suggested that **black cohosh** (*Cimicifuga racemosa*) may alleviate symptoms associated with menopause (Table 5.55). Tolerability was good in all trials.

CONDITIONS

Unfortunately, the lack of blinding and placebo controls of two trials limits the conclusiveness of the evidence.

Table 5.55 **RCTs of black cohosh for menopause**

Reference	Sample size	Interventions [dosage]	Result	Comment
Med Welt 1985;36: 871–874	60	A) Black cohosh [80 drops/d for 3 mo] B) Conjugated estrogens [0.625 mg] C) Diazepam [2 mg]	A no different to B or C on menopausal symptoms	Study not blinded
Thera-peuticon 1987; 1:23–31	80	A) Black cohosh [8 mg/d for 3 mo] B) Conjugated estrogens [0.625 mg] C) Placebo	A superior to B and C on menopausal symptoms	Double-blind trial; symptom scores reached normal levels
Zentralbl Gynäkol 1988;110: 611–618	60	A) Black cohosh [4 tabs/d for 6 mo] B) Estriol [1 mg] C) Conjugated estrogens [1.25 mg] D) Estriol [2 mg] & norethisterone acetate [1 mg]	A no different to B, C or D on menopausal symptoms	Study not blinded; sample was hysterectomized women with menopausal symptoms

A double-blind RCT (n=71) of **dong quai** (*Angelica sinensis*) found no superiority over placebo in reducing menopausal symptoms and no estrogenic effects after 6 months of treatment.[5]

The efficacy of oil of **evening primrose** (*Oenothera biennis*) for alleviating hot flushes was examined in a double-blind RCT (n=56).[6] No benefit over placebo was demonstrated for the frequency of night or daytime flushes.

Ginseng (*Panax ginseng*) was investigated in a double-blind RCT (n=384) for its effects on quality of life.[7] Results were no different to placebo for quality of life or hot flushes and no effects on vaginal cytology were observed.

Two double-blind, placebo-controlled RCTs (n=40) of **kava** (*Piper methysticum*) (300 mg daily for 2–3 months) suggested that it was effective in alleviating menopausal symptoms.[8,9]

Two double-blind RCTs of an isoflavone supplement derived from **red clover** (*Trifolium pratense*) found no superiority over placebo in alleviating menopausal symptoms.[10,11] However, in both trials the authors suggested that dietary isoflavone ingestion in the placebo group may have masked any effect of the intervention.

St John's wort (*Hypericum perforatum*) (900 mg daily for 3 months) produced positive results on psychological symptoms in an uncontrolled study[12] and in an RCT when combined with black cohosh.[13]

Relaxation

Three small RCTs have suggested that relaxation training can have positive effects on hot flush symptoms (Table 5.56). The results are inconsistent regarding the best type of relaxation method, with progressive muscle relaxation proving effective in two studies but no better than the control intervention in the other one where a breathing technique produced positive results.

Table 5.56 **RCTs of relaxation training for menopause**

Reference	Sample size	Interventions [regimen]	Result	Comment
J Consult Clin Psychol 1984; 52:1072–1079	14	A) Muscle relaxation [1 h/w for 6 w] B) EEG biofeedback	A superior to B in hot flush frequency	Hot flushes assessed by self-report 1 & 6 mo after treatment
Am J Obstet Gynecol 1992; 167:436–439	33	A) Paced respiration [1 h/fortnight for 16 w] B) Muscle relaxation C) EEG biofeedback	A superior to B & C in hot flush frequency	Hot flushes assessed by ambulatory monitoring of skin conductance for 24 h
J Psychosom Obstet Gynecol 1996; 17:202–207	45	A) Relaxation training [20 min/d for 7 w] B) Attention control C) Reading	A superior to B & C in hot flush intensity & depression/ anxiety	Hot flush assessed by daily charting; drop-out rate of over 25%

Spinal manipulation

An RCT (n=30) compared the effects of **osteopathy** (once weekly for 10 weeks) with sham treatment.[14] Superior results were reported for osteopathy on several menopausal symptoms including depression and hot flushes.

Supplements

Dietary **linseed, soy** and **wheat** reduced hot flushes in comparative RCTs[15,16] and further positive evidence for **soy** exists from RCTs versus placebo or normal diets (Table 5.57). The small body of evidence is encouraging with regard to the usefulness of soy for alleviating hot flushes, but is currently not compelling.

Vitamin E was reported useful for reducing hot flushes according to uncontrolled studies (e.g. [17]). However, a placebo-controlled trial found no specific effect of the treatment.[18]

CONDITIONS

Table 5.57 **Double-blind RCTs of soy supplementation for menopause**

Reference	Sample size	Interventions [dosage]	Result	Comment
Menopause 1997;4: 89–94	145	A) Soy drink [400 ml/d for 12 w] B) Regular diet	A superior to B for hot flush & vaginal dryness but not overall symptoms	Other phyto-estrogens were also part of intervention diet
Obstet Gynecol 1998;91: 6–11	104	A) Soy protein [60 g/d for 12 w] B) Placebo	A superior to B for hot flush frequency	Placebo response of 30%
Menopause 1999;6: 7–13	51	A) Soy protein [20 g/d single dose for 6 w] B) Soy protein [20 g/d 2 divided doses] C) Complex carbohydrates	B superior to C for hot flush severity & estrogenic symptoms; A no different to B or C on any symptoms	Crossover trial with no washout between interventions
Menopause 2000;7: 105–111	39	A) Soy extract [400 mg/d for 6 w] B) Placebo	A superior to B for hot flush frequency & severity	No effects on vaginal cytology

Other therapies

The results of case-control and uncontrolled studies suggest that aerobic **exercise** training is associated with a reduction in

Table 5.58
Summary of clinical evidence for menopause

Treatment	Weight of evidence	Direction of evidence	Serious safety concerns
Acupuncture	O	⬀	Yes (see p 29)
Herbal medicine			
Black cohosh	OO	⇧	Yes (see p 90)
Dong quai	O	⇩	Yes (see p 5)
Evening primrose oil	O	⇩	Yes (see p 104)
Ginseng	O	⇧	Yes (see p 88)
Kava	O	⇧	Yes (see p 129)
Red clover	O	⇩	Yes (see p 148)
St John's wort	O	⇧	Yes (see p 156)
Spinal manipulation			
Osteopathy	O	⇧	Yes (see p 65)
Relaxation	OO	⇧	No (see p 71)
Supplements			
Soy	OO	⇧	No (see p 144)
Vitamin E	O	⇩	No

menopausal symptoms.[19-21] Another study found no correlation between energy expenditure and menopausal symptoms.[22] Without RCT evidence, it is unclear whether exercise can have beneficial effects, but the existing studies suggest it has potential.

Overall recommendation

There is no compelling evidence for the efficacy of any complementary treatment for alleviating menopausal symptoms, particularly in comparison with hormone replacement therapy. However, black cohosh looks encouraging in this respect and has a favorable safety profile. Kava also looks promising and can be considered as an option. Soy may have potential, particularly for reducing hot flushes, so efforts to increase consumption of soy products in the diet may be worthwhile. Relaxation techniques also appear to have some benefits.

REFERENCES

1 Kass-Annese B. Alternative therapies for menopause. Clin Obstet Gynecol 2000;43:163–183

2 Wyon Y, Lindgren R, Hammar M, Lundeberg T. Acupuncture against climacteric disorders? Lower number of symptoms after menopause. Lakartidningen 1994;91:2318–2322

3 Kraft K, Coulon S. Effect of a standardised acupuncture treatment on complaints, blood pressure and serum lipids of hypertensive postmenopausal women. A randomized controlled clinical study. Forsch Komplementärmed 1999;6:74–79

4 Vorberg G. Therapie klimakterischer Beschwerden. Z Allg Med 1984;60:626–629

5 Hirata J D, Swiersz L M, Zell B, Small R, Ettinger B. Does dong quai have estrogenic effects in postmenopausal women? A double-blind placebo controlled trial. Fertil Steril 1997;68:981–986

6 Chenoy S, Hussain S, Tayob Y, O'Brien P M S, Moss M Y, Morse P F. Effect of oral gamolenic acid from evening primrose oil on menopausal flushing. Br Med J 1994;308:501–503

7 Wiklund I K, Mattsson L A, Lindgren R, Limoni C. Effects of a standardized ginseng extract on quality of life and physiological parameters in symptomatic postmenopausal women: a double-blind, placebo-controlled trial. Int J Clin Pharmacol Res 1999;19:89–99

8 Warnecke G, Pfaender H, Gerster G, Gracza E. Wirksamkeit von Kawa-Kawa-Extrakt beim klimakterischen Syndrom. Zeitschr für Phytotherapie 1990;11:81–86

9 Warnecke G. Psychosomatische Dysfunktionen im weiblichen Klimakterium: Klinische Wirksamkeit und Verträglichkeit von Kava-Extrakt WS 1490. Fortschr der Medizin 1991;109:119–122

10 Baber R J, Templeman C, Morton T, Kelly G E, West L. Randomized placebo-controlled trial of an isoflavone supplement and menopausal symptoms in women. Climacteric 1999;2:85–92

11 Knight D C, Howes J B, Eden J A. The effect of Promensil, an isoflavone extract, on menopausal symptoms. Climacteric 1999; 2:79–84

12 Grube B, Walper A, Wheatley D. St. John's wort extract: efficacy for menopausal symptoms of psychological origin. Adv Ther 1999;16:177–186

13 Boblitz N, Schrader E, Henneicke-von Zepelin H H, Wüstenberg P. Benefit of a fixed drug combination containing St John's wort and black cohosh for climacteric patients – results of a randomized clinical trial. Focus Alt Compl Ther 2000;5:85–86

14 Cleary C, Fox J P. Menopausal symptoms: an osteopathic investigation. Compl Ther Med 1994;2:181–186

15 Murkies A L, Lombard C, Strauss B J, Wilcox G, Burger H G, Morton M S. Dietary flour supplementation decreases post-menopausal hot flushes: effect of soy and wheat. Maturitas 1995;21:189–195

16 Dalais F S, Rice G E, Wahlqvist M L et al. Effects of dietary phytoestrogens in postmenopausal women. Climacteric 1998;1:124–129

17 McLaren H C. Vitamin E in the menopause. Br Med J 1949;2:1378–1382

18 Blatt M H G, Weisbader H, Kupperman H S. Vitamin E and climacteric syndrome. Arch Intern Med 1953;91:792–799

19 Hammar M, Berg G, Lindgren R. Does physical exercise influence the frequency of postmenopausal hot flushes? Acta Obstet Gynecol Scand 1990;69:409–412

20 Wallace J P, Lovell S, Talano C, Webb M L, Hodgson J L.Changes in menstrual function, climacteric syndrome and serum concentrations of sex hormones in pre and post-menopausal women following a moderate intensity conditioning program. Med Sci Sports Exer 1982:14:154

21 Slaven L, Lee C. Mood and symptom reporting among middle-aged women: the relationship between menopausal status, hormone replacement therapy and exercise participation. Health Psychol 1997;16:203–208

22 Wilbur J, Holm K, Dan A. The relationship of energy expenditure to physical and psychologic symptoms in women at midlife. Nurs Outlook l992;40:269–275

FURTHER READING

Seidl M M, Stewart D E. Alternative treatments for menopausal symptoms: systematic review of scientific and lay literature. Can Fam Physic 1998;44:1299–1308

Useful insight into the extent to which claims in lay literature are supported by clinical evidence

MIGRAINE

Synonyms

Vascular headache, bilious headache, sick headache, blind headache, hemicrania. May also be named according to associated symptom, e.g. hemiplegic, ophthalmoplegic and ophthalmic nerve migraines.

Definition

Episodic headache, often preceded by an aura, usually lasting 6–24 hours which is associated with transient visual, neurological and/or gastrointestinal disturbances.

CAM usage

Patients with this chronic complaint are very likely to seek help from CAM, the commonest forms being herbal medicine, spinal manipulation, acupuncture, homeopathy and reflexology.[1]

Clinical evidence

The available evidence relates mostly to prevention of migraine rather than treatment of an acute attack.

Acupuncture

A systematic review (Box 5.31) concluded cautiously in favor of acupuncture for prevention of migraine: the generally modest quality of studies prevented a firmer conclusion. In one study involving 85 migraineurs, acupuncture was compared with sham acupuncture and metoprolol in a double-dummy design.[2] Both groups improved in frequency and duration of attacks, with no significant difference between them. However, metoprolol was judged better on global assessment by patients. In an RCT involving 179 patients in the early stages of acute migraine, acupuncture reduced the number of patients who developed a full migraine within 48 hours compared with placebo sumatriptan; the effect was similar to sumatriptan.[3]

Box 5.31
Systematic review
Acupuncture for migraine
Cephalalgia 1999;19: 779–786

- Twenty-two RCTs involving 1042 subjects with chronic headache
- Fifteen RCTs in migraine alone
- Quality of studies was variable
- Pooled responder rate for placebo-controlled studies in migraine was 1.55 (CI 1.04 to 2.33)
- The single study of good quality showed no effect
- Conclusion: acupuncture has a role but the quality and amount of evidence is not fully convincing

Biofeedback
See Relaxation below.

Diet
Of 88 children with severe, frequent migraine, 93% improved on a low-allergen diet. The role of foods provoking migraine was established by double-blind challenge in 40 of the children.[4] Confirmation of the role of food allergy in causing migraine was provided by a study of 43 adults with migraine who were skin tested for allergies.[5] Those who were positive were significantly more likely to respond to dietary manipulation than those who were negative. Attacks were provoked in several cases (71%) by blinded food challenge but not by placebo. Clearly, if trigger foods such as chocolate, cheese, shellfish or red wine are identified, these should be avoided. No rigorous studies of other nutritional approaches are available.

Herbal medicine
A systematic review of **feverfew** (*Tanacetum parthenium*), (Box 5.32) found three positive studies but there are weaknesses in most of these and the evidence was not considered to be conclusive in favor of feverfew.

CONDITIONS

Box 5.32
Systematic review
Feverfew for migraine
Cochrane Library 2000

- Four RCTs including 196 subjects
- Results favored feverfew over placebo but had limitations, in particular short duration
- The study with the highest methodological quality was negative
- Conclusion: effectiveness not established beyond doubt

Homeopathy

A systematic review of homeopathy for chronic headache, mainly migraine (Box 5.33), found that the evidence suggests that this therapy is not superior to placebo.

Box 5.33
Systematic review
Homeopathy for migraine
J Pain Symptom Manage 1999;18: 353–357

- Four RCTs including 294 subjects
- One study also included patients with other forms of chronic headache
- One RCT, the lowest quality, found significant improvement in frequency, duration and intensity of attacks
- The remaining three RCTs were negative for attack frequency, severity and intensity, although in one, the neurologist's assessment favored homeopathy
- Conclusion: the effectiveness of homeopathy is not known

Relaxation and biofeedback

Overall, the evidence suggests that these therapies have benefits for adults with migraine, according to a metaanalysis (Box 5.34) but the conclusions must be cautious since truly appropriate controls are difficult to arrange. Moreover, the review included all prospective studies, whether controlled or not, and aggregated the responses for all groups receiving each therapy or control. This is likely to overstate the effect size.

Box 5.34
Metaanalysis
Relaxation/ biofeedback for migraine (adults)
Pain 1990;42:1–13

- Thirty-five prospective trials of relaxation and/or biofeedback (sample sizes not quoted)
- Simultaneous analysis of 25 trials of propranolol, for comparison
- Overall, effect size similar to propranolol: 43% reduction in headache activity (improvement as a percentage of baseline symptoms)
- Effect size for those who received placebo medication was 14% and for untreated group 0%
- Conclusion: evidence provides substantial support for effectiveness of relaxation/biofeedback and for propranolol

A 1995 NIH Technology Assessment Panel[6] found moderate evidence in support of the hypothesis that biofeedback is more effective than either relaxation or no treatment in relieving migraine headache. The evidence was less clear when biofeedback was compared with placebo. Some RCTs suggest that the response to relaxation and biofeedback may be largely due to a placebo effect. For example, 116 patients were randomized to receive one of three interventions involving attention (biofeedback, or biofeedback with cognitive therapy, or an attention control alone) or no additional treatment.[7] All three intervention groups improved more than the untreated controls, with no significant differences between the groups. The main response was a reduced frequency of attacks, with their duration largely unchanged.

Prospective studies in pediatric migraine point towards the effectiveness of biofeedback, either alone or in combination with relaxation, with a similar effect to propranolol, though the result is not supported by the evidence from controlled studies (Box 5.35).

Box 5.35
Metaanalysis
**Relaxation/
biofeedback for
migraine (children)**
Pain 1995;60:239–256

- Twenty-nine prospective investigations of behavioral interventions, mainly biofeedback and/or relaxation, involving 471 subjects

- Investigations of drug therapy (n=556) used for comparison

- Effect sizes (measured in standard deviations): biofeedback, 2.6; relaxation, 1.0; biofeedback combined with relaxation, 3.1; placebo, 0.6; waiting list, 0.6; propranolol, 2.8; ergotamine 1.6: clonidine, 1.5

- Further analysis restricted to controlled trials found no significant differences

- Conclusion: cautiously positive, lack of good-quality studies

Spinal manipulation
Two RCTs (Table 5.59) found no benefit from treating migraine with cervical manipulation.

Table 5.59 **RCTs of spinal manipulation for migraine**

Reference	Sample size	Interventions [regimen]	Result
Aust NZ J Med 1978;8: 589–593	85	A) Manipulation by physician or physiotherapist [8 w] B) Manipulation by chiropractor C) Mobilization (control)	No difference between A, B and C
J Manip Physiol Ther 1998;21: 511–519	218	A) Chiropractic manipulation [8 w] B) Amitriptyline	No difference between A and B

CONDITIONS

Other therapies

In an RCT involving 20 subjects with mixed migraine and tension headache over 4 months, **yoga** in addition to standard medication produced significant reduction in headache activity in contrast to standard medication alone.[8]

Table 5.60
Summary of clinical evidence for migraine

Treatment	Weight of evidence	Direction of evidence	Serious safety concerns
Acupuncture	OO	⬈	Yes (see p 29)
Biofeedback	OO	⬆	No (see p 42)
Diet	OO	⬆	No
Herbal medicine Feverfew	OO	⬈	Yes (see p 107)
Homeopathy	OO	⬂	No (see p 55)
Relaxation (children)	OO	⬇	No (see p 71)
(adults)	OO	⬆	
Spinal manipulation	OO	⬇	Yes (see pp 47, 65)

Overall recommendation

If food allergens can be identified, these should be excluded from the diet. The best choice for prevention of migraine appears to be biofeedback (either alone or with relaxation). Selection of practitioner may be important as the effect may be largely non-specific. Biofeedback appears to be at least as effective as the drugs it has been compared with and the same may be true of acupuncture, though the evidence is very limited. Feverfew has some evidence to support it and yoga looks promising though it has not been sufficiently tested. Like other self-help techniques, it needs long-term application and is more likely to be useful in patients who are enthusiastic. None of these therapies is associated with major risks and thus may be preferable to long-term use of conventional preventive drugs with limited effectiveness and recognized adverse effects. The role of CAM therapies in treatment of acute migraine attacks has not been investigated or compared with modern medications such as triptans.

REFERENCES

1 Eisenberg D M, Davis R, Ettner S L, Appel S, Wilkey S, Rompay M V. Trends in alternative medicine use in the United States, 1990–1997. JAMA 1998;280:1569–1575

2 Hesse J, Mogelvang B, Simonsen H. Acupuncture versus metoprolol in migraine prophylaxis: a randomised trial of trigger point inactivation. J Intern Med 1994;235:451–456

3 Melchart D, Thormaehlen J, Hager S, Liao J. Acupuncture versus sumatriptan for early treatment of acute migraine attacks – a

randomized controlled trial. Forsch
Komplementärmed Klass Naturheilkd 2000;7:53

4 Egger J, Carter C M, Wilson J, Turner M W,
Soothill J F. Is migraine food allergy? A
double-blind controlled trial of oligoantigenic
diet treatment. Lancet 1983;2:865–869

5 Mansfield L E, Vaughan T R, Waller S F,
Haverly R W, Ting S. Food allergy and adult
migraine: double-blind and mediator
confirmation of an allergic etiology.
Ann Allergy 1985;55:126–129

6 NIH Technology Assessment Statement.
Integration of behavioral and relaxation

approaches into the treatment of chronic pain
and insomnia. NIH Technology Assessment
Statement 1995;Oct 16–18:1–34

7 Blanchard E B, Appelbaum K A, Radnitz
G L et al. A controlled evaluation of thermal
biofeedback and thermal biofeedback combined
with cognitive therapy in the treatment of
vascular headache. J Consult Clin Psychol
1990; 58:216–224

8 Latha, Kaliappan K V. Efficacy of yoga therapy
in the management of headaches. J Indian
Psychol 1992;10:41–47

MULTIPLE SCLEROSIS

**Synonyms/
subcategories**

Disseminated, focal or insular sclerosis, demyelinating disease.

Definition

A common demyelinating disorder of the central nervous system,
causing patches of sclerosis (plaques) in the brain and spinal cord.

**Related
conditions**

None, but numerous other conditions can mimic the extremely
variable symptoms of multiple sclerosis (MS), particularly in the
early stages.

CAM usage

Survey data suggest that up to 64% of MS patients use CAM.[1]
Relaxation techniques, homeopathy, herbal medicines and
dietary treatments are amongst the most common modalities. In
our survey of CAM organizations (see p 3), the following
treatments were recommended: aromatherapy, hypnotherapy,
massage, reflexology and yoga.

**Clinical
evidence**

Feldenkrais method
In a small (n=20) crossover RCT, MS patients were allocated to
Feldenkrais or sham sessions for 8 weeks.[2] Patients reported less
stress and anxiety with Feldenkrais compared with sham.

Herbal medicine
At present the evidence to suggest that **cannabis** (*Cannabis
sativa*) reduces spasticity in MS patients is largely anecdotal
(e.g. [3]). No other herbal medicines have been reported to be
effective for MS.

Imagery
An RCT with ambulatory MS patients tested imagery versus no
treatment.[4] Its results demonstrated a significant reduction in
state anxiety, but no change in depression or physical symptoms associated with MS.

CONDITIONS

Magnetic field therapy

Two sham-controlled RCTs of magnetic field therapy for the symptoms of MS are available.[5,6] One trial (n=38) demonstrated an improvement in spasticity but not in other symptoms.[5] The other study (n=30) showed significant improvement in the combined rating for bladder control, cognitive function, fatigue level, mobility, spasticity and vision. There was, however, no change in the overall symptom score and some patients in the treatment group had increased headaches during the initial treatment phases.[8]

Massage

Twenty-four MS patients were randomized to receive either regular massage therapy or no treatment in addition to standard care.[7] At the end of the 5-week treatment period the former group had significantly lower anxiety levels and were less depressed. Moreover, they had improved self-esteem, body image and social functioning.

Neural therapy

The treatment was tested in a small (n=21) double-blind RCT against placebo.[8] A significantly larger proportion improved in the actively treated compared with the control group according to validated outcome scales measuring subjective symptoms.

Reflexology

Seventy-one MS patients were randomized to receive either 11 weeks of regular (foot) reflexology or non-specific (sham) massage of the calf.[9] Significant improvements were noted in terms of paresthesias, urinary symptoms, muscle strength and spasticity.

Supplements

Epidemiological studies (e.g. [10]) suggest the effectiveness of **linoleic acid** in MS. In the first RCT 87 patients with MS were randomized to receive twice-daily supplements of vegetable oil mixture containing either a total of 17.2 g linolate or 7.6 g oleate (control) for 2 years.[11] The results suggest a greater severity of clinical relapses in patients taking oleate than those receiving the linolate. The second study[12] involved 116 MS patients in an RCT of polyunsaturated fatty acids taken for 2 years. Patients were randomly allocated to one of four groups. Two groups received linoleic acid either as a spread (23 g of linoleic acid) or in naudicelle capsules (2.92 g of linoleic acid and 0.34 g of gamma-linoleic acid). Two control groups received oleic acid (16 g and 4 g daily). Rates of clinical deterioration and frequencies of attacks were not significantly different between treated and control groups. Exacerbations were marginally shorter and less severe in patients receiving the higher dose of linoleic acid than controls. In the third RCT,[13] 96 patients were randomized to receive either a dose of 17 g/day of linoleic acid or 21 g/day of oleic acid. The trial results showed no therapeutic benefit from the use of linoleic acid during the 30-month period.

An RCT investigated the effects of eicosapentaenic (EPA) and docosahexaenic (DHA) acids on the symptoms of MS patients.[14] Three hundred and twelve MS patients were randomized into taking 20 capsules of fish oil daily, containing 18% EPA and 12% DHA, or taking 20 capsules of olive oil daily. In the treatment group, 66 patients got worse and 79 were unchanged or got better. In the control group, 82 patients were worse and 65 were unchanged or better. These differences were not statistically significant.

Overall recommendation

There is some encouraging evidence that several CAM modalities alleviate the symptoms of MS. In as far as these are not associated with risks, they can be endorsed for the use of patients who are keen to try CAM14 and are probably best used as adjunctive forms of treatment. Whether food supplements like linoleic acid delay the course of the disease is unclear at present. Compared with conventional treatments, CAM might prove useful for improving quality of life of MS patients. None of the CAM treatments offers the prospect of a cure for MS.

Table 5.61
Summary of clinical evidence for multiple sclerosis

Treatment	Weight of evidence	Direction of evidence	Serious safety concerns
Feldenkrais	O	↗	No (see p 80)
Herbal medicine			
Cannabis	O	⇒	Yes (see p 5)
Imagery	O	↗	No (see p 80)
Magnetic field therapy	OO	↗	No (see p 80)
Massage	O	↗	No (see p 60)
Neural therapy	O	↗	Yes (see p 81)
Reflexology	O	⇧	No (see p 68)
Supplements			
Linoleic acid	OO	⇒	No
EPA/DHA	O	⇩	No

CONDITIONS

REFERENCES

1 Winterholler M, Erbguth F, Neudorfer B. Use of alternative medicine by patients with multiple sclerosis – users characterization and patterns of use. Fortschr Neurol Psychiatr 1997;65:555–561

2 Johnson S K, Frederick J, Kaufman M et al. A controlled investigation of body work in multiple sclerosis. J Alt Compl Med 1999; 5:237–243

3 Brenneisen R, Egli A, Elsohly M A, Henn V, Spiess Y. The effect of orally and rectally administered Δ^9-tetrahydrocannabinol on spasticity: a pilot study with 2 patients. Int J Clin Pharmacol Therapeut 1996;34:446–452

4 Maguire B L. The effects of imagery on attitudes and moods in multiple sclerosis patients. Alt Ther Health Med 1996;2:75–79

5 Nielson J F, Sinkjaer T, Jakobsen J. Treatment of spasticity with repetitive magnetic stimulation; a double-blind placebo-controlled study. Multiple Sclerosis 1996;2:227–232

6 Richards T L, Lappin M S, Acosta-Urquidi J et al. Double-blind study of pulsing magnetic field effects on multiple sclerosis. J Alt Compl Med 1997;3:21–29

7 Hernandez-Reif M, Field T, Scafidi F et al. Multiple sclerosis patients benefit from massage therapy. J Bodywork Movement Ther 1998;2:168–174

8 Gibson R G, Gibson S L M. Neural therapy in the treatment of multiple sclerosis. J Alt Compl Med 1999;5:543–552

9 Siev-Ner I, Gamus D, Lermer-Gevea L et al. Reflexology treatment relieves the symptoms of multiple sclerosis: a randomized controlled study. Focus Alt Compl Ther 1997; 2:196

10 Agranoff B W, Goldberg D. Diet and the geographical distribution of multiple sclerosis. Lancet 1974;2:1061–1066

11 Millar J H D, Zilkha K J, Langman M J S et al. Double-blind trial of linoleate supplementation of diet in multiple sclerosis. Br Med J 1973;1:765–768

12 Bates D, Fawcett P R W, Shaw D A et al. Polyunsaturated fatty acids in treatment of acute remitting multiple sclerosis. Br Med J 1978;2:1390–1391

13 Paty D W. Double-blind trial of linoleic acid in multiple sclerosis. Arch Neurol 1983;40:693–694

14 Bates D, Cartlidge N E F, French J M et al. A double-blind controlled trial of long chain n-3 polyunsaturated fatty acids in the treatment of multiple sclerosis. J Neurol Neurosurg Psychiatr 1989;52:18–22

NAUSEA AND VOMITING

Definition

Vomiting is the ejection of matter through the mouth from the stomach and nausea is the inclination to vomit or the sensation associated with vomiting. Nausea and vomiting associated with pregnancy, surgery, chemotherapy and motion will be considered.

CAM usage

Acupuncture and acupressure are commonly used for nausea in early pregnancy, commercial acupressure wrist-bands for seasickness and various CAM methods may be used as adjuncts in cancer therapy.

Clinical evidence

Acupuncture

Stimulation at the relevant point (known as PC6) by acupuncture, acupressure wrist-bands and electrical apparatus are often regarded as so similar that they can be combined in reviews. A systematic review combined 33 RCTs and CCTs of acupuncture and related forms of stimulation, mostly given as an adjunct to standard treatment, for postoperative, early pregnancy or chemotherapy-induced nausea and vomiting.[1] Twenty-seven trials were positive: in four negative trials the acupuncture was given after the emetic stimulus and under general anesthetic. Subsequent reviews have reached a cautiously positive conclusion for nausea of pregnancy (Box 5.36) and a strongly positive conclusion for postoperative nausea and vomiting (Box 5.37).

Box 5.36
Systematic review
Acupoint stimulation for nausea and vomiting (pregnancy)
Obstet Gynecol 1998; 91:149–155

- Seven RCTs included 686 women
- Quality not assessed; problems with blinding noted in some studies
- Six positive, one showed no effect
- Conclusion: women appear to benefit, though this has not been fully demonstrated to be more than a placebo effect

Box 5.37
Metaanalysis
Acupoint stimulation for nausea and vomiting (postoperative)
Anesth Analg 1999;88: 1362–1369

- Nineteen studies involving 1679 participants
- Overall quality score was average
- Four studies in children: all negative
- Acupuncture better than placebo for early nausea and vomiting (but not late)
- Acupuncture is comparable to standard antiemetic medication (for early or late nausea and vomiting)
- Conclusion: 20–25% of adults would benefit

For chemotherapy-induced nausea, the five CCTs in the original review[1] were all positive. In subsequent RCTs, electrical stimulation of PC6 reduced the severity of nausea induced by chemotherapy in a double-blind RCT among 42 gynecological cancer patients[2] and manual pressure by the patient on one of two points reduced the incidence and severity of nausea in 17 women undergoing a 10-day chemotherapy program.[3]

In motion sickness (Table 5.62), two out of three RCTs investigating acupuncture stimulation in the laboratory for experimentally induced symptoms were positive. A controlled laboratory trial in 18 subjects[4] found no benefit from wrist-bands in comparison with hyoscine. One poorly designed, controlled partial crossover trial of an electrical device used by nine subjects in rough seas suggested a positive effect but placebo effects were not satisfactorily controlled for.[5]

In nausea occurring in hospice care, a small crossover study with six patients found no effect of acupressure wrist-bands.[6]

Biofeedback

After early promising case studies, an RCT compared electromyographic and galvanic response biofeedback with relaxation and no treatment for nausea in 81 patients undergoing cancer chemotherapy.[7] Biofeedback was not effective compared with relaxation. Another RCT found no effect of biofeedback compared with placebo feedback or no treatment in laboratory-induced motion sickness.[8]

CONDITIONS

Table 5.62 **RCTs of acupoint stimulation for nausea and vomiting (motion sickness)**

Reference	Sample size	Interventions [regimen]	Result	Comment
Aviat Space Environ Med 1991;62:776–778	36	A) Acupressure [bilateral wrist band for 15 min] B) Placebo stimulation	No difference	Double-blind: experimentally induced nausea
Aviat Space Environ Med 1995;66:631–634	64	A) Acupressure [unilateral finger pressure 1 Hz for 12 min] B) Dummy-point acupressure C) Placebo acupressure D) No treatment	A superior to all other groups	Experimentally induced nausea
Gastroenterology 1992;102:1854–1858	45	A) Electrical stimulation [unilateral 10 Hz for 15 min] B) Sham stimulation C) Control	A superior to both other groups	Experimentally induced nausea

Herbal medicine

The small number of studies of **ginger** (*Zingiber officinale*) for nausea of various causes contained in a systematic review (Box 5.38) are uniformly positive and suggest that ginger is more effective than placebo and about as effective as metoclopramide.

Box 5.38
Systematic review
Ginger for nausea and vomiting
Br J Anaesth 2000;84: 367–371

- Six RCTs involving 480 patients

- Overall study quality good

- Postoperative nausea and vomiting: positive in two studies, positive trend in one other

- Seasickness and morning sickness (see p 113): superior to placebo

- One study for chemotherapy-induced nausea positive but details incomplete

- Conclusion: ginger is a promising antiemetic herbal remedy, but insufficient data for firm conclusions

Peppermint oil was superior to placebo and no treatment when given preoperatively in an RCT.[9]

Hypnotherapy

Self-hypnosis has been described as helpful for both anticipatory and post-chemotherapy nausea and vomiting in children and adolescents and several controlled trials support this view.

For example, an RCT in 20 children found that hypnosis training prevented anticipatory nausea and reduced the need for antiemetic medication.[10-12] Two of these studies provide evidence that the effect is greater than that of attention alone: in an RCT with 30 children and adolescents, hypnosis training was more effective than no treatment and therapist contact (attention control) in preventing anticipatory nausea before chemotherapy.[11] The second found both hypnotherapy and distraction/relaxation better than attention control for nausea in 54 pediatric cancer patients.[12] Hypnotherapy may be less effective in adults according to one RCT, but the intervention used may have been little more than relaxation.[13] Hypnotherapy was found to be effective against postoperative nausea and vomiting in women undergoing breast surgery.[14]

Relaxation

On balance, the evidence from about a dozen RCTs shows that relaxation is effective in preventing nausea and vomiting before, during and after chemotherapy (Table 5.63). Research from one center was summarized by the principal investigator,[15] who found that relaxation appears to be more effective if it is learnt before treatment with chemotherapy starts. An RCT involving 60 cancer patients found that the related technique of systematic desensitization (relaxation learned as a response to nausea) was more effective than counseling and no treatment.[16]

Table 5.63 **RCTs of relaxation for nausea and vomiting (anticipatory and post-chemotherapy nausea)**

Reference	Sample size	Interventions	Result	Comment
Cognitive Ther Res 1986;10: 421–466	92	A) Relaxation B) Systematic desensitization C) Counseling D) No intervention	A and B superior to C and D	B better than A for anticipatory nausea
Cancer Nurs 1997;20:342–349	60	A) Relaxation B) Attention control	A superior	
J Consult Clin Psychol 1987; 55:732–737	50	A) Relaxation by professional therapist B) Relaxation by trained volunteer C) Relaxation by audiotape D) Standard treatment	A superior to all other groups	
Pain 1995;63: 189–198	94	A) Usual treatment B) Therapist support C) Relaxation & imagery D) as C) plus cognitive training	No differences between groups	

Supplements

A systematic review of **vitamin B$_6$** (Box 5.39) in pregnancy drew a cautiously positive conclusion.

Box 5.39
Systematic review
**Vitamin B$_6$ for
nausea and
vomiting (nausea
of pregnancy)**
Cochrane Library 1998

- Two RCTs involving 416 women
- Pyridoxine (vitamin B$_6$) 75 mg or 30 mg/day respectively
- Quality not specifically reported
- No effect on vomiting
- Results suggest an effect on nausea, but insufficient evidence for firm conclusions

Other therapies

A single RCT of 33 patients suggests that **music** may have some benefit in the management of chemotherapy nausea in addition to standard therapy.[17]

Table 5.64
**Summary of
clinical evidence
for nausea and
vomiting**

Treatment	Weight of evidence	Direction of evidence	Serious safety concerns
Nausea of pregnancy			
Acupoint stimulation	OOO	⬈	Yes (see p 29)
Herbal medicine Ginger	O	⬆	Yes (see p 113)
Supplements Vitamin B$_6$	O	⬆	Yes (see p 5)
Postoperative nausea and vomiting			
Acupoint stimulation	OOO	⬆	Yes (see p 29)
Herbal medicine Ginger Peppermint	OO O	⬆ ⬆	Yes (see p 113) Yes (see p 142)
Hypnotherapy	O	⬆	Yes (see p 58)
Nausea and vomiting induced by chemotherapy			
Acupoint stimulation	OO	⬆	Yes (see p 29)
Biofeedback	O	⬇	No (see p 42)
Hypnotherapy	OO	⬈	Yes (see p 58)
Music	O	⬆	No (see p 81)
Relaxation	OO	⬈	No (see p 71)
Motion sickness			
Acupoint stimulation	OO	⬈	Yes (see p 29)
Biofeedback	O	⬇	No (see p 42)
Herbal medicine Ginger	O	⬆	Yes (see p 113)

Overall recommendation

For nausea and vomiting of pregnancy, where no conventional drug therapy is acceptable, vitamin B_6 has a role. Acupressure is known to be useful and safe, but the effect may be due to placebo. Ginger, although probably effective, is contraindicated.

For nausea and vomiting in other circumstances, some forms of CAM appear to offer a role as adjuncts to conventional therapies. In postoperative nausea and vomiting, conventional therapies are effective but expensive and have known adverse effects; acupressure bands are cheap, safe and easy to administer, so both they and ginger are recommended.

For nausea induced by chemotherapy, effective conventional drugs will usually be available because of the high incidence and severity of symptoms. However, both hypnotherapy and relaxation appear to have a useful preventive role in children, for the nausea and vomiting before, during and after chemotherapy. The place of hypnotherapy for adults is less certain. Acupuncture/acupressure are also useful.

For motion sickness, ginger and acupuncture are worth using since conventional drugs, although effective, may have adverse effects.

REFERENCES

1 Vickers A. Can acupuncture have specific effects on health? A systematic review of acupuncture antiemesis trials. J Roy Soc Med 1996;89:303–311

2 Pearl M L, Fischer M, McCauley D L, Valea F A, Chalas E. Transcutaneous electrical nerve stimulation as an adjunct for controlling chemotherapy-induced nausea and vomiting in gynecologic oncology patients. Cancer Nurs 1999;22:307–311

3 Dibble S L, Chapman J, Mack K A, Shih A-S. Acupressure for nausea: results of a pilot study. Oncol Nurs Forum 2000;27:41–47

4 Bruce D G, Golding J F, Hockenhull N, Pethybridge R J. Acupressure and motion sickness. Aviat Space Environ Med 1990; 61:361–365

5 Bertolucci L E, DiDario B. Efficacy of a portable acustimulation device in controlling seasickness. Aviat Space Environ Med 1995;66:1155–1158

6 Brown S, North D, Marvel M K, Fons R. Acupressure wrist bands to relieve nausea and vomiting in hospice patients: do they work? Am J Hospice Palliat Care 1992;9:26–29

7 Burish T G, Jenkins R A. Effectiveness of biofeedback and relaxation training in reducing the side effects of cancer chemotherapy. Health Psychol 1992; 11:17–23

8 Jozsvai E E, Pigeau R A. The effect of autogenic training and biofeedback on motion sickness tolerance. Aviat Space Environ Med 1996;67:963–968

9 Tate S. Peppermint oil: a treatment for postoperative nausea. J Adv Nurs 1997;26:543–549

10 Jacknow D S, Tschann J M, Link M P, Boyce W T. Hypnosis in the prevention of chemotherapy-related nausea and vomiting in children: a prospective study. J Develop Behav Ped 1994;15:258–264

11 Hawkins P J, Liossi C, Ewart B W, Hatira P, Kosmidis V H, Varvutsi M. Hypnotherapy for control of anticipatory nausea and vomiting in children with cancer: preliminary findings. Psycho-Oncology 1995;4:101–106

12 Zeltzer L K, Dolgin M J, LeBaron S, LeBaron C. A randomized, controlled study of behavioral intervention for chemotherapy distress in children with cancer. Pediatrics 1991;88:34–42

13 Syrjala K L, Cummings C, Donaldson G W. Hypnosis or cognitive behavioral training for the reduction of pain and nausea during cancer treatment: a controlled clinical trial. Pain 1992;48:137–146

14 Enqvist B, Bjorklund C, Engman M, Jakobsson J. Preoperative hypnosis reduces postoperative vomiting after surgery of the breasts. A prospective, randomized and

blinded study. Acta Anaesthes Scand 1997;41:1028–1032

15 Burish T G, Tope D M. Psychological techniques for controlling the adverse side effects of cancer chemotherapy: findings from a decade of research. J Pain Symptom Manage 1992;7:287–301

16 Morrow G R, Morrell C. Behavioral treatment for the anticipatory nausea and vomiting induced by cancer chemotherapy. New Engl J Med 1982;307:1476–1480

17 Ezzone S, Baker C, Rosselet R, Terepka E. Music as an adjunct to antiemetic therapy. Oncol Nurs Forum 1998;25:1551–1556

NECK PAIN

Synonym

Mechanical neck disorder.

Definition

Pain in the cervical region, with or without referral to the shoulder and arm. The symptom may arise from a broad range of conditions involving muscle, joint, disc, ligament or degenerative disorders. It may also occur with diffuse connective tissue diseases including rheumatoid arthritis, arthritis associated with spondylitis and a number of other systemic conditions.

CAM usage

According to survey data from the US,[1] 57% of people with neck pain used CAM in the previous 12 months, two-thirds visiting a practitioner. Manual therapies are commonly used, as is acupuncture. Approximately 30% of chiropractic practice consists of patients with a primary complaint of neck pain.

Clinical evidence

Acupuncture

Despite clinical reports that neck pain often responds well to acupuncture, the results of a systematic review of RCTs (Box 5.40) do not provide evidence that it is superior to placebo. A subsequent RCT of 40 subjects found acupuncture at appropriate points superior to acupuncture at inappropriate points in respect of some measures, though the results are not clear-cut because heat treatment was also given.[2]

Box 5.40
Systematic review
Acupuncture for neck pain
Rheumatology 1999;38: 143–147

- Fourteen RCTs involving 724 subjects with neck pain from various causes

- Seven studies were of good quality

- Acupuncture was superior to waiting list (one study), either no different from or superior to physiotherapy (three studies) and no different from placebo acupuncture (four out of five studies)

- Conclusion: no evidence that acupuncture is superior to placebo

Electromagnetic therapy

There is some evidence from a systematic review of RCTs from one research team that this treatment may be effective (Box 5.41) but confirmation is required from other centers.

Box 5.41
Systematic review
Electromagnetic therapy (pulsed) for neck pain
Cochrane Library 1998

- Two RCTs involving 60 subjects
- Both good quality
- Short-term pain reduction compared with placebo, but not at 6 weeks' follow-up
- Data insufficient to allow an estimate of the effect size

Low-dose laser

A systematic review and metaanalysis (Box 5.42) found no effect from low-level laser therapy.

Box 5.42
Metaanalysis
Low-dose laser for neck pain
Cochrane Library 1998

- Three RCTs with 138 patients
- Quality was moderate
- Data were combined to calculate effect size for improvement in function: 0.8 (CI −4.07 to 9.67)
- Conclusion: not better than placebo

Spinal manipulation

A systematic review (Box 5.43) was cautious in its conclusion since many RCTs used manipulation in combination with other therapies.

Box 5.43
Systematic review
Spinal manipulation and mobilization for neck pain
Br Med J 1996;313: 1291–1296

- Nine RCTs involving 508 patients
- Quality varied from poor to good
- Two RCTs of manual treatment alone: one positive, one negative
- Seven RCTs of manual treatment in combination with other interventions overall positive; pooled effect size for reduction of pain −0.6 (CI −0.9 to −0.4)
- No conclusion drawn because of insufficient data

In three subsequent RCTs, one involving 323 patients with either back or neck pain found no difference in outcome or costs between physiotherapy and chiropractic manipulation during 12 months follow-up.[3] In the second, manipulation was compared with intensive training for neck muscles and with physiotherapy in 119 patients.[4] All groups improved over 12 months, with no difference between them. In a third RCT in 76 subjects with neck or back pain, spinal manipulation was claimed to be superior to acupuncture and to antiinflammatory drugs.[5] However, because of considerable practical difficulties in the conduct of the study, the results must be considered unreliable. Thus, there is evidence that combined physical approaches that include spinal manipulation are effective for neck pain, but insufficient evidence to recommend manipulation as a sole therapy.

Table 5.65
Summary of clinical evidence for neck pain

Treatment	Weight of evidence	Direction of evidence	Serious safety concerns
Acupuncture	OO	↘	Yes (see p 29)
Electromagnetic therapy	O	⇧	No
Low-level laser	OO	⇩	No
Spinal manipulation	OO	↗	Yes (see pp 47, 65)

Overall recommendation

Conventional methods for managing neck pain either have little supporting evidence (physiotherapy, cervical collars) or may have serious adverse effects (e.g. NSAIDs). Complementary therapies are therefore potentially important, but are not better supported by evidence of efficacy. The data on electromagnetic therapy look promising but the method is not widely available. Spinal manipulation appears to be possibly effective but has been associated with serious adverse events including strokes and fatalities. The incidence is rare but not precisely known. Therefore the safety of cervical manipulation compared with that of NSAIDs cannot be accurately known and remains a question of judgement. Since acupuncture to the neck is associated with a risk of pneumothorax, it can only be recommended when given by a well-qualified practitioner.

REFERENCES

1 Eisenberg D M, Davis R, Ettner S L, Appel S, Wilkey S, Rompay M V. Trends in alternative medicine use in the United States, 1990–1997. JAMA 1998;280:1569–1575

2 Birch S, Jamison R N. Controlled trial of Japanese acupuncture for chronic myofascial neck pain: assessment of specific and nonspecific effects of treatment. Clin J Pain 1998;14:248–255

3 Skargren E I, Oberg B E, Carlsson P G, Gade M. Cost and effectiveness analysis of chiropractic and physiotherapy treatment for low back and

neck pain. Six-month follow-up. Spine 1997;22:2167–2177

4 Jordan A, Bendix T, Nielsen H, Hansen F R, Host D, Winkel A. Intensive training, physiotherapy, or manipulation for patients with chronic neck pain. A prospective, single-blinded, randomized clinical trial. Spine 1998;23:311–318

5 Giles L G, Muller R. Chronic spinal pain syndromes: a clinical pilot trial comparing acupuncture, a nonsteroidal anti-inflammatory drug, and spinal manipulation. J Manip Physiol Ther 1999;22:376–381

OSTEOARTHRITIS

Synonyms/ subcategories
Degenerative arthritis, degenerative arthrosis, degenerative joint disease, hypertrophic arthritis, osteoarthrosis, gonarthrosis, coxarthrosis.

Definition
Degenerative disease of joints, usually defined by pathological or radiological criteria rather than clinical features: characterized by erosion of articular cartilage, either primary or secondary to trauma or other conditions, with remodeling of underlying bone and mild synovitis. In severe disease, joint space narrowing and osteophyte formation occur.

This chapter deals primarily with peripheral joint arthritis. For spinal joints, see sections on neck pain and back pain.

CAM usage
In a US survey, 27% of people who described themselves as suffering from 'arthritis' had used CAM in the previous 12 months,[1] a third of them seeing a therapist. Acupuncture, massage, manipulation and homeopathy are the therapies most commonly used.

Clinical evidence

Acupuncture
Acupuncture is widely used for treating the pain of osteoarthritis (OA). A rigorous comparison with standard care in 73 patients showed acupuncture produces overall beneficial symptomatic improvement which is still significant 4 weeks after the end of treatment.[2] However, rigorous comparisons with placebo have failed to demonstrate that its efficacy is superior to that of placebo acupuncture (Box 5.44).

Box 5.44
Systematic review
Acupuncture for osteoarthritis
Scand J Rheumatol 1997;26:444–447

- Thirteen CCTs involving 436 subjects with OA of any joint
- Seven positive and six negative
- No difference from placebo in four out of five studies
- Older and smaller studies are more likely to be positive
- Conclusion: no evidence that acupuncture is superior to placebo acupuncture

CONDITIONS

Herbal medicine

In a double-blind RCT of good quality, **devil's claw** (*Harpagophytum procumbens*) taken for 3 weeks was compared with placebo in a sample of 50 subjects.[3] The herbal preparation was significantly better than placebo for pain reduction. In a second study, 89 patients with OA were treated for 2 months with devil's claw or placebo. Again, the herb produced a significant reduction in pain and increase in mobility, with no adverse events recorded.[4]

Ginger (*Zingiber officinale*) is a common constituent of herbal mixtures for arthritis and of Ayurvedic medicine for rheumatic diseases, but in a three-arm crossover study in 75 patients comparing ginger with ibuprofen and placebo for OA, there was only a non-significant trend in favor of ginger over placebo in pain or dysfunction.[5] Ibuprofen was significantly superior to both.

Gitadyl is a proprietary preparation containing feverfew, American aspen and milfoil. In a crossover RCT of 35 subjects, its analgesic effects were not significantly different from those of a non-steroidal antiinflammatory drug, but it caused fewer gastrointestinal symptoms.[6]

The efficacy of **Phytodolor** (a proprietary preparation which contains *Populus tremula*, *Fraxinus excelsior* and *Solidago virgaurea*) in painful arthritic conditions has been demonstrated by a number of studies. For example, 108 inpatients with joint pain gained greater pain relief with either Phytodolor or piroxicam over 4 weeks than with placebo (quoted in[7]).

A proprietary preparation which is known as **Rumalex** and contains five herbs (willow bark, guaiacum resin, black cohosh, sarsaparilla and poplar bark) was demonstrated to have mild analgesic effects compared with placebo in an RCT involving 82 subjects.[8]

Tipi (*Petiveria alliacea*) is commonly used in rheumatic diseases but in a short RCT in patients with OA, showed no benefit compared with placebo.[9]

In an RCT involving 78 inpatients with OA of knee or hip, standardized **willow bark** (*Salix* spp) extract produced greater pain relief than placebo over the 14-day trial period, supported by global assessments by patient and physician (quoted in[7]).

A mixture of extracts of **Withania somnifera, Boswellia serrata** and **Curcuma longa** was shown to be superior to placebo in a crossover RCT involving 3 months' treatment, as measured by pain severity and disability score.[10]

Homeopathy

A systematic review (Box 5.45) found four trials of either oral or topically applied homeopathy, which were promising but insufficient to draw any conclusions for clinical practice.

Box 5.45
Systematic review
Homeopathy for osteoarthritis
Br Homeopath J 2001;
90:37–43

- Four RCTs involving 406 patients with OA

- All trials of high quality

- Two positive and one negative comparison with conventional oral drugs

- Topical homeopathic gel no different effect from conventional non-steroidal gel

- Evidence inconclusive because of small volume

Supplements

Avocado–soybean unsaponifiables (ASU) were compared with placebo in a 6-month RCT in patients with OA of the knee or hip. The ASU preparation was superior in both pain and functional measures.[11] In another double-blind RCT involving 164 patients, the effect of ASU on reducing the use of standard NSAIDs was compared with placebo and found to have statistically significant benefit.[12]

Chondroitin sulfate (Box 5.46) and glucosamine (Box 5.47) both appear to be effective in OA and to have fewer adverse effects than NSAIDs. Yet another metaanalysis[13] has looked at similar data for both supplements and concluded that, although the effect sizes seen in the published studies are likely to be exaggerated by publication bias and quality issues, some degree of effectiveness appears probable for both preparations.

Green-lipped mussel (*Perna canaliculus*) was investigated in a double-blind controlled trial which included 28 rheumatoid and 38 OA patients, on a waiting list for joint surgery.[14] Full results are not given but 38% of those who received mussel improved compared with 14% of the placebo group (not statistically significant). A further study by the same group[15] compared

Box 5.46
Metaanalysis
Chondroitin sulfate for osteoarthritis
J Rheumatol 2000;27:
205–211

- Seven studies (703 patients) with duration of ⩾3 months included

- Pain scores decreased progressively to 42% over the first 6 months of therapy (compared with 80% in placebo). Increased dosage did not result in better effectiveness

- Required daily dose of analgesic and NSAID medications was reduced

- Conclusion: evidence of clinically relevant efficacy of chondroitin sulfate on pain and function of knee and hip OA, at least when given as an adjunct to standard analgesic and NSAID medications

CONDITIONS

Box 5.47
Metaanalysis
Glucosamine for osteoarthritis
Arthritis Rheum 1998; 41:S198

- OA of any site. Peripheral joints and cervical spine included
- Eight RCTs, 810 patients
- Glucosamine oral 1.5 g/day and/or IM injection 400 mg two or three times a week
- Study quality: six were of good quality
- Result: glucosamine was significantly better than placebo in seven studies. Other studies suggest glucosamine is not significantly different in effectiveness from NSAIDs. Few adverse effects or study withdrawals reported, and less frequently than with NSAIDs

different preparations of the mussel, again including patients with either rheumatoid or osteoarthritis. There were significant improvements in various outcomes in both groups. The evidence that green-lipped mussel has any effect in OA is suggestive but not convincing.

Other therapies

Bee venom is subject to popular interest at times but was not found to be effective in a controlled trial in chronic arthritis.[16]

Significant numbers of subjects noted a symptomatic improvement with **copper** compared with aluminum bracelets in a controlled trial but the high drop-out rate makes this evidence highly unreliable.[17]

Dietary changes are often recommended for osteoarthritis, either complete approaches or particular components such as wheat germ. However, no clinical studies were found.

Massage and **manipulation** are widely used for OA and although one literature review[18] reports a favorable opinion, their effectiveness has not been investigated in controlled trials.

In view of the use of **relaxation** in chronic pain generally, it is surprising that there are no controlled trials into the effects of relaxation and other mind–body approaches to the pain of OA. **Therapeutic touch (healing)** showed a trend to greater effectiveness for reducing OA pain in 82 elderly subjects than progressive muscle relaxation and was more effective at reducing distress.[19]

Yoga has been studied in a small (n=17) RCT, aimed specifically at testing the effect on osteoarthritic hands.[20] There were significant improvements, compared with untreated controls, in hand pain during activity and in tenderness of finger joints.

Overall recommendation

There is a reasonable amount of evidence to recommend devil's claw, chondroitin sulfate and glucosamine, and perhaps avocado-soybean unsaponifiables, for their analgesic effect.

Acupuncture treatment is clearly better than no treatment but has not been demonstrated to be better than placebo. These therapies have good safety profiles, particularly in comparison with the high incidence of serious adverse effects from NSAIDs. None of these CAM therapies has been shown to have any disease-modifying properties.

Table 5.66
Summary of clinical evidence for osteoarthritis

Treatment	Weight of evidence	Direction of evidence	Serious safety concerns
Acupuncture	OO	⬀	Yes (see p 29)
Herbal medicine			
Devil's claw	OO	⇧	Yes (see p 101)
Ginger	O	⇨	Yes (see p 113)
Tipi	O	⇩	Yes (see p 5)
Willow bark	O	⇧	Yes (see p 163)
Homeopathy	O	⬀	No (see p 55)
Supplements			
Avocado-soybean unsaponifiables	O	⇧	Yes (see p 5)
Chondroitin	OO	⇧	Yes (see p 96)
Glucosamine	OO	⇧	Yes (see p 117)
Green-lipped mussel	O	⬀	Yes (see p 5)

REFERENCES

1 Eisenberg D M, Davis R, Ettner S L, Appel S, Wilkey S, Rompay M V. Trends in alternative medicine use in the United States, 1990–1997. JAMA 1998;280:1569–1575

2 Berman B M, Singh B B, Lao L et al. A randomized trial of acupuncture as an adjunctive therapy in osteoarthritis of the knee. Rheumatology 1999;38:346–354

3 Guyader M. Les polantes antirheumatismales. Etudes historique et pharmcologique, et etude clinique du nebulisat d'Harpagophytum procumbens DC chez 50 patients arthrosiques suivis en service hospitalier [dissertation]. Paris: Universite Pierre et Marie Curie, 1984

4 Lecomte A, Costa J P. Harpagophytum dans l'arthrose: etudes en double insu contre placebo. 37°2 Le Magazine 1992;15:27–30

5 Bliddal J, Rosetzsky A, Schlichting P et al. A randomized, placebo-controlled, cross-over study of ginger extracts and ibuprofen in osteoarthritis. Osteoarthritis Cartilage 2000;8:9–12

6 Ryttig K, Schlamowitz P V, Warnoe 0, Wilstrup F. Gitadyl versus ibuprofen in patients with osteoarthrosis. The result of a double-blind, randomized cross-over study. Ugeskrift for Laeger 1991;153:2298–2299

7 Ernst E. Phyto-anti-inflammatories: a systematic review of randomized, placebo-controlled, double-blind trials. Rheum Dis Clin: Compl Alt Ther Rheum Dis II 2000;26:13–27

8 Mills S M, Jacoby R K, Chacksfield M et al. Effect of a proprietary herbal medicine on the relief of chronic arthritic pain: a double-blind study. Br J Rheumatol 1996;35:874–878

9 Bosi Ferraz M, Borges Pereira R, Iwata N M, Atra E. Tipi. A popular analgesic tea: a double-blind cross-over trial in arthritis. Clin Exper Rheumatol 1991;9:205–212

10 Kulkarni R R, Patki P S, Jog V P et al. Treatment of osteoarthritis with a herbomineral formulation: a double-blind, placebo-controlled, cross-over study. J Ethnopharmacol 1991;33:91–95

11 Maheu E, Mazieres B, Valat J P et al. Symptomatic efficacy of avocado/soybean unsaponifiables in the treatment of osteoarthritis of the knee and hip. Arthritis Rheum 1998;41:81–91

CONDITIONS

12 Blotman F, Maheu E, Wulwik A, Caspard H, Lopez A. Efficacy and safety of avocado/soybean unsaponifiables in the treatment of symptomatic osteoarthritis of the knee and hip. Revue Du Rhumatisme (English edition) 1997;64:825–834

13 McAlindon T E, LaValley M P, Gulin J P, Felson D T. Glucosamine and chondroitin for treatment of osteoarthritis. JAMA 2000;283:1469–1475

14 Gibson R G, Gibson S L M, Conway V, Chappell D. *Perna canaliculus* in the treatment of arthritis. Practitioner 1980;224:955–960

15 Gibson S L M, Gibson R G. The treatment of arthritis with a lipid extract of *Perna canaliculus*: a randomised trial. Compl Ther Med 1998;6:122–126

16 Hollander J. Bee venom in the treatment of chronic arthritis. Am J Med Sci 1941; 201:796–801

17 Whitehouse M W, Walker W R. Copper and inflammation. Agents Actions 1978; 8:85–90

18 Gottlieb M S. Conservative management of spinal osteoarthritis with glucosamine and chiropractic treatment. J Manip Physiol Ther 1997;20:400–414

19 Eckes Peck S D. The effectiveness of therapeutic touch for decreasing pain in elders with degenerative arthritis. J Holistic Nurs 1997;15:176–198

20 Garfinkel M S, Schumacher H R, Husain A, Levy M, Reshetar R A. Evaluation of a yoga based regimen for treatment of osteoarthritis of the hands. J Rheumatol 1994;21:2341–2343

FURTHER READING

Panush R S (ed). Complementary and alternative therapies for rheumatic diseases. Rheum Dis Clin North Am I 1999;25(4) and II 2000;26(1)
Several opinion pieces as well as evidence-based chapters on a wide range of therapies.

OVERWEIGHT

Synonyms   Corpulence, corpulency.

Definition   An abnormal increase of fat, particularly in the subcutaneous connective tissues. Overweight and obesity are also defined according to body mass index (BMI), which is body weight in kilogram divided by the square of height in meters. Overweight: $23.9–29.9 \, kg/m^2$; obesity: $30 \, kg/m^2$ and over.[1,2]

CAM usage   Complementary therapies commonly used by those attempting to lose weight include acupuncture, dietary supplements and herbal medicine.

Clinical evidence

Acupuncture/acupressure

A systematic review on the subject found no clear evidence for effectiveness (Box 5.48). Two of the reviewed trials report beneficial effects for the reduction of hunger, while two others do not support the notion that acupuncture/acupressure reduces body weight. It is concluded that claims of specific effects of acupuncture/acupressure for weight loss are not based on the results of rigorous clinical studies. In a subsequently published RCT 60 overweight patients were treated with either electroacupuncture or sham acupuncture twice daily for 4 weeks.[3] The authors report that the number of patients who lost weight as well as the mean weight loss were significantly greater in the acupuncture group.

Box 5.48
Systematic review
**Acupuncture/
acupressure for
overweight**
Wien Klin Wochenschr
1997;109:60–62

- Four sham-controlled RCTs including 270 subjects

- Heterogeneous in terms of treatment modality and design

- Two trials assessed hunger (positive) and two body weight (negative) as the primary endpoint

- Methodological quality higher in the two negative trials

Herbal medicine

One double-blind RCT assessed 70 obese subjects who received one of three **Ayurvedic herbal formulations** or indistinguishable placebo for 3 months.[4] All patients entered into the trial were at least 20% in excess of their ideal body weight and non-diabetic. The authors report that patients in the treatment group experienced a significant weight loss compared with those in the placebo group.

Whether **guar gum,** a plant-based dietary fiber derived from the Indian cluster bean (*Cyamopsis tetragonolobus*), is an option for this condition has been assessed by a metaanalysis (Box 5.49). The results of this study suggested, contradictory to other reports,[5,6] that guar gum is not effective for reducing body weight.

Box 5.49
Metaanalysis
**Guar gum for
overweight**
Am J Med 2001
(in press)

- Twenty double-blind, placebo-controlled RCTs including 392 patients; metaanalysis of 11 trials

- Trial quality satisfactory

- Two trials report positive results

- Metaanalysis suggests no beneficial effect (weighted mean difference: −0.04 kg, CI −2.22 to 2.14)

A double-blind RCT investigated the effects of **malabar tamarind** (*Garcinia cambogia*) extract in 135 overweight individuals.[7] These received either 1 g of *Garcinia cambogia* extract (50% hydroxycitrate) three times daily or placebo for 12 weeks. The results suggest no beneficial effect on weight loss beyond that observed with placebo. A combination preparation containing 400 mg *Garcinia cambogia* (50% hydroxycitrate) and 25 mg caffeine (guarana and green tea) was assessed in a double-blind RCT, which found no significant effects compared with placebo.[8]

Maté extract was assessed in a small (n=12) double-blind RCT, which reported a rise in respiratory quotient indicating an increase in the proportion of fat oxidized.[9] Other extracts, such as

CONDITIONS

Corylus avellana, Crithmum maritinum, Ephedra sinica and guarana, were reported in the same study to have no such effects.

Supplements

A metaanalysis of RCTs of **chitosan** found some positive evidence on the subject (Box 5.50). It concluded, however, that due to methodological limitations of the available data, the effectiveness of chitosan for weight reduction is not established beyond reasonable doubt. Two double-blind RCTs[10,11] conducted after the metaanalysis also suggested that chitosan has no beneficial effect for this indication. Overall, there is no convincing evidence that chitosan is beneficial for lowering body weight.

Box 5.50
Metaanalysis
Chitosan for overweight
Perfusion 1998;11: 461–465

- Five double-blind RCTs including 386 subjects
- Trial quality was good
- Treatment period was 28 days in all trials
- Hypocaloric diet (1000–2000 kcal/day) administered in all trials
- It was concluded that the effectiveness is not established beyond reasonable doubt

Overall recommendation

Conventional interventions consisting of diet modification, increased physical activity and lifestyle changes are the most effective measures to achieve weight loss. There are few encouraging findings from complementary approaches, but some exist for an Ayurvedic herbal formulation. There is no compelling evidence for the effectiveness of any other complementary therapy. Thus, at present, none of these treatments can be recommended for weight loss.

Table 5.67
Summary of clinical evidence for overweight

Treatment	Weight of evidence	Direction of evidence	Serious safety concerns
Acupuncture/ acupressure	OO	⇨	Yes (see p 29)
Herbal medicine			
Ayurveda	O	⇧	Yes (see p 52)
Guar gum	OOO	⇩	Yes (see p 122)
Malabar tamarind	O	⇩	Yes (see p 169)
Supplements			
Chitosan	OO	⇘	Yes (see p 94)

REFERENCES

1 Hill T, Roberts J. Changing the thresholds of body mass index that indicates obesity affects health targets. Br Med J 1996;313:815–816

2 World Health Organization. Obesity: preventing and managing the global epidemic. Geneva: World Health Organization, 1998

3 Richards D, Marley J. Stimulation of auricular acupuncture points in weight loss. Aust Fam Physician 1998;27(suppl 2):S73–77

4 Paranjpe P, Patki P, Patwardhan B. Ayurvedic treatment of obesity: a randomised double-blind, placebo-controlled clinical trial. J Ethnopharmacol 1990;29:1–11

5 Pizzorno J E, Murray M T (eds). Textbook of natural medicine. London: Churchill Livingstone, 1999, pp 1434–1436

6 Murray M T (ed). Encyclopedia of nutritional supplements. Rocklin: Prima Health, 1996, 317–319

7 Heymsfield S B, Allison D B, Vasselli J R, Pietrobelli A, Greenfield D, Nunez C. Garcinia cambogia (hydroxycitric acid) as a potential antiobesity agent. JAMA 1998;280:1596–1600

8 Rothacker D Q, Waitman B E. Effectiveness of a Garcinia cambogia and natural caffeine combination in weight loss – a double-blind, placebo-controlled pilot study. Int J Obes 1997;21 (suppl 2):53

9 Martinet A, Hostettmann K, Schutz Y. Thermogenic effect of commercially available plant preparations aimed at treating human obesity. Phytomedicine 1999;6:231–238

10 Wuolijoki E, Hirvela T, Ylitalo P. Decrease in serum LDL cholesterol with microcrystalline chitosan. Methods Find Exper Clin Pharmacol 1999;21:357–361

11 Pittler M H, Abbot N C, Harkness E F, Ernst E. Randomised, double blind trial of chitosan for body weight reduction. Eur J Clin Nutr 1999;53:379–381

FURTHER READING

Rosenbaum M, Leibel R L, Hirsch J. Obesity. New Engl J Med 1997;337:396–407
A thorough review of the current understanding of the pathogenesis of obesity.

PREMENSTRUAL SYNDROME

Synonyms/ subcategories

Late luteal phase dysphoric disorder, premenstrual dysphoric disorder, premenstrual tension.

Definition

The regular occurrence of physical, behavioral and psychological symptoms during the luteal phase of the menstrual cycle which disappear within a few days of the onset of menstruation, causing disruption to personal and occupational functioning.

CAM usage

Surveys from the US and UK reported the complementary therapies most popular with premenstrual syndrome (PMS) sufferers as exercise, vitamins/supplements, meditation, massage, homeopathy and chiropractic.[1,2]

Clinical evidence

Biofeedback

Vaginal temperature feedback (12 weekly sessions) was compared with no treatment in two identically reported RCTs with 30 women.[3] Biofeedback was reported to alleviate both physiological and affective symptoms. Several shortcomings in the procedures and discrepancies in the reporting of these trials cast doubt on the validity of the findings.

Herbal medicine

For chaste tree (*Vitex agnus castus*) extract there are several uncontrolled studies with positive results including a large (n=1634) study in which 81% rated themselves 'much better'.[4]

CONDITIONS

However, the results of two double-blind RCTs (Table 5.68) do not suggest that it is an effective treatment.

Table 5.68   **Double-blind RCTs of chaste tree for premenstrual syndrome**

Reference	Sample size	Interventions [dosage]	Result	Comment
Compl Ther Med 1993; 1:73–77	217	A) Chaste tree [1800 mg/d] B) Placebo	A no different to B	Postal study; other treatments not excluded
Phytomedicine 1997;4:183–189	127	A) Chaste tree [3.5–4.2 mg/d] B) Vitamin B$_6$ [200 mg/d]	A no different to B	Sample size lacked statistical power; efficacy of control intervention (B$_6$) unclear

A systematic review of **evening primrose** (*Oenothera biennis*) oil included uncontrolled studies as well as randomized and placebo-controlled trials (Box 5.51). None of the trials had large samples. The conclusion drawn from the available evidence was that evening primrose oil is of little, if any, value for PMS.

Box 5.51
Systematic review
Evening primrose oil for premenstrual syndrome
Controlled Clin Trials 1996;17:60–68

- Eleven trials of any design (four RCTs) including 455 patients
- Trial quality generally low
- Three most rigorous trials had negative results
- Concluded little, if any, value

Ginkgo (*Ginkgo biloba*) (160 mg daily for 2 months) was investigated in a double-blind placebo-controlled RCT with 163 women.[5] The results suggested it may be helpful for breast pain, but not other PMS symptoms.

A small uncontrolled pilot study (n=19) of **St John's wort** (*Hypericum perforatum*) (300 mg daily for 2 months) reported improvements on all types of PMS symptoms, particularly those relating to mood.[6] This herb has not yet been tested in RCTs for this condition.

Homeopathy

Two double-blind, placebo-controlled RCTs of classical homeopathy have been conducted. In the first trial, stringent exclusion criteria led to the sample being too small (n=10) for meaningful results.[7] The other study included 105 patients monitored for 3 months,[8] at which point symptom scores were significantly lower in the homeopathy group. There was also less use of tranquillizers and analgesics and fewer work days lost than in the placebo group.

Massage
An RCT (n=24) of massage therapy for women with premenstrual dysphoric disorder (PMDD) reported some improvements in symptoms immediately after massage sessions and after one month of treatment. However, the mood symptoms that are central to PMDD were not significantly lowered at one month. Relaxation was used as a control, but intergroup analyses were not conducted.[9]

Reflexology
An RCT (n=35) of reflexology treatment (once weekly for 2 months) produced superior results on both somatic and psychological PMS symptoms than sham reflexology, which involved treating points unrelated to premenstrual symptoms.[10] No replication of this study has taken place.

Relaxation
Progressive muscle relaxation training (twice weekly for 3 months) alleviated physical symptoms of PMS in an RCT (n=46) compared with the control interventions of reading and charting symptoms.[11] For women with severe symptoms, there were also improvements in emotional symptoms.

Spinal manipulation
A crossover RCT (n=25) of **chiropractic** manipulation (2–3 times premenstrually for 3 months) reported superior results to a sham device.[12] However, improvements were greatest with whichever intervention was received first so results may have simply reflected a placebo response.

Supplements
Calcium supplementation has been demonstrated to be superior to placebo for most types of PMS symptom in two double-blind RCTs (Table 5.69). The second of these trials is impressive in terms of size and rigor and provides promising evidence in favor of calcium.

Table 5.69 **Double-blind RCTs of calcium for premenstrual syndrome**

Reference	Sample size	Interventions [dosage]	Result	Comment
J Gen Intern Med 1989;4: 183–189	33	A) Calcium [1000 mg/d for 3 mo] B) Placebo	A superior in 3 of 4 symptom subgroups	Crossover trial; high drop-out rate; non-compliance
Am J Obstet Gynecol 1998; 179:444–452	466	A) Calcium [1200 mg/d for 3 mo] B) Placebo	A superior in all symptom subgroups	Trial rigorous but not all other treatments excluded

CONDITIONS

Two small double-blind RCTs of **magnesium** supplements have indicated some benefits over placebo (Table 5.70). However, the type of symptoms that improved was different in each study and the data are not compelling.

Table 5.70 **Placebo-controlled, double-blind RCTs of magnesium for premenstrual syndrome**

Reference	Sample size	Interventions [dosage]	Result	Comment
Obstet Gynecol 1991;78:177–181	28	A) Magnesium [360 mg/d for 2 mo] B) Placebo	A superior overall & for 'negative affect' symptom	Unusual lack of placebo response
J Wom Health 1998;7:1157–1165	38	A) Magnesium [200 mg/d for 2 mo] B) Placebo	A only superior for fluid retention subgroup	Crossover trial; other treatments allowed

Potassium was investigated as a therapy in a non-randomized, placebo-controlled trial.[13] The results showed no effect on PMS symptoms or premenstrual weight gain.

The RCT evidence for **vitamin B$_6$** has been subjected to two systematic reviews. One concluded that there is no evidence of efficacy.[14] The other pooled the data, reporting a greater effect than placebo for overall symptoms and premenstrual depression, but cautioned that conclusions are limited due to the low quality of most trials (Box 5.52). The authors advised that doses in excess of 100 mg per day were not justified due to neurological adverse effects.

Box 5.52
Metaanalysis
Vitamin B$_6$ for premenstrual syndrome
Br Med J 1999;318: 1375–1381

- Nine double-blind, placebo-controlled RCTs including 940 patients
- Three used a multinutrient supplement containing vitamin B$_6$
- Trial quality generally low
- Superior to placebo (odds ratio 2.32; CI 1.95 to 2.54)
- Conclusions limited due to low quality of trials

Vitamin E has been investigated in two double-blind, placebo-controlled RCTs.[15,16] Although both show positive results for some PMS symptoms, the overall evidence is ambiguous.

Other therapies

There are no RCTs on the subject of **exercise** and PMS. However, preliminary evidence from questionnaire studies, non-randomized trials and case control studies suggest aerobic exercise training may help prevent or alleviate premenstrual symptoms (e.g. [17–20]).

Table 5.71
**Summary of
clinical evidence
for premenstrual
syndrome**

Treatment	Weight of evidence	Direction of evidence	Serious safety concerns
Biofeedback	O	⬈	No (see p 42)
Herbal medicine			
Chaste tree	O	⬆	Yes (see p 92)
Evening primrose oil	OO	⬆	Yes (see p 104)
Ginkgo	O	⬆	Yes (see p 115)
St John's wort	O	⇧	Yes (see p 156)
Homeopathy	O	⇧	No (see p 55)
Massage	O	⬈	No (see p 60)
Reflexology	O	⇧	No (see p 68)
Relaxation	O	⇧	No (see p 71)
Spinal manipulation			
Chiropractic	O	⬈	Yes (see p 47)
Supplements			
Calcium	OO	⇧	No
Magnesium	O	⬈	Yes (see p 5)
Potassium	O	⇩	Yes (see p 5)
Vitamin B_6	OO	⬈	Yes (see p 5)
Vitamin E	O	⇨	No

**Overall
recommendation**

The evidence is not convincing for any complementary treatment. However, given that some have few risks, that conventional treatments are limited and that there is a substantial placebo response in PMS, such treatments may be worth considering. Supplementation with vitamin B_6, calcium or magnesium has been shown to be beneficial in some women. Other interventions where the preliminary evidence looks promising include aerobic exercise and relaxation. These can be encouraged as part of a healthy lifestyle for all women.

REFERENCES

1 Singh B, Berman B, Simpson R, Annechild A. Incidence of premenstrual syndrome and remedy usage: a national probability sample study. Alt Ther Health Med 1998;4:75–79

2 Corney R H, Stanton R. A survey of 658 women who report symptoms of premenstrual syndrome. J Psychosom Res 1991;35:471–482

3 Van Zak D B. Biofeedback treatments for the premenstrual and premenstrual affective syndromes. Int J Psychosom 1994; 41:53–60

4 Loch E G, Selle H, Boblitz N. Treatment of premenstrual syndrome with a phytopharmaceutical formulation containing Vitex agnus castus. J Wom Health Gender-Based Med 2000;9:315–320

5 Tamborini A, Taurelle R. Intérêt de l'extrait standardisé de Ginkgo biloba (Egb 761) dans la prise en charge des symptômes congestifs du syndrome prémenstruel. Rev Fr Gynécol Obstét 1993;88:447–457

6 Stevinson C, Ernst E. A pilot study of Hypericum for premenstrual syndrome. Br J Obstet Gynecol 2000;107:870–876

7 Chapman E H, Angelica J, Spitalny G, Strauss M. Results of a study of the

CONDITIONS

homeopathic treatment of PMS. J Am Inst Homeopath 1994;87:14–21

8 Yakir M, Kreitler S, Bzizinsky A, Bentwich Z, Vithoulkas G. Homeopathic treatment of premenstrual syndrome – repeated study. Proceedings of the Annual Conference of the International Homoeopathic League. Budapest, Hungary, May 2000

9 Hernandez-Reif M, Martinex A, Field T, Quintero O, Hart S, Burman I. Premenstrual symptoms are relieved by massage therapy. J Psychosom Obstet Gynecol 2000; 21:9–15

10 Oleson T, Flocco W. Randomized controlled study of premenstrual symptoms treated with ear, hand and foot reflexology. Obstet Gynecol 1993;82:906–907

11 Goodale I L, Domar A D, Benson H. Alleviation of premenstrual syndrome symptoms with the relaxation response. Obstet Gynecol 1990;75:649–655

12 Reeves B D, Garvin J E, McElin T W. Premenstrual tension: symptoms and weight changes related to potassium therapy. Am J Obstet Gynecol 1971;109:1036–1041

13 Kleijnen J, Ter Riet G, Knipschild P. Vitamin B_6 in the treatment of the premenstrual syndrome – a review. Br J Obstet Gynaecol 1990;97:847–852

14 London R S, Sundaram G S, Murphy L, Goldstein P J. The effect of α-tocopherol on premenstrual symptomology: a double-blind study. J Am Col Nutr 1983;2:115–122

15 London R S, Murphy L, Kitlowski K E, Reynolds M A. Efficacy of α-tocopherol in the treatment of premenstrual syndrome. J Reprod Med 1987;32:400–402

16 Walsh M J, Polus B I. A randomized, placebo-controlled clinical trial on the efficacy of chiropractic therapy on premenstrual syndrome. J Manip Physiol Ther 1999; 22:582–585

17 Choi P Y L, Salmon P. Symptom changes across the menstrual cycle in competitive sportswomen, exercisers and sedentary women. Br J Clin Psychol 1995;34:447–460

18 Aganoff J A, Boyle G J. Aerobic exercise, mood states and menstrual cycle symptoms. J Psychosom Res 1994;38:183–192

19 Steege J F, Blumenthal J A. The effects of aerobic exercise on premenstrual symptoms in middle aged women: a preliminary study. J Psychosom Res 1993;37:127–133

20 Prior J C, Vigna Y, Sciarretta D, Alojada N, Schulzer M. Conditioning exercise decreases premenstrual symptoms: a prospective controlled 6 month trial. Fertil Steril 1987;47:402–408

FURTHER READING

Carter J, Verhoef M J. Efficacy of self-help and alternative treatments of premenstrual syndrome. Women's Health Issues 1994; 4:130–137
Critique of the clinical evidence for some popular non-prescription remedies.

RHEUMATOID ARTHRITIS

Synonyms Arthritis deformans, arthritis nodosa, nodose rheumatism.

Definition A systemic disease affecting the connective tissue, with inflammation of the joints as its dominant clinical manifestation.

Related conditions Other rheumatic diseases such as ankylosing spondylitis.

CAM usage As with most chronic conditions, rheumatoid arthritis (RA) is associated with a high level of CAM usage. In particular, patients often try herbal treatments and other nutritional supplements.[1] Modifications of the regular diet are also frequent (e.g. vegetarianism); most of these approaches are, however, conventional therapeutic options. In our survey of CAM organizations (see p 3) the following treatments were recommended for arthritis: aromatherapy, homeopathy, hypnotherapy, magnet therapy, massage, nutrition, reflexology and yoga.

Clinical evidence

Acupuncture

Even though acupuncture is often advocated for RA, relatively few rigorous clinical trials have been published. A review of acupuncture for all types of inflammatory rheumatoid diseases concluded that, due to methodological weaknesses of the primary studies, firm conclusions were not possible.[2] This was confirmed by a formal systematic review (Box 5.53). Even though this article is not recent, its conclusion is still valid.

Box 5.53
Systematic review
Acupuncture for rheumatoid arthritis
Sem Arthr Rheum 1985; 14:225–231

- Eight CCTs were included

- Five of these reported that acupuncture was effective for pain control

- One study claimed that acupuncture had antiinflammatory effects

- Methodological flaws were abundant

- Conclusion: it is imperative that satisfactory trials be conducted

Diet

Various (mostly conventional) dietary approaches have been tried for RA, usually with little success. Several trials from Scandinavia show encouraging effects for fasting followed by a vegetarian diet. A systematic review included four such studies.[3] The metaanalysis of these data suggests long-term improvements in pain and related outcomes. Both fasting and strict vegetarian diets are associated with the risk of malnutrition, thus adequate medical supervision is essential.

Herbal medicine

An **Ayurvedic** herbal mixture of *Withania somnifera*, *Boswellia serrata*, *Zingiber officinale* and *Curcuma longa* has been tested in a double-blind RCT with 182 patients suffering from chronic RA.[4] Patients were given either the herbal mixture or placebo for 16 weeks. Of multiple endpoints, only joint swelling showed a significant intergroup difference in therapeutic response.

Blackcurrant (*Ribes nigrum*) seeds contain high levels of gamma-linolenic acid (GLA) which exerts antiinflammatory activity through interfering with prostaglandin metabolism. An RCT was conducted of blackcurrant seed oil (15 capsules/day) versus placebo for 25 weeks.[5] Even though the 34 RA patients showed objective signs of reduced disease activity, the clinical response was not significantly better in the experimental compared with the placebo group.

CONDITIONS

Borage (*Borago officinalis*) is also a rich source of GLA. Two RCTs have been published, one with 37 RA patients suffering from active synovitis,[6] the other with 56 patients with active RA.[7] In both studies significant clinical benefits were observed in the experimental compared with the placebo groups.

Boswellia (*Boswellia serrata*) is used in Ayurvedic medicine and has been shown to have antiinflammatory activity by reducing leukotriene synthesis. One preliminary report of a placebo-controlled RCT showed that 3600 mg of extract daily was not effective in reducing pain or increasing function in 37 patients with RA.[8]

Evening primrose (*Oenothera biennis*) oil capsules containing 540 mg of GLA were tested in a three-armed RCT against 240 mg of eicosapentaenic acid (i.e. fish oil) plus 540 mg of GLA or placebo in 49 RA patients.[9] The results show a reduction of NSAID consumption in both experimental groups but no significant change in clinical outcomes.

Feverfew (*Tanacetum parthenium*) has been tested in one RCT for RA; 41 RA patients were randomized to receive either 70–86 mg chopped dried feverfew leaves per day or placebo for 6 weeks.[10] The results show no benefit in terms of subjective symptoms or objective signs of feverfew over placebo.

Garlic (*Allium sativum*) extract was given at a daily dose of 300 mg to 15 RA patients for 4–6 weeks while the control group was treated with conventional therapy;[11] 87% of the garlic-treated patients showed a 'good partial' response. This study requires replication through an RCT.

In an uncontrolled experiment, 28 RA patients were treated with ginger (*Zingiber officinale*).[12] Apparently 75% of the patients responded with pain relief and a reduction in swelling. Controlled studies are needed to confirm this result.

Several European herbal mixtures have been tested in clinical trials with positive results for RA patients. Of these preparations, only Phytodolor (a German proprietary medicine containing extracts of *Populus tremula*, *Fraxinus excelsior* and *Solidago virgaurea*) has been submitted to independently replicated clinical trials (Box 5.54).

Thunder god vine (*Tripterygium wilfordii* Hook) is recommended in traditional Chinese medicine for a large range of conditions. Two RCTs suggest it has antiinflammatory properties and is effective in reducing the objective signs and subjective symptoms of RA.[13,14]

Homeopathy

A recent review summarized three RCTs, including 226 patients, of homeopathic treatments of RA.[15] The odds ratio was 2.04 in favor of homeopathic remedies over placebo. No single homeopathic remedy emerged as more effective than another.

Box 5.54
Systematic review
**Phytodolor for
rheumatoid
arthritis**
J Natural Med 1999;
2:3–8

- Ten RCTs met the inclusion criteria. Six were conducted against placebo, four against reference medication

- Total sample size was 1035

- Most studies included patients with various rheumatic diseases

- The quality of these trials was, on average, good

- The results imply that Phytodolor is superior to placebo and equally effective as standard NSAIDS in alleviating arthritic pain and restoring function

- Conclusion: Phytodolor is a safe and effective treatment of musculoskeletal pain

Hypnotherapy

Most clinical trials on this topic suggest that hypnotherapy can be useful in pain management. In particular, pain perception seems to be influenced positively.[16] However, methodological shortcomings abound and no rigorous RCTs exist specifically for RA.

Relaxation

Several relaxation techniques are being advocated for RA. Muscle relaxation training was demonstrated to be superior to no intervention in an RCT with 68 RA patients.[17] They received 30 min twice weekly for 10 weeks and subsequently showed improvement in both function and well-being. A recent systematic review of all RCTs on relaxation for chronic pain arrived at cautiously positive conclusions.[18]

Spiritual healing

Several RCTs of various forms of spiritual healing have been published.[19] The question of whether spiritual healing alleviates arthritic pain more than placebo does not find a uniform answer in these studies. Firm recommendations are therefore not possible at present.

Supplements

Fish oil is rich in eicosapentaenic acid and docosahexaenic acid which have antiinflammatory activity through interfering with prostaglandin metabolism. Several RCTs have shown clinical benefit of regular fish oil supplementation in RA.[20] The overall effect size is, however, usually modest. Interestingly, alpha-linolenic acid (e.g. from **flaxseed oil**), which is the precursor of these omega-3 polyunsaturated fatty acids, does not seem to have the same clinical effects.[21]

Green-lipped mussel (*Perna canaliculus*) was tested in an RCT in which 30 RA patients took either 1150 mg/day

CONDITIONS

green-lipped mussel powder or 210 mg/day lipid extract of the green-lipped mussel;[22] 76% of the patients had a positive clinical response with no difference between the groups. As the trial did not include a placebo control group, it is not possible to determine whether the two treatments were equally ineffective or effective.

In an open pilot study 20 RA patients received 20 mcg or 1000 mcg **selenium** orally for 4 weeks.[23] At the end of this treatment phase both immunological and clinical outcome variables suggested a positive effect. This trial requires replication in a rigorous RCT.

Table 5.72
Summary of clinical evidence for rheumatoid arthritis

Treatment	Weight of evidence	Direction of evidence	Serious safety concerns
Acupuncture	OO	⇨	Yes (see p 29)
Diet			
Fasting & vegetarianism	OO	⇧	Yes (see p 6)
Herbal medicine			
Blackcurrant	O	⇲	Yes (see p 5)
Borage	OO	⇧	Yes (see p 167)
Boswellia	O	⇲	Yes (see p 5)
Evening primrose	O	⇗	Yes (see p 104)
Feverfew	O	⇩	Yes (see p 107)
Garlic	O	⇗	Yes (see p 109)
Ginger	O	⇗	Yes (see p 113)
Phytodolor	OOO	⇧	Yes (see p 5)
Thunder god vine	OO	⇧	Yes (see p 5)
Homeopathy	OO	⇗	No (see p 55)
Hypnotherapy	O	⇗	Yes (see p 58)
Relaxation	OO	⇧	No (see p 71)
Spiritual healing	O	⇨	No (see p 73)
Supplements			
Alpha-linolenic acid	O	⇩	Yes (see p 5)
Fish oil	OOO	⇧	Yes (see p 5)
Flaxseed oil	O	⇩	Yes (see p 5)
Green-lipped mussel	O	⇨	Yes (see p 5)
Selenium	O	⇧	Yes (see p 5)

Other therapies

An observational study suggested that **aromatherapy** massage increases the well-being of patients with RA.[24] Children with juvenile RA received **massage** therapy from their parents 15 min daily for 30 days.[25] Subsequently, a decrease in self-reported and physician-assessed pain was noted. Some encouraging but mostly anecdotal evidence exists to suggest that **yoga** might benefit RA patients.[26] Unfortunately this hypothesis has so far not been tested in rigorous clinical trials.

Overall recommendation

No disease-modifying complementary treatment of RA exists. The evidence for CAM as a symptomatic therapy is mixed. Given the high rates of adverse effects of synthetic drugs used for RA, the following CAM modalities would seem to be reasonable therapeutic options: borage, fish oil, Phytodolor, thunder god vine, relaxation techniques. With all of these therapies the effect size is usually moderate to small. Thus such CAM treatments would normally be reasonable adjuvant treatments rather than true therapeutic alternatives.

REFERENCES

1 Resch K L, Hill S, Ernst E. Use of complementary therapies by individuals with 'arthritis'. Clin Rheumatol 1997;16:391–395

2 Lautenschlager J. Acupuncture in treatment of inflammatory rheumatoid diseases. Zeitschr für Rheumatol 1997;56:8–20

3 Müller H, Wilhelmi de Toledo F, Resch K L. A systematic review of clinical studies on fasting and vegetarian diets in the treatment of rheumatoid arthritis. Forsch Komplementärmed Klass Naturheilkd 2000;7:48

4 Chopra A, Lavin P, Patwardhan B, Chitre D. Randomized double blind trial of an Ayurvedic plant derived formulation for treatment of rheumatoid arthritis. J Rheumatol 2000;27:1365–1372

5 Leventhal L J, Boyce E G, Zurier R B. Treatment of rheumatoid arthritis with blackcurrant seed oil. Br J Rheumatol 1994;33:847–852

6 Leventhal L J, Boyce E G, Zurier R B. Treatment of rheumatoid arthritis with gammalinolenic acid. Ann Intern Med 1993; 119:867–873

7 Zurier R B, Rossett R G, Jacobson E W et al. Gamma-linolenic acid treatment of rheumatoid arthritis. Arthritis Rheum 1996;39:1808–1817

8 Sander O, Herborn G, Rau R. Is H15 (resin extract of Boswellia serrata, 'incense') a useful supplement to established drug therapy of chronic polyarthritis? Results of a double-blind pilot study. Zeitschr Rheumatol 1998; 57:11–16

9 Belch J J F, Ansell D, Madhok R et al. Effects of altering dietary essential fatty acids on requirements for non-steroidal anti-inflammatory drugs in patients with rheumatoid arthritis: a double blind placebo controlled study. Ann Rheum Dis 1988; 47:96–104

10 Pattrick M, Heptinstall S, Doherty M. Feverfew in rheumatoid arthritis: a double blind, placebo controlled study. Ann Rheum Dis 1989;48:547–549

11 Denisov L N, Andrianova I V, Timofeeva S S. Garlic effectiveness in rheumatoid arthritis. Tereapevticheskii Arkhiv 1999;71:55–58

12 Srivastaya K C, Mustafa T. Ginger (Zingiber officinale) in rheumatism and musculoskeletal disorders. Medical Hypotheses 1992; 39:342–348

13 Tao X L, Sun Y, Dong Y et al. A prospective, controlled, double-blind, cross-over study of tripterygium wilfordii hook F in treatment of rheumatoid arthritis. Chin Med J 1989; 102:327–332

14 Li R L, Liu P L, Wu X C. Clinical and experimental study on sustained release tablet of Tripterygium wilfordii in treating rheumatoid arthritis. Chung-Kuo Chung Hsi I Chieh Ho Tsa Chih 1996;16:10–13

15 Jonas W, Linde L, Ramirez G. Homeopathy and rheumatic disease. Rheum Dis Clin North Am 2000;26:117–123

16 Weissenberg M. Cognitive aspects of pain and pain control. Int J Clin Exper Hypnosis 1998; 46:44–61

17 Lundgren S, Stenstrom C H. Muscle relaxation training and quality of life in rheumatoid arthritis. A randomized controlled clinical trial. Scand J Rheumatol 1999;28:47–53

18 Carroll D, Seers K. Relaxation for the relief of chronic pain: a systematic review. J Adv Nurs 1998;27:476–487

19 Astin J A, Harkness E, Ernst E. The efficacy of 'distant healing': a systematic review of randomized trials. Ann Intern Med 2000; 132:903–910

20 McCarthy G M, Kenny D. Dietary fish oil and rheumatic diseases. Semin Arthritis Rheum 1992;21:368–375

21 Nordstrom D C E, Honkanen V E A, Nasu Y, Antila E, Friman C, Konttinen Y T. Alpha-linolenic acid in the treatment of rheumatoid arthritis: a double-blind, placebo-controlled and randomized study: flaxseed vs safflower seed. Rheumatol Int 1995;14:231–234

22 Gibson S L M, Gibson R G. The treatment of arthritis with a lipid extract of Perna canaliculus: a randomized trial. Compl Ther Med 1998;6:122–126

23 Maleitzke R, Gottl K H. Treatment of rheumatoid arthritis with selenium. Therapiewoche 1996;46:1529–1532

24 Brownfield A. Aromatherapy in arthritis: a study. Nurs Standard 1998;13:34–35

25 Field T, Hernandez-Reif M, Seligman S et al. Juvenile rheumatoid arthritis: benefits from massage therapy. J Paediatr Psychol 1997; 22:607–617

26 Haslock I, Monro R, Nagarathna R, Nagendra H R, Raghuram N V. Measuring the effects of yoga in rheumatoid arthritis. Br J Rheumatol 1994;33:787–788

SMOKING CESSATION

Synonyms Nicotine withdrawal, nicotine dependence.

Definition Desire to stop smoking.

CAM usage Acupuncture and hypnotherapy are the CAM therapies most commonly used for smoking cessation.

Clinical evidence

Acupuncture

Acupuncture appears to be more helpful for smoking cessation than doing nothing (waiting list), but this seems to be a placebo, or non-specific, effect since a metaanalysis found acupuncture not to be superior to placebo acupuncture (Box 5.55).

Box 5.55
Metaanalysis
Acupuncture for smoking cessation
Cochrane Library 1999

- Twenty sham-controlled RCTs involving 2069 smokers
- Quality varied from poor to good
- Variety of acupuncture techniques used
- Acupuncture was not superior to sham acupuncture at any time point. The odds ratio for immediate outcomes was 1.22 (CI 0.99 to 1.49)
- No single technique was superior
- No clear evidence of effects beyond placebo

Electrostimulation

One hundred and one smokers were randomized to daily electro-stimulation for 5 days or placebo stimulation.[1] There was no difference between the groups in terms of withdrawal symptoms or successful cessation.

Exercise

A systematic review of nine RCTs of exercise as an adjunct to a smoking cessation program included only two with large sample sizes. One of these showed superiority of exercise over a behavioral program (Box 5.56).

Box 5.56
Systematic review
Exercise-based interventions for smoking cessation
Cochrane Library 2000

- Eight RCTs of exercise as an adjunct to a smoking cessation program

- 744 smokers, follow-up periods of at least 6 months

- Control groups received multisession cognitive behavioral program only

- Six trials had fewer than 25 people in each treatment arm

- Only one trial (in 281 women) showed adjunctive exercise superior to program alone

- Conclusion: insufficient evidence to reach conclusion

Hypnotherapy

There are many anecdotal reports of individuals stopping smoking with the help of hypnotherapy and rates of abstinence achieved in uncontrolled studies vary between 4% and 88%. A systematic review found no reliable evidence that hypnotherapy is more effective for smoking cessation than the various control methods, which are themselves unproven (Box 5.57).

Box 5.57
Systematic review
Hypnotherapy for smoking cessation
Cochrane Library 1998

- Nine RCTs comparing hypnotherapy with a variety of control procedures in 677 smokers, follow-up period of 6 months

- Quality poor: no validation of successful cessation

- Different methods and regimens of hypnotherapy

- Conflicting results when compared with no treatment or advice

- Conclusion: no evidence of effectiveness when compared with rapid smoking or other psychological treatment

Relaxation

Relaxation has not been rigorously investigated for smoking cessation itself, but an RCT tested the effect of relaxation with

CONDITIONS

imagery on relapse prevention in 76 recently successful participants in a smoking cessation program. Relaxation imagery over the following 3 months resulted in reduced stress and improved abstinence, compared with no additional treatment.[2]

Other therapies

A small (n=20) study using **self-massage** of hand and ear compared with no massage suggested that it may be effective in reducing stress and cigarette consumption but its role in quitting is unknown.[3]

The use of **restricted environmental stimulation therapy** (REST) involving 12- or 24-hour residence in special chambers with repeated recorded messages has produced quit rates of 20% or more in smokers in uncontrolled studies (e.g. [4]), but no controlled studies are available. A similar therapy involving time spent with restricted sensory input in **flotation** tanks showed no benefit compared with various control methods.[5]

Table 5.73
Summary of clinical evidence for smoking cessation

Treatment	Weight of evidence	Direction of evidence	Serious safety concerns
Acupuncture	OOO	⇩	Yes (see p 29)
Electrostimulation	O	⇩	Yes (see p 6)
Exercise	OO	⇨	Yes (see p 5)
Hypnotherapy	OO	⇩	Yes (see p 58)
Relaxation	O	⇧	No (see p 71)

Overall recommendation

Conventional techniques of smoking cessation including nicotine replacement or medication with buproprion achieve higher quit rates than anything CAM has to offer and are the most cost effective of all medical interventions. However, specialist clinics, multiple interventions and continuing support add to the success and therefore CAM may have an adjunctive role in particular circumstances. It seems reasonable to argue that, because of the importance of smoking cessation, any safe form of intervention that smokers find helpful can be permitted, even if the evidence points to no more than a placebo effect. Patients should be advised of the nature of the evidence and any precautions that are necessary. Relaxation with imagery looks promising for relapse prevention, although the benefit of personal contact should not be underestimated.

REFERENCES

1 Pickworth W B, Fant R V, Butschky M F, Goffman A L, Henningfield J E. Evaluation of cranial electrostimulation therapy on short-term smoking cessation. Biol Psychiatr 1997;42:116–121

2 Wynd C A. Relaxation imagery used for stress reduction in the prevention of smoking relapse. J Adv Nurs 1992;17:294–302

3 Hernandez-Reif M, Field T, Hart S. Smoking cravings are reduced by self-massage. Prev Med 1999;28:28–32

4 Suedfeld P, Baker-Brown G. Restricted environmental stimulation therapy of smoking: a parametric study. Addict Behav 1987;12:263–267

5 Forgays D G. Flotation rest as a smoking intervention. Addict Behav 1987;12:85–90

FURTHER READING

Hughes J R, Fiester S, Goldstein M et al. Practice guideline for the treatment of patients with nicotine dependence. Am J Psychol 1996; 153(10 suppl):1–31

A useful guide to the range of therapies available for smoking cessation and their appropriate application to the individual.

STROKE

Synonyms/ subcategories	Apoplexy, cerebral infarct, cerebral infarction, cerebral thrombosis, cerebral hemorrhage, cerebral embolism, cerebrovascular accident, intracranial hemorrhage, subarachnoid hemorrhage.
Definition	A clinical syndrome characterized by rapidly developing symptoms and/or signs of focal and at times global loss of cerebral function, with symptoms lasting more than 24 hours or leading to death, with no apparent cause other than that of vascular origin. For completeness, sudden onset of headache and isolated signs of meningism, without focal or global neurological dysfunction, is included as stroke due to subarachnoid hemorrhage.
Related conditions	Reversible ischemic neurological deficit (RIND), transient ischemic attack (TIA).
CAM usage	In the West, no single form of CAM is in particularly common use for the management of stroke recovery; rather, usage is either experimental or depends on personal recommendation. In the East, acupuncture and Chinese herbs are widely used for the treatment of stroke patients. No specific role has been identified for CAM in stroke prevention.
Clinical evidence	*Acupuncture* A systematic review (Box 5.59) located several studies which found that acupuncture was superior to no additional therapy, but placebo-controlled RCTs suggest that this effect may not be specifically due to needling but to other factors such as the extra attention received. *Diet* It seems logical that those diets that are cardioprotective, e.g. high intake of fruit and vegetables, complex carbohydrates and oily fish or the Mediterranean diet, are also protective against stroke (e.g. [1]). Vegetarians had a lower death rate from all causes, including cerebrovascular disease, than non-vegetarians in a cohort of 11 000 health-conscious British people followed

CONDITIONS

Box 5.58
Systematic review
Acupuncture for stroke
J Neurol 2001 (in press)

- Nine RCTs involving 538 patients with acute, subacute or chronic stroke

- Only two studies were of good quality

- Six studies suggested that acupuncture is effective: the two good-quality studies were negative

- Conclusion: evidence is suggestive but far from compelling

up for 17 years.[2] In the Framingham Study,[3] a cohort of 832 healthy men experienced a significant decrease in the risk of stroke for each increase in vegetable and fruit intake. A systematic review (Box 5.59) found a convincing inverse correlation between vitamin C intake or blood marker of vitamin C intake and death from stroke (in contrast to a negative association with coronary artery disease). One possible mechanism could be through the effect on mild hypertension. An RCT of 459 hypertensive adults found that increasing the intake of fruits and vegetables lowered the blood pressure, though not as much as a diet both rich in fruit and vegetables and low in fats.[4]

Box 5.59
Systematic review
Dietary vitamin C for stroke
J Cardiovasc Risk 1996; 3:513–521

- Studies quantifying dietary intake of vitamin C or measuring biological markers of vitamin C status

- Two ecological studies found strong correlation (-0.68 and -0.38)

- One case-control study (47 cases, 44 controls) found no correlation

- Seven prospective cohort studies (110 506 persons); two found significant protective association

- The evidence suggests a protective effect: caution because of the limitations of nature, duration and accuracy of these data

A retrospective epidemiological study found a slightly higher incidence of stroke in men with the highest level of reported fish consumption[5] but no direct evidence exists. The possible roles of increased exercise and reduced smoking in stroke prevention have not been defined.

Herbal medicine

Garlic (*Allium sativum*) is known to have a small but definite effect on serum cholesterol concentrations and it is also believed to reduce platelet aggregation. Its role in stroke prevention has never been tested clinically. However, promising results were obtained in a placebo-controlled RCT in 60 adolescent volunteers with increased platelet aggregation who were at risk of cerebral ischemic episodes.[6] Daily ingestion of 800 mg of powdered garlic for 4 weeks was associated with a reduction in platelet aggregation, which reverted to previous values after the garlic was stopped.

In a placebo-controlled RCT in 50 patients with cerebral insufficiency following surgery for subarachnoid hemorrhage, ginkgo (*Ginkgo biloba*) at a dose of 150 mg per day for 12 weeks produced improvements in attention, reaction time and short-term memory.[7] An intravenous preparation of ginkgo was given to 20 patients in an observational study in acute stroke;[8] 10 patients recovered completely or almost completely. There were no adverse effects recorded, but no conclusions on its use in acute stroke can be drawn until controlled trials have been performed. The role of ginkgo in prevention has not been investigated.

Homeopathy

Two double-blind RCTs of **arnica** (*Arnica montana*) given immediately after stroke found no difference in mortality, survival or functioning over a 3-month period in comparison with placebo.[9,10]

Meditation

There is some evidence that transcendental meditation may lower mild hypertension (e.g. [11]), though a review concluded that earlier positive claims were based on studies which found little difference between meditation and sham techniques.[12] In one RCT comparing meditation with relaxation in 73 elderly persons living in retirement homes, meditation was associated with lower blood pressure and improved survival at 3 years, from a figure of 65% for the relaxation group to 100% for the meditation group.[13] The study did not record death from stroke itself. An RCT in which 138 hypertensive subjects either learnt transcendental meditation or received standard health education found that in those who meditated for at least 6–9 months, the thickness of the intimal lining of the carotid arteries was reduced, compared with controls.[14] The effects on clinical outcomes such as stroke itself were not measured and longer term follow-up is necessary before drawing conclusions.

Supplements

In a large RCT in Italy involving 11324 patients who had survived recent myocardial infarction, supplementation with **n-3 PUFA** produced a clinically relevant decline in cardiovascular deaths including stroke.[15]

In an RCT among 29 584 Chinese, principally aimed at reducing cancer rates, supplementation with a combination of **selenium, vitamin A** and **vitamin E** was found to be associated with a lower incidence of stroke over 5 years.[16] The bioavailability of selenium is often low in Western diets.[17]

Other therapies

Listening to **music** with a strong rhythmic pulse can be set to match gait tempo in order to improve rehabilitation. Measurements of gastrocnemius EMG show improvements in laboratory studies but no CCTs exist and this therapy is still limited to individual academic or clinical centers that are particularly interested.[18]

Table 5.74
Summary of clinical evidence for stroke

Treatment	Weight of evidence	Direction of evidence	Serious safety concerns
Acupuncture	OOO	⤴	Yes (see p 29)
Diets			
Vegetarian (prevention)	O	⤴	No
Herbal medicine			
Garlic (prevention)	O	⤴	Yes (see p 109)
Ginkgo	O	⤴	Yes (see p 115)
Homeopathy	O	⇩	No (see p 55)
Meditation	O	⤴	Yes (see p 80)
Supplements			
n3-PUFA (prevention)	O	⇧	No

Overall recommendation

The single factor known to improve the outcome after acute stroke is admission to a specialist stroke unit. However, since no individual conventional therapy has been demonstrated unequivocally to improve rehabilitation, it may be a matter of personal preference and individual judgement whether to use the various CAM therapies available. It appears likely that the additional attention given as part of an individualized, hands-on treatment may in itself act as a stimulant and aid recovery.

Although the evidence for prevention of stroke is less complete than for prevention of ischemic heart disease, it is justifiable to recommend diets high in vegetables, fruits and fish intake, together with supplementation by selenium where dietary intake of this mineral is insufficient.

REFERENCES

1 Bradley S, Shinton R. Why is there an association between eating fruit and vegetables and a lower risk of stroke? J Human Nutr Dietet 1998;11: 363–372

2 Key T J A, Thorogood M, Appleby P N, Burr M L. Dietary habits and mortality in 1100 vegetarians and health conscious people: results of a 17 year follow up. Br Med J 1996;313:775–779

3 Gillman M W, Cupples A, Gagnon D et al. Protective effect of fruits and vegetables on development of stroke in men. JAMA 1995; 273:1113–1117

4 Appel L J, Moore T J, Obarzanek E et al.
   A clinical trial of the effects of dietary
   patterns on blood pressure. New Engl J Med
   1997;336:1117–1124

5 Orencia A J, Daviglus M L, Dyer A R et al.
   Fish consumption and stroke in men: 30-year
   findings of the Chicago Western Electric
   Study. Stroke 1996;27:204–209

6 Kiesewetter H, Jung F, Jung E M, Mroweitz C,
   Koscielny J, Wenzel E. Effect of garlic on
   platelet aggregation in patients with increased
   risk of juvenile ischemic attack. Eur J Clin
   Pharmacol 1993;45:333–336

7 Maier-Hauff K. LI 1370 nach zerebraler
   Aneurysma-Operation. Münch Med
   Wochenschr 1991;133(suppl 1):S34–S37

8 Buttner T, Ruhmann S, Przuntek H. The
   treatment of acute cerebral ischemia.
   Ginkgo: free radical scavenger and PAF
   antagonist. Therapiewoche
   1994;44:1394–1396

9 Savage R H, Roe P F. A double blind trial to
   assess the benefit of Arnica montana in acute
   stroke illness. Br Homeopath J 1977;
   66:207–220

10 Savage R H, Roe P F. A further double-blind
   trial to assess the benefit of Arnica montana
   in acute stroke illness. Br Homeopath J
   1978;67:210–222

11 Wenneberg S R, Schneider R H, Walton K G
   et al. A controlled study of the effects of
   transcendental meditation programme on
   cardiovascular reactivity and ambulatory
   blood pressure. Int J Neurosci 1997;89:15–28

12 Eisenberg D M, Delbanco T L, Berkey C S
   et al. Cognitive behavioral techniques for
   hypertension: are they effective? Ann Intern
   Med 1993;118:964–972

13 Alexander C N, Langer E J, Davies J L et al.
   Transcendental meditation, mindfulness, and
   longevity: an experimental study with the
   elderly. J Pers Soc Psychol 1989;57:950–964

14 Castillo-Richmond A, Schneider R H,
   Alexander C N et al. Effects of stress reduction
   on carotid atherosclerosis in hypertensive
   African Americans. Stroke 2000;31:568–573

15 Valagussa F, Franzosi M G, Geraci E et al.
   Dietary supplementation with N-3
   polyunsaturated fatty acids and vitamin E
   after myocardial infarction: results of the
   GISSI-Prevenzione trial. Lancet 1999;
   354:447–455

16 Mark S D, Wang W, Fraumeni J F Jr et al. Do
   nutritional supplements lower the risk of
   stroke or hypertension? Epidemiology
   1998;9:9–15

17 Rayman M P. Dietary selenium: time to act.
   Br Med J 1997;314:387–388

18 Purdie H. Music therapy in
   neurorehabilitation: recent developments and
   new challenges. Crit Rev Phys Med Rehabil
   1997;9:205–217

TINNITUS

Definition

A persistent or intermittent ringing, hissing or other noise in the ears in the absence of external stimuli.

CAM usage

According to a Swedish survey of tinnitus sufferers, acupuncture and relaxation were the most commonly used complementary therapies.[1]

Clinical evidence

Acupuncture

A systematic review of six RCTs of acupuncture or electro-acupuncture found no convincing evidence of effectiveness (Box 5.60). Two open trials comparing acupuncture to other interventions reported some beneficial effects, but four sham-controlled trials had negative results. Methodological limitations restrict the conclusiveness of the results but current evidence suggests that acupuncture has no specific benefit in tinnitus.

CONDITIONS

Box 5.60
Systematic review
Acupuncture for tinnitus
Arch Otolaryngol 2000; 126:489–492

- Six RCTs including 185 patients
- Trials of acupuncture (4) and electroacupuncture (2)
- Trial quality generally low
- Four sham-controlled trials had negative results
- Concluded that efficacy was not demonstrated

Biofeedback

Positive results for biofeedback have been reported in RCTs when compared with no treatment,[2] sham feedback[3] and other treatments.[3,4] However, another RCT (n=26) found no difference between groups receiving biofeedback, 'counterdemand' biofeedback (where patients were told to expect no treatment for the first 5 weeks) or no treatment.[5] The lack of rigor of most studies along with inconsistent results prevents conclusions about the efficacy of biofeedback for tinnitus.

Herbal medicine

A systematic review of five RCTs of **ginkgo** (*Ginkgo biloba*) compared with placebo or pharmacologic treatment concluded that the evidence was favorable, but not fully conclusive, due to a small number of trials and methodological limitations (Box 5.61).

Box 5.61
Systematic review
Ginkgo for tinnitus
Clin Otolaryngol 1999; 24:164–167

- Five RCTs including 541 patients
- Methodological quality generally mixed
- Results consistently positive with one exception that used low dose of ginkgo
- Concluded evidence is favorable, but not fully conclusive

Homeopathy

A double-blind RCT (n=28) of a homeopathic remedy called 'Tinnitus' found no superiority over placebo for intensity or intrusiveness of tinnitus or audiological measures.[6]

Hypnotherapy

Three RCTs have suggested that hypnotherapy or self-hypnosis is comparable or superior to counseling or masking interventions in reducing subjective tinnitus symptoms (Table 5.75). Taking into account some methodological limitations, the evidence can be considered encouraging.

Relaxation

RCTs have suggested that relaxation training may be superior to no treatment[7,8] and as effective as cognitive techniques,[9,10] but

Table 5.75 **RCTs of hypnotherapy for tinnitus**

Reference	Sample size	Interventions [regimen]	Result	Comment
Scand Audiol 1990;19: 245–249	36	A) Self-hypnosis [4 × 50 min] B) Auditory stimulus C) Waiting list	Tinnitus totally disappeared in 73% of A and 24% of B	Audiological tests showed no change
Audiology 1993;32: 205–212	45	A) Self-hypnosis [50 min per w for 5 w] B) Masking C) Attention control	Improvement in tinnitus severity was significant with A, partial with C and none with B	No analysis of intergroup differences
J Laryngol Otol 1996; 110:117–120	86	A) Hypnotherapy [3 sessions] B) Counseling [1 session]	A no different to B on tinnitus severity or loudness but superior on sense of improvement	More therapist contact with hypnosis

in most cases placebo effects can not be discounted. In one trial (n=30) the improvements with two forms of relaxation were no different to that of the control group.[11] On balance the evidence seems to suggest that relaxation may reduce the annoyance of tinnitus, but benefits appear to be quite modest and short term.

Supplements

A double-blind crossover RCT (n=30) of **melatonin** found no overall superiority over placebo, although a subgroup analysis indicated better results in patients with bilateral than unilateral tinnitus.[12]

Negative findings for **zinc** supplementation were reported from a double-blind, placebo-controlled RCT with 48 patients.[13] However, patients all had normal serum zinc levels before treatment.

Yoga

Yoga proved much less helpful than cognitive-behavioral therapy and no better than a self-monitoring control group on psychoacoustic measures and symptom ratings in an RCT lasting 3 months with 43 patients.[14]

Overall recommendation

There is no convincing evidence for the efficacy of any complementary therapy. However, given the lack of effective conventional treatment options and the placebo responsiveness observed with tinnitus, therapies that have few risks may be worthy of consideration. Ginkgo may have some promise as a treatment and both relaxation and hypnosis are associated with some improvements.

CONDITIONS

Table 5.76
Summary of clinical evidence for tinnitus

Treatment	Weight of evidence	Direction of evidence	Serious safety concerns
Acupuncture	OO	⇩	Yes (see p 29)
Biofeedback	O	⇨	No (see p 42)
Herbal medicine Ginkgo	OO	⬀	Yes (see p 115)
Homeopathy	O	⇩	No (see p 55)
Hypnotherapy	OO	⬀	Yes (see p 58)
Relaxation	O	⬀	No (see p 71)
Supplements Melatonin	O	⇩	Yes (see p 133)
Zinc	O	⇩	Yes (see p 5)
Yoga	O	⇩	Yes (see p 77)

REFERENCES

1 Andersson G. Prior treatments in a group of tinnitus sufferers seeking treatment. Psychother Psychosom 1997;66:107–110
2 White T P, Hoffman S R, Gale E N. Psychophysiological therapy for tinnitus. Ear Hearing 1986;7:397–399
3 Podoshin L, Ben-David Y, Fradis M et al. Idiopathic subjective tinnitus treated by biofeedback, acupuncture and drug therapy. Ear Nose Throat J 1991;70:284–289
4 Erlandsson S I, Rubinstein B, Carlsson S G. Tinnitus: evaluation of biofeedback and stomatognathic treatment. Br J Audiol 1991;25:151–161
5 Haralambos G, Wilson P H, Platt-Hepworth S, Tonkin J P, Hensley R, Kavanagh D. EMG biofeedback in the treatment of tinnitus: an experimental evaluation. Behav Res Ther 1987;25:49–55
6 Simpson J J, Donaldson I, Davies W E. Use of homeopathy in the treatment of tinnitus. Br J Audiol 1998;32:227–233
7 Lindberg P, Scott B, Melin L, Lyttkens L. The psychological treatment of tinnitus: an experimental evaluation. Behav Res Ther 1989;27:593–603
8 Scott B, Lindberg P, Melin L, Lyttkens L. Psychological treatment of tinnitus. An experimental group study. Scand Audiol 1985;14:223–230
9 Jakes S C, Hallam R S, Rachman S, Hinchcliffe R. The effects of reassurance, relaxation training and distraction on chronic tinnitus sufferers. Behav Res Ther 1986; 24:497–507
10 Davies S, McKenna L, Hallam R S. Relaxation and cognitive therapy: a controlled trial in chronic tinnitus. Psychol Health 1995;10:129–143
11 Ireland C E, Wilson P H, Tonkin J P, Platt-Hepworth S. An evaluation of relaxation training in the treatment of tinnitus. Behav Res Ther 1985;23:423–430
12 Rosenberg S I, Silverstein H, Rowan P T, Olds M J. Effect of melatonin on tinnitus. Laryngoscope 1998;108:305–310
13 Paaske P B, Pedersen C B, Kjems G, Sam I L. Zinc in the management of tinnitus. Placebo-controlled trial. Ann Otol Rhinol Laryngol 1991;100:647–649
14 Kroner-Herwig B, Hebing G, Van Rijn-Kalkmann U, Frenzel A, Schilkowsky G, Esser G. The management of chronic tinnitus – comparison of a cognitive-behavioural group training with yoga. J Psychosom Res 1995;39: 153–165

FURTHER READING

Dobie R A. A review of randomized clinical trials in tinnitus. Laryngoscope 1999; 109:1202–1211
A non-systematic but reasonably comprehensive critical review of rigorous research of all treatments for tinnitus.

UPPER RESPIRATORY TRACT INFECTION

Synonyms Common cold, upper respiratory infection.

Definition Inflammation of upper respiratory tract including nose (rhinitis), pharynx (pharyngitis) and larynx (laryngitis) due to viruses or bacteria.

CAM usage A survey of the home-based remedies used by various ethnic populations in the US reported herbal medicine, dietary supplements and spiritual approaches as the most common complementary therapies.[1]

Clinical evidence

Exercise

Epidemiological studies have suggested that regular exercise at a moderate intensity is associated with low risk of upper respiratory tract infection, compared with moderate risk for sedentary individuals and high risk with the intense training of elite athletes.[2] The findings from three RCTs suggest that adopting an exercise regime may result in shorter or fewer infections (Table 5.77).

Table 5.77 **RCTs of preventive effects of exercise for upper respiratory tract infection**

Reference	Sample size	Interventions [regimen]	Result	Comment
Int J Sports Med 1990;11: 467–473	36	A) Brisk walking [5×45 min/w for 15 w] B) No intervention	Shorter duration of symptoms with A than B; no difference in frequency of infections	Negative correlation between cardiovascular fitness & duration of infections
Med Sci Sports Exerc 1993;25: 823–831	32	A) Brisk walking [5×40 min/w or 12 w] B) Callisthenics	Lower incidence of infections with A than B	Participants were all females >67 years
Med Sci Sports Exerc 1998;30: 679–686	91	A) Brisk walking [5×45 min/w for 12 w] B) Callisthenics C) Walking & diet D) Diet & callisthenics	Shorter duration of symptoms with A & C than B & D	Participants were all obese females

Herbal medicine

A non-randomized trial[3] and two RCTs (Table 5.78) have suggested that **Andrographis paniculata** taken in the first stages of a cold reduces the severity and duration of symptoms compared with placebo. Tolerability appears to be good from these studies.

Table 5.78 **Double-blind RCTs of Andrographis paniculata for upper respiratory tract infection**

Reference	Sample size	Interventions [dosage]	Result	Comment
Phytomed 1997; 3:315–318	50	A) Andrographis paniculata [3×340 mg/d for 5 d] B) Placebo	A superior to B in symptom relief & days of sick leave	Reduction of sick leave was 0.75 d
Phytomed 1999; 6:217–223	158	A) Andrographis paniculata [3×400 mg/d for 5 d] B) Placebo	A superior to B on several symptoms at 2 & 4 d	No adverse events reported

A review of controlled trials of **Chinese herbs** included 10 on upper respiratory tract infections.[4] Most trials reported superiority over antibiotics, but poor methodological quality rendered the evidence unconvincing. The safety of these herbs was not addressed.

A systematic review of RCTs of **echinacea** (*Echinacea angustifolia, purpurea, pallida*) extracts (Box 5.62) found mainly positive results for both prevention and treatment of colds, but inconsistencies in the evidence and probable publication bias prevented clinical recommendations. This review included all species of echinacea and did not attempt to differentiate between them. A subsequent RCT (n=95) of treatment with echinacea tea reported a shorter duration of symptoms than with placebo.[5]

Box 5.62
Systematic review
Echinacea for upper respiratory tract infection
Cochrane Library 1998

- Sixteen RCTs including 3396 patients
- Trials of prevention (8) and treatment (8)
- Included combination or monopreparations of any species
- Comparison with placebo, no treatment or other intervention
- Trial quality ranged from good to poor
- Concluded that evidence was generally positive, but insufficient for firm conclusions.

Steam inhalation of **German chamomile** (*Matricaria recutita*) was reported to have a dose-dependent effect on symptoms of the common cold in a placebo-controlled trial.[6]

An RCT of patients receiving a flu vaccine (n=227) reported that compared with placebo, **ginseng** (*Panax ginseng*) (100 mg daily for 12 weeks) reduced the frequency of colds and flu and increased immune activity.[7]

Homeopathy

Several RCTs have investigated the therapeutic effects of various homeopathic remedies and combinations, with conflicting outcomes. Two trials reported similar results to acetylsalicylic acid,[8,9] while from placebo-controlled studies, there have been both negative[10] and positive[11,12] results. The value of homeopathy for this indication remains unclear.

Supplements

From a systematic review of 30 mostly large-scale controlled trials of high-dose ($\geqslant 1$ g daily) **vitamin C** (Box 5.63), it was concluded that there was no consistent evidence of a prophylactic effect. However, as a treatment, vitamin C shortened the duration of colds by about half a day.

Box 5.63
Systematic review
Vitamin C for respiratory tract infection
Cochrane Library 1997

- Thirty placebo-controlled trials including > 8000 patients (children & adults)
- Trial quality generally mixed
- No evidence of protective effect
- Modest reduction of duration of symptoms (8–9%) when taken for treatment purposes

A systematic review of double-blind, placebo-controlled RCTs of treatment with **zinc** lozenges (Box 5.64) found no overall evidence that the duration of colds was shortened. Two other systematic reviews had similar conclusions[13,14] and a subsequent large RCT in children (n=249) reported a negative finding.[15] However, a recent smaller trial in adults (n=50) had positive results.[16] The evidence for zinc is therefore inconsistent at present.

Box 5.64
Systematic review
Zinc for upper respiratory tract infection
Cochrane Library 1999

- Seven double-blind, placebo-controlled RCTs including 754 patients
- Trial quality generally good
- Positive results from two trials
- Overall, results suggested no superiority over placebo
- Adverse effects associated with zinc administration

A large-scale placebo-controlled RCT (n=725) reported a preventive role of supplementation with **trace elements** (zinc

CONDITIONS

and selenium) in elderly institutionalized patients, but not with **vitamins** (beta-carotene, vitamin C, vitamin E).[17]

Other therapies

Self-performed nasal **acupressure** provided significant relief of nasal congestion compared with no intervention in a small (n=20) RCT.[18]

A non-randomized trial (n=50) reported that regular **sauna bathing** (once or twice weekly for 6 months) resulted in a lower incidence of colds, although no difference in their duration or severity, than no intervention.[19]

Table 5.79 Summary of clinical evidence for upper respiratory tract infection

Treatment	Weight of evidence	Direction of evidence	Serious safety concerns
Exercise (prevention)	OO	⇧	Yes (see p 5)
Herbal medicine			
Andrographis paniculata	OO	⇧	Yes (see p 166)
Chinese herbs	O	⤴	Yes (see p 52)
Echinacea			
(prevention)	OOO	⤴	Yes (see p 102)
(treatment)	OOO	⤴	Yes (see p 102)
German chamomile	O	⇧	Yes (see p 111)
Ginseng (prevention)	O	⇧	Yes (see p 88)
Homeopathy	OO	⇨	No (see p 55)
Supplements			
Vitamin C			
(prevention)	OOO	⇩	No
(treatment)	OOO	⇧	No
Zinc	OOO	⤵	Yes (see p 5)

Overall recommendation

There is a lack of compelling evidence for the effectiveness of complementary therapies in relieving symptoms of upper respiratory tract infections. However, given that conventional options are limited, echinacea is probably worth considering and it appears that large doses of vitamin C may have a small therapeutic effect. *Andrographis paniculata* also looks promising, although evidence is currently insufficient for recommendations. For the prevention of infections, echinacea may be useful and regular exercise of a moderate intensity appears to reduce the risk.

REFERENCES

1 Pachter L M, Sumner T, Fontn A, Sneed M, Bernstein B A. Home-based therapies for the common cold among European American and ethnic minority families. Arch Pediatr Adolesc Med 1998;152:1083–1088

2 Peters E M. Exercise, immunology and upper respiratory tract infections. Int J Sports Med 1997;18:S69–S77

3 Hancke J, Burgos R, Caceres D, Wikman G. A double-blind study with a new monodrug

Kan Jang: decrease of symptoms and improvement in the recovery from common colds. Phytother Res 1995;9:559–562

4 Liu C, Douglas R M. Chinese herbal medicines in the treatment of acute respiratory infections: a review of randomised and controlled clinical trials. Med J Aust 1998; 169:579–582

5 Lindenmuth G F, Lindenmuth E B. The efficacy of echinacea compound herbal tea preparation on the severity and duration of upper respiratory and flu symptoms: a randomized, double-blind placebo-controlled study. J Alt Compl Med 2000;6:327–334

6 Saller R, Beschomer M, Hellenbrecht D, Buhring M. Dose dependency of symptomatic relief of complaints by chamomile steam inhalation in patients with common cold. Eur J Pharm 1990;183:728–729

7 Scaglione F, Cattaneo G, Alessandria M, Cogo R. Efficacy and safety of the standardized ginseng extract G115 for potentiating vaccination against common cold and/or influenza syndrome. Drugs Exper Clin Res 1996;22:65–72

8 Maiwald L, Weinfurtner T, Mau J, Connert W D. Treatment of common cold with a combination homoeopathic preparation compared with acetylsalicylic acid. Controlled randomised single-blind study. Drug Res 1988; 38:578–582

9 Gassinger C A, Wuenstel G, Netter P. Controlled clinical trial for testing the efficacy of the homoeopathic drug eupatorium perfoliatum D2 in the treatment of common cold. Drug Res 1981;31:732–736

10 De Lange De Klerk E S M, Blommers J, Kuik D J, Bezemer P D, Feenstra L. Effect of homoeopathic medicines on daily burden of symptoms in children with recurrent upper respiratory tract infections. Br Med J.1994; 309:1329–1332

11 Diefenbach M, Schilken J, Steiner G, Becker H J. Homeopathic therapy in respiratory tract diseases. Evaluation of a clinical study in 258 patients. Zeitschr für Allgemeinmedizin 1997;73:308–314

12 Ferley J P, Zmirou D, D'Adhemar D, Balducci F. A controlled evaluation of a homeopathic preparation in the treatment of influenza-like syndromes. Br J Clin Pharmacol 1989; 27:329–335

13 Galand M L, Hagmeyer K O. The role of zinc lozenges in treatment of the common cold. Ann Pharmacother 1998;32:63–69

14 Jackson J L, Peterson C, Lesho E. A meta-analysis of zinc salts lozenges and the common cold. Arch Intern Med 1997; 157:2373–2376

15 Macknin M L, Piedmonte M, Calendine C, Janosky J, Wald E. Zinc gluconate lozenges for treating the common cold in children. JAMA 1998;279:1962–1967

16 Prasad A S, Fitzgerald J T, Beck F W J, Chandrasekar P H. Duration of symptoms and plasma cytokine levels in patients with the common cold treated with zinc acetate. Ann Intern Med 2000;133:245–252

17 Girodon F, Galan P. Monget A L et al and the MIN.VIT.AOX Geriatric Network. Impact of trace elements and vitamin supplementation on immunity and infections in institutionalized elderly patients: a randomized controlled trial. Arch Intern Med 1999;159:748–754

18 Takeuchi H, Jawad M S, Eccles R. Effects of nasal massage of the 'yingxiang' acupuncture point on nasal airway resistance and sensation of nasal airflow in patients with nasal congestion with acute upper respiratory tract infection. Am J Rhinol 1999; 13:77–79

19 Ernst E, Pecho E, Wirz P, Saradeth T. Regular sauna bathing and the incidence of common colds. Ann Med 1990;22: 225–227

FURTHER READING

Nieman D C. Exercise and immune function: recent developments. In: Shanahan J (ed) Exercise for health. Hong Kong: Adis International, 2000
A concise overview of the evidence on the relationship between exercise and immune function.

General topics

Complementary and Alternative Medicine: A Canadian Perspective

Heather Boon
Marja J Verhoef

Introduction

Complementary and alternative medicine (CAM) has become an important Canadian health-care issue driven primarily by the large numbers of patients who seek CAM products and therapies. This chapter will first present an overview of the extent of CAM use in Canada and characteristics of CAM use. This will be followed by a discussion of the perceptions of Canadian physicians with respect to CAM and an update on the integration of CAM topics into the educational programs of Canadian health-care professionals. The chapter will conclude with an overview of the current regulation of CAM products and practitioners in Canada.

Use of CAM by Canadians

CAM use in the general population

The first Canadian survey of CAM use was conducted in 1990 for the Canada Health Monitor.[1] The survey showed that 20% of Canadians had used CAM during the 6 months preceding the survey. Two recent Canada-wide surveys report higher rates of CAM use. The Fraser Institute survey found that half of the respondents reported use of CAM in the 12 months immediately preceding the survey and that almost three-quarters (73%) reported use of CAM at some time during their lives.[2] An Angus Reid poll conducted at approximately the same time found that 42% of the Canadians surveyed had used CAM.[3]

In general, use of CAM is greatest among residents of British Columbia (BC), the most westerly Canadian province, where 84% of respondents reported use of CAM at least once in their lives. Use decreases by region as one moves east to the Atlantic provinces where only 69% of respondents reported using CAM at some time during their lives. Use during the past 12 months ranged from 60% in BC to 45% in the Atlantic provinces.[2] The most common forms of CAM used were similar to those identified in 1990 and include: chiropractic (36%); massage (23%); relaxation techniques (23%); prayer (21%); herbal therapies (17%); special diet programs (12%); folk remedies (12%) and acupuncture (12%).[2]

On average, Canadians reported using CAM products or therapies 4.4 times in the year prior to the survey, most often to prevent future illness occurring or to maintain health and vitality (81% in total). For the remainder, CAM was most commonly used during the past 12 months to treat back and neck problems (71%)*; gynecological problems (70%)*; anxiety attacks (69%)*; difficulty walking (67%)*; frequent headaches (65%)*; and digestive problems (63%)*. Canadians appear to believe that use of CAM together with conventional medicine is more beneficial than using either alone.[2] More than half (56%) of Canadians reporting CAM use did not disclose this use to their physicians.[2,4]

According to the Fraser Institute survey, the age group most likely to report use of CAM products or therapies was 18–24 year olds;[2] however, the Angus Reid group found that use was more common among 35–54 year olds.[3] Canadians with some postsecondary education were slightly more likely to report CAM use.[2] Income did not appear to be correlated with use in one survey;[2] however, in the other, Canadians with higher incomes were more likely to report CAM use.[3]

While both surveys generate interesting data, they should be considered with caution. The response rate in the Fraser Institute survey was only 26% so the results may be biased. The response rate for the Angus Reid poll was not reported. In addition, the surveys used very different definitions of CAM. The Fraser Institute survey questionnaire is based on that used by Eisenberg et al[5] and includes forms of CAM that are considered by many to be standard care, such as lifestyle diets. In the Angus Reid poll, CAM is assessed by asking about 'medicines and practices which include things like acupuncture, homeopathy, herbology, macrobiotics, chiropractic and other therapies which are not usually prescribed by conventional doctors'.[3]

CAM use in specific populations

Several studies of CAM use in specific Canadian populations with chronic diseases have been conducted. Some examples are included in Table 6.1.1. Age, education and income were significantly related to CAM use in breast cancer and HIV-infected patients.[4,6] Younger patients, those with higher education and higher income were more likely to use CAM. In brain tumor patients, age and income were also significantly related to CAM use, but education was not[7] and for inflammatory bowel disease (IBD) only patients' education was significant.[8] This appears to show considerable consistency with characteristics associated with CAM use in the general population. Disease- and treatment-related variables were of importance in all four studies. Among breast cancer patients, CAM users were more likely to have attended a support group and to have had chemotherapy as part of their conventional treatment protocol for breast cancer than non-users. Brain tumor patients who used CAM were more likely to be on sick or disability leave and to have received conventional treatments than non-users. Disease activity,

* Percentages are of those suffering from each condition

GENERAL TOPICS

Table 6.1.1 **Examples of studies of CAM use in specific populations**

Reference	Sample	% Use	Type of treatments (top 4)
Boon et al 2000[4]	422 Breast cancer	67% (ever) (62% products, 39% practitioners)	Products: vitamins/minerals (50%) herbs (25%) green tea (17%) special foods/diets (15%) Practitioners: chiropractors (29%) herbalists (7%) acupuncturists/TCM practitioners (7%) naturopathic practitioners (6%)
Verhoef et al 1999[7]	167 Brain tumor	24% (past year)	Herbs (65%) Mind–body (33%) Animal/vegetable derived (25%) Vitamins (20%)
Hilsden et al 1998[8]	134 Inflammatory bowel disease	33% (past year)	Vitamins (65%) Herbs (40%) Dietary treatments (16%) Physical therapies (30%)
Ostrow et al 1997[6]	657 HIV infected	39% (ever)	Dietary supplements (30%) Herbs/other medicinal therapies (22%) Tactile therapies (22%) Relaxation techniques (20%)

disease duration, previous surgery and hospitalization and a history of steroid use were significantly associated with CAM use among IBD patients and having greater physical pain was related to use among HIV-infected patients. The latter results seem to imply that patients who have more serious disease or have already tried conventional treatment(s) are more likely to use CAM. All studies suggest that most patients reporting CAM use do not reject conventional Western medicine, but see CAM therapies as an additive approach.

Participants in the brain tumor study were followed up 6–9 months after the first interview. While the percentage of patients using CAM had only slightly increased, there were major changes in the type and number of CAM therapies and practices patients used. Only 20% of users were using the same number and type of therapies at the time of the follow-up. In addition, some patients stopped using, while other patients started using CAM. Due to attrition, the numbers at follow-up were quite small. Therefore, these findings need to be tested in further research.

Almost half of breast cancer and brain tumor patients who reported use of CAM indicated that their physicians knew about this treatment choice (46% and 45% respectively). Sixty-two percent of IBD patients reported telling their doctors.

Common reasons for using CAM reported by patients included boosting the immune system, increasing quality of life, dealing with side effects of conventional medicine, preventing recurrences, gaining a feeling of control over disease management and doing something when no conventional options were left.[4,6-8] Patients also expressed beliefs in the uniqueness of the individual and holistic approaches to health and health care.[8,9] The most common barriers to CAM use have been identified as cost, lack of information, fear of harm from the product or therapy, lack of time to devote to CAM and lack of access to CAM. Fear of physicians' reactions to CAM use does not appear to be a significant deterrent.[4,10]

Perceptions of physicians regarding CAM

Several studies have investigated Canadian physicians' perceptions of CAM. Table 6.1.2 presents the results of studies of general practitioners in three provinces: Alberta, Ontario and Quebec.[11,12] These studies show that despite limited knowledge of CAM, substantial proportions of general practitioners considered CAM to be useful and were referring patients to CAM practitioners.

Guidelines for physician referrals to complementary practitioners are in different stages of development across Canadian provinces. A critical factor in determining whether or not a referral can be made within College guidelines is whether or not the CAM discipline is regulated at the statutory level. Currently,

Table 6.1.2 **General knowledge, opinions and behaviors of Canadian general practitioners concerning complementary therapies (%)[11,12]**

Variable	Province		
	Alberta	**Ontario**	**Quebec**
Knows a lot/a considerable amount about:			
Chiropractic	25	32	10
Acupuncture	20	31	11
Hypnosis	25	21	8
Perceives as useful to very useful:			
Chiropractic	79	77	78
Acupuncture	70	75	70
Hypnosis	65	65	50
Desires more education in CAM	43	63	48
Refers to CAM practitioners	44	65	77
Practices some form of CAM	14	17	13

GENERAL TOPICS

there is much variation in which disciplines are regulated across provinces (see p 369). With respect to practicing CAM, six of the 10 provinces (British Columbia, Alberta, Saskatchewan, Manitoba, Ontario and Quebec) have formal statements regarding physician practice of CAM. Of the six, five have issued general policy statements while one (Saskatchewan) appears to be developing practice guidelines for specific therapies. Newfoundland is in the process of developing policy guidelines and the remaining three have nothing in place (New Brunswick, Nova Scotia and Prince Edward Island).

Other Canadian studies have focused on physicians' perspectives on CAM therapies used by patients with cancer. These studies appear to show that physicians are unfamiliar with many CAM cancer therapies and often identify their own patients as a key source of information about these therapeutic options.[11] In these surveys, physicians identified the need for objective information that is easily accessible. Providing patients' conventional care was not compromised, most physicians indicated that they would be supportive of patients' decisions to use CAM.[13] However, in general there was little interest in initiating communication about CAM, with most seeing such discussions as poor use of their time. On the other hand, physician interest in CAM has been demonstrated by the initiation of CAM sections in a number of provincial medical associations (Ontario, Nova Scotia, British Columbia) and by the establishment of the Canadian Complementary Medical Association (CCMA) in 1996, a national organization of physicians who support the use of combined complementary and conventional approaches.

Investigation of Canadian medical students' attitudes towards CAM suggests that they believe that physicians need some knowledge about common CAM therapies. The majority of the medical students surveyed wanted additional education about CAM topics.[14,15] Perceived usefulness of CAM was found to be correlated with the students' level of knowledge about a specific CAM therapy.[14] Chiropractic, massage therapy and herbal medicine were the most well known and considered the most useful by fourth-year medical students at the University of Western Ontario.[14] Chiropractic, acupuncture and massage therapy were the best-known CAM therapies identified by first-year medical students at the University of Calgary.[15]

Inclusion of CAM in conventional training programs

A recent survey of Canadian medical schools found that 81% (13 schools) currently offer some form of CAM education and that the remaining three schools plan to incorporate CAM instruction into the curriculum in the future. Two-thirds (69%) of those schools currently teaching undergraduate medical students about CAM do so in a separate, required course. Many schools also reported elective or selective courses in CAM (46%) or independent study experiences (54%). Topics most commonly discussed include acupuncture (77%), homeopathy (69%), herbal medicine (62%), chiropractic (46%) and naturopathic medicine, traditional Chinese medicine or biofeedback (38%). The majority of schools do not currently provide instruction on the actual practice of CAM.[16]

Discussion of CAM is being integrated into the curricula of other health professional programs across Canada. In Ontario, other health-care professionals (i.e. pharmacy, nursing, occupational therapy and physiotherapy) appear to have more hours of instruction about CAM than medical students. In a comparative study, final-year pharmacy students reported more knowledge of herbal medicine and homeopathy than other final-year health professional students; final-year physiotherapy students reported more knowledge of acupuncture, chiropractic and massage therapies than all other faculties; and final-year nursing students reported the highest knowledge of therapeutic touch. More than two-thirds of all student groups surveyed, except medicine, expressed interest in receiving training to practice some form of CAM as part of their undergraduate training.[14]

Regulation of CAM in Canada

In Canada, CAM products are regulated by the federal government and all health-care practitioners, including CAM practitioners, are regulated by individual provinces. The result is that although the regulation of CAM products is standardized across Canada, regulation of CAM practitioners varies widely from province to province. Thus, a group of practitioners may be regulated in one province, but not in others. The current situation is summarized below.

CAM products

Regulation of CAM products (now called natural health products) is currently in transition in Canada. Thus it is necessary to describe the current regulatory system, the transition process and recommendations for the new regulatory system. At present, all products legally for sale in Canada are regulated as either foods or drugs as stipulated by the Food and Drugs Act. Some natural health products are currently considered to be foods (e.g. supplements such as glucosamine), others are classified as drugs (e.g. homeopathic products) and still others may be either foods or drugs depending on whether they meet specific criteria and whether they make health claims (e.g. herbal products). Some specific products have been identified by Health Canada as not acceptable for sale in Canada in any category.[17] Currently, the manufacturer of any product marketed as a food (which includes many herbal products and a variety of non-herbal supplements) may not print any medicinal claims on the label of the product. In addition, cautions, adverse effects and other warnings are not required on foods.

GENERAL TOPICS

In Canada, homeopathic products are currently classified as drugs and thus are given drug identification numbers or DINs[18] and must meet good manufacturing[19] and labeling standards.[20] However, they do not go through the same approval process with respect to providing evidence for safety and efficacy that is required of other pharmaceutical products.[18] At present, manufacturers of multi-ingredient, low-dilution (8CH or less) homeopathic preparations may make therapeutic claims on the label provided that the indication is suitable for self-diagnosis and self-treatment and corresponds to a self-limiting condition. All indications must be supported by a minimum of two traditional homeopathic references to be approved by Health Canada.[21]

Some herbal products are classified as drugs in a special category called Traditional Herbal Medicines. Traditional Herbal Medicines must be intended for self-medication use only, all the active ingredients must be herbal and the therapeutic indication must be supported by herbal reference texts at the dose provided.[22] Manufacturers of Traditional Herbal Medicines are allowed to make approved medicinal claims on product labels; however, the products must also indicate that they are for use by adults only (some exceptions exist), should not be used in pregnancy or lactation (unless use in these populations is supported by the herbal literature) and the term 'natural' may only be used to describe a product sold in its original state (i.e. without processing or refinement).[22] Labeling standards currently exist for chamomile, echinacea root, ephedra, feverfew leaf, peppermint and valerian. In addition, all Traditional Herbal Medicines must adhere to good manufacturing practices.[23] No products for sale in Canada as non-prescription products (i.e. sold directly to the public without consultation with a health-care provider) may suggest that they are treatments for conditions listed in Schedule A of the Food and Drugs Act which includes such conditions as arthritis, asthma and cancer.

Given the confusing and often inconsistent regulation of natural health products that currently exists in Canada, an Advisory Panel on Natural Health Products was established which provided a report to the Standing Committee on Health in 1998. In March 1999, the Federal Minister of Health accepted all 53 recommendations made by the Standing Committee on Health, including the creation of a new Federal Office of Natural Health Products. The mission of the new Office is to 'ensure that all Canadians have ready access to natural health products that are safe, effective and of high quality, while respecting freedom of choice and philosophical and cultural diversity' (p i).[24] The new Office of Natural Health Products is responsible for developing: a working definition of 'natural health product'; site licensing requirements for manufacturers; guidelines for importing natural health products into Canada for personal use; a natural health product licensing system that establishes criteria for safety, quality and therapeutic claims; product licensing monographs and good manufacturing requirements. Clearly, there is much work to be done before new regulations can be implemented and at this time it is not possible to predict when this new regulation system will be enacted.

CAM practitioners Regulation of CAM practitioners differs in each province; however, most CAM practitioners (e.g. herbalists, homeopathic practitioners, reflexologists, Reiki practitioners and many others) are not regulated by the state in any manner. This means that anyone, with any level of experience and training, may practice these modalities. This situation results in a 'buyer beware' atmosphere for consumers. Other practices, such as chiropractic, massage therapy, naturopathic medicine and acupuncture, are regulated to some extent in some provinces, but not in others. The provinces in which each of these practices is regulated will be identified and the regulations in one or two provinces will be reviewed to provide examples of the regulatory environment for CAM practitioners across the country.

Chiropractors Chiropractors are currently regulated in all Canadian provinces. Each province has its own Chiropractic Act; however, in all provinces, the minimum licensure requirements include:

- graduation from an accredited chiropractic college
- a minimum of 3 years pre-professional university/college studies
- passing scores on national examinations administered by the Canadian Chiropractic Examining Board
- passing scores in provincial licensing examinations.

Some provinces also require minimum age, period of residency within the province and evidence of good moral character. There are currently two chiropractic training facilities in Canada: the Canadian Memorial Chiropractic College in Toronto, Ontario, and the chiropractic program at the Université du Québec à Trois-Rivières (UQTR).

The actual legislation that governs chiropractic practice varies from province to province. Ontario and Saskatchewan will be used as examples to explore the regulations in more detail. In Ontario chiropractors are regulated under the Regulated Health Professions Act (1991) and the Chiropractic Act (1991) with a scope of practice defined as the diagnosis, treatment and prevention of disorders arising from the spine, other joints and related tissues. Chiropractors in Ontario are authorized to use the title 'Doctor'. Chiropractic is considered a primary health-care profession so patients may self-refer for chiropractic care. Chiropractic has been a self-regulated profession in the province of Saskatchewan since 1943 and is currently regulated under the Chiropractic Act (1994). In Saskatchewan, chiropractors have the right to diagnose, refer

GENERAL TOPICS

directly to medical specialists, use, refer and request hospital privileges for access to diagnostic X-ray services and treat patients in hospital on the request of the attending physician.

Reimbursement for chiropractic treatment also varies from province to province. Currently, chiropractic services are included, and partially government funded, in the provincial health-care plans of Ontario, Manitoba, Saskatchewan, Alberta and British Columbia. Patients must pay directly for chiropractic services in the other Canadian provinces.

Massage therapists

Massage therapists are only regulated in Ontario and British Columbia. The practice is not regulated in other regions of Canada and so the title 'massage therapist' is only protected in Ontario and British Columbia. The scope of practice of massage therapists in Ontario is defined under the Regulated Health Professions Act (1991) as: 'The assessment of the soft tissue and joints of the body and the treatment and prevention of physical dysfunction and pain of the soft tissues and joints by manipulation to develop, maintain, rehabilitate or augment physical function, or relieve pain'. Most massage therapists are self-employed although they work in a variety of different settings including massage therapy clinics, chiropractic offices, community health clinics, rehabilitation centers, health spas, health and fitness clubs, nursing homes and hospitals. The majority of patients self-refer to massage therapists but physicians and chiropractors may recommend a patient to seek massage therapy.

Massage therapy is not currently included in any provincial health insurance plan. However, it is covered by a variety of policies offered by private insurance companies including Sun Life, Blue Cross, and Liberty Health. In addition, the Workplace Safety and Insurance Board will pay for massage therapy for workers injured on the worksite. Some third-party payers require a written 'referral' from a physician in order for a patient to be reimbursed for the cost of massage therapy treatment.[25]

Naturopathic practitioners

Naturopathic practitioners are currently regulated in four* provinces (British Columbia, Saskatchewan, Manitoba and Ontario). Practitioners in regulated provinces must attend 4 years of full-time education at an approved training institution and then complete provincial and national licensing examinations. The national licensing examination (Naturopathic Physicians Licensing Examination or NPLEX) is used by all licensed jurisdictions in North America and is managed by the North American Board of Naturopathic Examinations (NABNE). Approved training institutions include the Canadian College of Naturopathic Medicine (in Toronto, Ontario), Bastyr University (in Seattle, Washington), National College of Naturopathic Medicine (in Portland, Oregon) and Southwest College of Naturopathic Medicine and Health Sciences (in Scottsdale, Arizona).

* Regulation in Alberta is currently pending

In Ontario, naturopathic practitioners have been regulated under the Drugless Practitioners Act since 1925. They are currently under review by the Health Professions Regulatory Advisory Council for possible inclusion under the Regulated Health Professions Act, the umbrella legislation under which all health-care professions in Ontario will eventually be regulated. Neither naturopathic medicine visits nor products are currently reimbursed by the Ontario Health Insurance Plan (OHIP). However, many private insurance companies offer plans to employers or individuals that include coverage of naturopathic consultations.

In British Columbia, the Naturopathic Physicians Act was passed in 1936, giving naturopathic practitioners their own unique Act in that province. This Act defines naturopathy as 'the art of healing by natural methods as taught in schools of naturopathy'. In British Columbia, naturopathic consultations are partially reimbursed by the provincial government under the Medical Services Plan (MSP).

Acupuncture

Regulation of traditional Chinese medicine and acupuncture also varies from province to province. Acupuncture is currently regulated in British Columbia, Alberta and Quebec. In Alberta, acupuncturists are one of 14 'designated health disciplines' and are regulated under the Health Disciplines Act. For the purposes of this Act, acupuncture is defined as 'the stimulation of an acupuncture point on or near the surface of the body by the insertion of needles to normalize physiological functions or the flow of Chi for the treatment of discomfort of the body and means the techniques of needle acupuncture, electro-acupuncture, acupressure and moxibustion'. The Act also stipulates that acupuncturists may not treat a patient unless the person has already consulted with a physician (or dentist for dental conditions). Acupuncturists in Alberta may not inform patients that acupuncture 'cures' any disease nor may they advise patients to discontinue any treatment prescribed by a physician or dentist. Finally, patients whose conditions do not improve after 6 months of acupuncture treatment must be referred to a physician (or dentist if appropriate).

The practice of acupuncture is currently regulated in British Columbia and in June 1999 the provincial government announced that new legislation will be introduced to regulate traditional Chinese medicine practitioners as well. This will include changing the name of the College of Acupuncturists of British Columbia to the College of Traditional Chinese Medicine and Acupuncture Practitioners of British Columbia. Legislation has not yet been passed to enact this decision. Similarly, in Ontario the Health Professions Regulatory Advisory Council is currently reviewing applications for the regulation of traditional Chinese medicine/acupuncture practitioners. Their final report to the Ontario Minister of Health was expected in December 2000.

Summary and discussion

Complementary and alternative medicine is used by a growing number of Canadians. Most individuals have not turned their backs on conventional Western medicine, but choose CAM to supplement conventional care. Health-care providers generally acknowledge that the high use of CAM among Canadians necessitates their learning something about the most common CAM therapeutic options their patients are using. As long as conventional care is not jeopardized, physicians are generally supportive of patients' decisions to use CAM. An example of physicians' interest is the newly established Canadian Complementary Medicine Association. However, despite the widespread use of CAM among Canadians, regulation of CAM products and therapies is somewhat haphazard. CAM products are regulated federally and the regulations are currently undergoing a major revision and restructuring by the newly created Office of Natural Health Products. CAM practitioners are largely unregulated. For those that are regulated, regulations are applied provincially and standards vary across the country. Many provinces are currently reassessing the regulatory status of CAM practitioners within their jurisdictions.

Finally, it should be noted that Canadian researchers, physicians, CAM practitioners and administrators established an Integrative Medicine and Health Network in 1999.[26] This has been instrumental in placing CAM on the agenda of the Canadian Institutes of Health Research (the new federal agency through which Canadian medical research is funded). In addition, Health Canada's Health Systems Division is mandated to examine the impact of CAM on the health system and the implications for health system renewal.[27] In general, these initiatives are occurring in an atmosphere of collaboration among stakeholders. Given the widespread use of CAM in Canada, increasing attempts to regulate products and practitioners and to integrate CAM with conventional care seem likely.

REFERENCES

1 Berger E. The Canada Health Monitor. Survey No. 4. Toronto: Price-Waterhouse, 1990

2 Ramsay C, Walker M, Alexander J. Alternative medicine in Canada: use and public attitudes. Public Policy Sources Number 21. Vancouver: The Fraser Institute, 1999

3 CTV/Angus Reid Group. Use of alternative medicines and practices. Winnipeg: Angus Reid Group, 1997

4 Boon H, Stewart M, Kennard M A et al. The use of complementary/alternative medicine by breast cancer survivors in Ontario: prevalence and perceptions. J Clin Oncol 2000; 18:2515–2521

5 Eisenberg D M, Kessler R C, Foster C, Norlock F E, Calkins D R, Delbanco T L. Unconventional medicine in the United States: prevalence, costs and patterns of use. New Engl J Med 1993;328:246–252

6 Ostrow M J, Cornelisse P G, Heath K V et al. Determinants of complementary therapy use in HIV-infected individuals receiving antiretroviral or anti-opportunistic agents. J Acq Immune Defic Syndr Human Retrovirol 1997;15:115–120

7 Verhoef M J, Hagen N, Pelletier G, Forsyth P. Alternative therapy use in neurologic disease. Use in brain tumour patients. Neurology 1999;52:617–622

8 Hilsden R J, Scott C M, Verhoef M J. Complementary medicine use by patients with inflammatory bowel disease. Am J Gastroenterol 1998;93:697–701

9 Pawluch D, Cain R, Gillett J. Ideology and alternative therapy use among people living with HIV/AIDS. Health Can Soc 1994;2:63–84

10 Boon H, Brown J B, Gavin A, Kennard M A, Stewart M. Breast cancer survivors' perceptions of complementary/alternative medicine (CAM): making the decision to use or not to use. Qual Health Care 1999; 9:639–653

11 Bourgeault I L. Physicians' attitudes toward patients' use of alternative cancer therapies. Can Med Assoc J 1996;155:1679–1685

12 Verhoef M J, Sutherland L R. Alternative medicine and general practitioners: opinions and behaviour. Can Fam Physician 1995; 41:1005–1011

13 Gray R E, Fitch M, Greenberg M et al. Physician perspectives on unconventional cancer therapies. J Palliat Care 1997;13:14–21

14 Baugniet J, Boon H, Ostbye T. Complementary/alternative medicine: comparing the view of medical students with students in other health care professions. Fam Med 2000;32:178–184

15 Duggan K, Verhoef M J, Hilsden R J. First-year medical students, and complementary and alternative medicine: attitudes, knowledge and experiences. Ann Roy Coll Physicians Surgeons Canada 1999;32:157–160

16 Ruedy J, Kaufman D M, MacLeod H. Alternative and complementary medicine in Canadian medical schools: a survey. Can Med Assoc J 1999;160:816–817

17 Drugs Directorate (Bureau of Nonprescription Drugs). Medicinal herbs in traditional herbal medicines. Ottawa: Drugs Directorate (Bureau of Nonprescription Drugs), 1995

18 Drugs Directorate. Drugs Directorate guidelines. Homeopathic preparations: application for drug identification numbers. Ottawa: Health Canada, 1990

19 Drugs Directorate. Good manufacturing practices. Supplementary guidelines for homeopathic preparations. Ottawa: Health Canada, 1996

20 Drugs Directorate. Labelling standard. Homeopathic preparations. Ottawa: Health Canada, 1995

21 Therapeutics Products Programme. Indications for use – multi-ingredient low dilution homeopathic preparations (revised). Ottawa: Health Canada, 1998

22 Drugs Directorate. Drugs Directorate guideline. Traditional herbal medicines (revised). Ottawa: Health Canada, 1995

23 Drugs Directorate. Good manufacturing guidelines for the manufacture of herbal medicinal products. Final version. Ottawa: Drugs Directorate, 1996

24 Transition Team of the Office of Natural Health Products. A fresh start: final report of the ONHP Transition Team. Ottawa: Office of Natural Health Products, 2000

25 Leach E. Personal communication. (Ontario Massage Therapists Association) July 2000

26 Best A, Balon J. Design for a Canadian Office for Complementary and Alternative Health Care. A White Paper for the Interim Governing Committee of the Canadian Institutes of Health Research. Integrative Medicine and Health Network (unpublished), 1999

27 Simpson J E. Attention to complementary and alternative practices and therapies. Ottawa: Health Canada, 1999

6.2

Complementary and Alternative Medicine Use in the United States: Epidemiology and Trends 1990–2000

David Eisenberg

Terminology

Alternative (aka complementary, unconventional, unorthodox, integrative) therapies encompass a broad spectrum of practices and beliefs.[1] From the standpoint of medical sociology, they may be defined '... as practices that are not accepted as correct, proper or appropriate or are not in conformity with the beliefs or standards of the dominant group of medical practitioners in a society'.[2] Two national surveys conducted in the United States have functionally defined alternative (aka complementary, integrative) therapies as 'interventions neither taught widely in U.S. medical schools nor generally available in U.S. hospitals'.[3,4] Ernst et al[5] contend that complementary medicine is diagnosis, treatment and/or prevention which complements mainstream medicine by contributing to a common whole, by satisfying a demand not met by orthodoxy or by diversifying the conceptual frameworks of medicine. Anecdotally, a patient with cancer who attributed her survival to a combination of conventional surgery, chemotherapy, radiation therapy and regular use of complementary and alternative medical interventions offered the following definition: 'Complementary and alternative therapies are those therapies which, for the past 20 years, I have had to pay for out-of-pocket and never felt comfortable discussing with my physicians'.

It is useful to be reminded that the term 'alternative' medicine was not in common use until the United States Senate Committee on Appropriations, under the Chairmanship of Senator Tom Harkin, established the Office of Alternative Medicine in 1992. Since that time, US federal documents and requests for applications involving the National Institutes of Health have included the term 'alternative' medicine and, as of the mid-1990s, 'complementary and alternative medicine' (CAM) has been the phraseology used in all US federal publications. While the term 'integrative medicine' is gaining popularity in the USA and is being used with increased frequency by investigators across a range of medical institutions and universities, the term 'CAM' is currently used by US governmental agencies to describe this field of inquiry. For the purpose of this chapter, CAM will be used throughout.

A 10-year retrospective of CAM trends in the United States: a brief journey in time

It is an interesting exercise to reflect on milestones involving CAM use, public awareness, professional interest, resource development and policy in the United States between 1990 and 2000.

It can be argued that a watershed moment was the creation of the Office of Alternative Medicine in the 1992–93 federal legislative session. As mentioned earlier, Senator Thomas Harkin chaired the Subcommittee on Appropriations and, with consensus from his democratic and republican peers, wrote legislation and held hearings that led to the creation of the Office of Alternative Medicine within the Office of the Director of the National Institutes of Health. The budget of this new office in 1992 was $2 million.

In January 1993, the *New England Journal of Medicine* published the first US national survey of CAM therapy prevalence, costs and patterns of use (see detailed discussion below).[4] Data from this survey confirmed the enormous extent to which CAM therapies and services were, for better or worse, part of the intrinsic fabric of US health care. Controversies emanating from this initial survey increased the resolve of proponents and antagonists alike to become increasingly involved in and committed to research and the formation of responsible health policy.

By 1995, the NIH Office of Alternative Medicine had funded an initial 10 centers whose mandate was principally to identify research opportunities and help shape a national research agenda. By the mid 1990s, the Office of Alternative Medicine budget had risen from $2 million per year to $20 million per year.

In 1998, the NIH established the National Center for Complementary and Alternative Medicine, thereby replacing the Office of Alternative Medicine with a center which had the authority to both prioritize and fund projects and programs deemed important by its governmentally chartered advisory council. Before this date, all funding of CAM projects had to be done in partnership with existing NIH centers and institutes. The budget for the new National Center for Complementary and Alternative Medicine was $50 million per year.

1998 was also a watershed year for editorial comment regarding the field of CAM as a whole. In a now classic editorial by Drs Angell and Kassirer, then editors of the *New England Journal of Medicine*, the statement was made, 'It's time to stop giving alternative medicine a free ride'.[6] Angell and Kassirer went on to say: 'There cannot be two kinds of medicine – conventional and alternative. There is only medicine that has been adequately tested and medicine that has not, medicine that works and medicine that may or may not work'.[6]

In November 1998, the *Journal of the American Medical Association* and all nine AMA speciality journals published that month were devoted to the topic of CAM. These publications included a total of 80 peer-reviewed manuscripts including

18 RCTs.[7] In the editorial of the November 11th issue of the *JAMA*, then Editor-in-Chief George Lundberg MD stated, 'There is no alternative medicine'.[8] In contrast to the *New England Journal of Medicine*, *JAMA* editors argued that the scientific evaluation of CAM practices was the medical community's shared responsibility. An editorial by Frank Davidoff MD of the *Annals of Internal Medicine* concluded:

'Changing our practices in recognition of those gaps may be painful, but, if done carefully, there is no reason to believe that such changes would compromise scientific care. The real issue for conventional medicine here is not how to manage our patients' involvement in alternative care; it is rather, in T.S. Eliot's phrase, how to learn from alternative practices in an effort to regain the knowledge we have lost in information'.[9]

By 1999, the National Center for Complementary and Alternative Medicine had funded a range of new centers and phase III clinical trials and its budget had increased to $68.5 million per year. During this same year, large pharmaceutical corporations in the United States (and globally) began to advertise herbal medical products and nutraceuticals. Examples included items produced by American Home Products, Whitehall Robbins, Warner Lambert, Bayer Pharmaceuticals, Johnson & Johnson and Bristol-Myers Squibb.

In March 2000, President Clinton signed an executive order to establish a White House Commission on Complementary and Alternative Medicine Policy.[10] The role of the Presidential Commission is to address issues of:

- training and education
- coordination of research
- provision of useful information
- guidance for appropriate access and delivery of CAM services.

In 2000, the Federation of State Medical Boards created a committee to evaluate policy pertaining to the regulation of licensed physicians who provide CAM services and/or co-manage patients with CAM providers. The Josiah Macy Foundation, historically known for its pursuit of medical education reform, focused its annual conference on the topic of CAM education and the American Association of Medical Colleges has established a special interest group in CAM education. The National Center for Complementary and Alternative Medicine currently supports more than 200 studies involving CAM therapies. (Additional information on the NCCAM can be found at http://www.aamc.org/ and http://www.fsmb.org/)

Lastly, the number of private corporations, including Internet companies, seeking to develop content and services involving CAM practices continues to grow at a remarkable pace. Taken as a whole, this rapid evolution between 1990 and 2000 suggests that CAM prevalence, costs and patterns of use will remain areas of intense interest and debate well into this next century.

The epidemiology of CAM in the United States

Results from nationally representative surveys

Eisenberg et al published the first national survey of CAM prevalence, costs and patterns of use, summarizing data representative of 1990.[4] This initial survey consisted of telephone interviews with 1539 adults (response rate 67%). In a national sample of adults 18 years of age or older, respondents were asked to report any serious or bothersome medical conditions and details of their use of conventional medical services. Interviewers then inquired about their use of 16 complementary/alternative medical therapies. Principal findings from this initial survey included the observation that one in three respondents (34%) reported using at least one unconventional therapy during the past year; a third of CAM users saw one or more professional providers for CAM treatments. CAM therapy use was highest amongst non-black persons age 25–49 who had relatively more education and higher incomes. The majority used CAM therapies for chronic as opposed to life-threatening conditions.

Extrapolations to the US population suggested that in 1990 Americans made an estimated 425 million visits to providers of CAM therapy. This number exceeded the number of visits to all US primary care physicians (388 million). Expenditures associated with use of CAM therapies in 1990 amounted to approximately $13.7 billion, three quarters of which ($10.3 billion) were paid out of pocket. This figure was comparable to the amount spent out of pocket annually for all hospitalizations in the United States. The authors concluded that the frequency of use of CAM therapies in the United States was far higher than previously reported. They suggested that medical doctors ask their patients about their use of CAM therapies whenever obtaining a medical history.[4]

In the absence of a follow-up national survey, it was temporarily unclear as to whether the observations made in 1990 were representative of a 'hidden mainstream' which had, unbeknownst to the medical establishment, plateaued or, alternatively, represented the first point on a curve suggestive of increased prevalence and expenditures involving CAM services. For this reason, a follow-up national survey was conducted by Eisenberg et al in 1997, funded by the US National Institutes of Health with co-funding from the John E Fetzer Institute and the American Society of Actuaries.

In 1998, Eisenberg et al reported the results of this follow-up national survey of CAM prevalence, costs and patterns of use, having incorporated all of the initial 16 CAM therapies surveyed

GENERAL TOPICS

in their earlier study of 1990.[3] Results from the follow-up national survey are summarized below.

The design of the follow-up national survey was similar to that of the initial national survey, reflective of the utilization rates in 1990. Specifically, the 1997 survey included a telephone survey of nationally representative random households as well as a questionnaire comparable to that used in the 1990 survey. A total of 2055 adults (response rate 60%) completed the survey in 1997.

As shown in Figure 6.2.1, the use of at least one of 16 CAM therapies increased from 34% in 1990 to 42% in 1997. Therapies which increased the most included herbal medicines, massage, high-dose vitamins, self-help groups, folk remedies, energy healing and homeopathy. The probability that CAM users also sought professional services of CAM providers increased from 36% in 1990 to 46% in 1997. In both surveys, alternative therapies were used most frequently for chronic conditions including back problems, anxiety, depression and headaches.

Figure 6.2.1
Adult US population using alternative therapy in the past 12 months (from reference [3]).

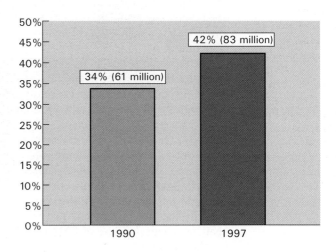

As shown in Figure 6.2.2, there was no significant change in disclosure rates between the two survey years; 40% of CAM therapies were disclosed to physicians in 1990 as compared with 39% in 1997.

As shown in Figure 6.2.3, extrapolations to the US population suggested that there had been a 47% increase in the total visits to CAM providers from 427 million in 1990 to 629 million in 1997, thereby exceeding total visits to all US primary care physicians by more than 200 million visits per year.

As shown in Figure 6.2.4, more than half of the 629 million annual visits were attributed to professional services rendered by chiropractors and massage therapists. Interestingly, neither of

Figure 6.2.2
**Disclosure rates to
medical doctors
(from reference³).**

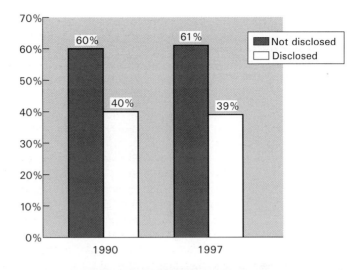

Figure 6.2.3
**Trends in annual
visits to
practitioners of
alternative
therapies versus
visits to primary
care physicians,
1997 versus 1990.
Data from the
National
Ambulatory
Medical Care
Survey from
1996⁴⁶ and 1990.⁴⁷**

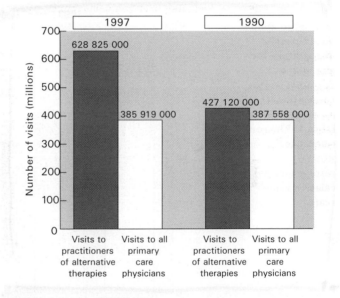

these modalities is routinely discussed in US schools of medicine, nursing or pharmacy.

The survey also estimated that in 1997 15 million adults took prescription medications concurrently with herbal remedies and/or high-dose vitamins. This represented 18% of all prescription drug users. This observation anticipated the more recent descriptions of clinically significant adverse drug–herb interaction.[11-14]

Estimated expenditures for CAM professional services increased by 45% between 1990 and 1997 and were conservatively estimated at $21 billion with at least $12 billion paid out of pocket. This amount (as shown in Figure 6.2.5) exceeded the 1997 out-of-pocket expenditures for all US hospitalizations.

GENERAL TOPICS

Figure 6.2.4
Alternative practitioner visits, 1997 (from reference [3]).

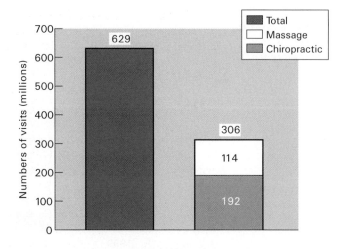

Figure 6.2.5
Estimated annual out-of-pocket expenditure for alternative therapies versus conventional medical services, USA, 1997 (from reference [48]). RBRVS, resource-based relative value scale.

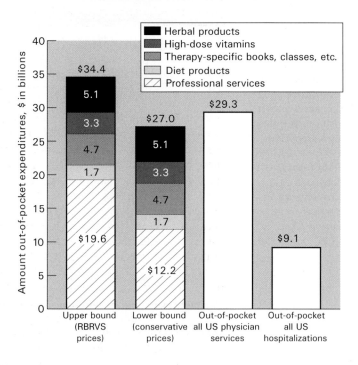

Furthermore, total 1997 out-of-pocket expenditures relating to CAM therapies were conservatively estimated at $27 billion (and less conservatively at $34 billion), which is comparable to the out-of-pocket expenditures for all US physician services. Eisenberg et al concluded that CAM therapy use and expenditures had increased substantially between 1990 and 1997 and attributed this primarily to an increase in the number of adults seeking CAM therapies rather than increased visits per user.

In a study by Paramore,[15] data were analyzed from a general probability sample of 3450. The results indicated that approximately 10% of the US population (an estimated 25 million persons) saw a professional in 1994 for at least one of four therapies: chiropractic, relaxation techniques, therapeutic massage or acupuncture. The study also observed that users of CAM therapies made almost twice as many visits to conventional medical providers as were made by non-users. In addition, the majority of persons seeking professional care from CAM providers also saw medical doctors during the reference year. These findings are consistent with those of the two surveys by Eisenberg et al mentioned earlier.

Astin reported results from a survey of 1035 individuals randomly selected from a convenience panel of individuals who had agreed to participate in mail surveys and who lived throughout the United States.[16] This survey investigated possible predictors of alternative (CAM) health-care use which included: more education; poor health status; a holistic orientation to health; having had a transformational experience that changed the person's world view; any of the following health problems: anxiety; back problems; chronic pain; urinary tract problems; and classification in a cultural group identifiable by their commitment to environmentalism, commitment to feminism and interest in spirituality and personal growth psychology. Astin reported that dissatisfaction with conventional care was not a predictor of alternative (CAM) use. In addition, only 4.4% of those surveyed reported relying primarily on alternative (CAM) therapies. Astin concluded that: 'The majority of alternative medicine users appear to be doing so not so much as a result of being dissatisfied with conventional medicine, but largely because they find these health care alternatives to be more congruent with their own values, beliefs and philosophical orientation towards health and life'.[16]

An article by Druss & Rosenbeck[17] investigated the association between use of unconventional (CAM) therapies and conventional care in a national sample taken from the 1996 medical expenditure panel survey (n=16068 adults). The authors reported that in 1996, an estimated 6.5% of the US population visited both CAM providers and conventional medical providers. Fewer than 2% used only CAM services, 60% used only conventional care and 32% used neither. Comparison of those respondents who used only conventional medical care with those who used both types of care revealed that the latter had significantly more outpatient physician visits during the reference year and used more of all types of preventive medical services except mammography. Individuals in the top quartile of number of physician visits were more than twice as likely as those in the bottom quartile to have used unconventional (CAM) therapies during the previous year. The authors concluded that, from a health services perspective, practitioner-based unconventional (CAM) therapies appear to serve more as a complement than an alternative to conventional medicine.[17]

CAM use among adults aged 65 and older

By utilizing data from the same nationally representative random telephone survey, Foster et al measured the prevalence, costs and patterns of CAM therapy use by people aged 65 or older.[18] This sample included 311 respondents aged 65 and older, all of whom were participants in the larger national survey (n=2055) by Eisenberg et al.[3]

The results of this analysis included the observation that 30% of adults aged 65 and older used at least one CAM therapy during the previous 12 months. This was compared with 46% of CAM users under the age of 65 (p < 0.001). Nineteen percent of older adults saw a provider of CAM therapies during the previous 12 months (compared with 26% of those under age 65). Interestingly, the most commonly used CAM modalities among adults aged 65 and older were:

- chiropractic (11%)
- herbal remedies (8%)
- relaxation techniques (5%)
- high-dose or megavitamins (5%).

Older adults who saw their physician(s) more frequently were also more likely to use CAM therapies. Importantly, 6% reported taking both herbs and prescription drugs simultaneously. Among older adults who used CAM services, 57% made no mention of their use of any CAM modality to their physician.

Foster et al concluded that among those aged 65 and older, 30% reported using CAM therapies during the previous year (amounting to an estimated 10 million adults) and 19% visited a CAM provider.[18] Extrapolating to the US adult population, this would suggest an estimated 63 million office visits to CAM providers by persons over the age of 65. The two most commonly used CAM therapies were chiropractic and herbal remedies, both of which may be problematic in older patients. As such, the authors suggested that physicians ask all patients including those over the age of 65 about their use of individual CAM interventions. When caring for individuals aged 65 and older, physicians should ask specific questions about their use of chiropractic and herbal remedies.

The relationship between income and alternative medicine use

Utilizing the same national database as Eisenberg et al, Foster et al examined the effect of income on CAM use.[19] Questions included out-of-pocket expenses for CAM therapies. For analytic purposes, income was grouped approximately into quartiles (income less than $20 000; $20 000–$29 999; $30 000–$49 999; greater than or equal to $50 000). Foster et al found that those in the lower income groups were more likely to be female, non-white and have fewer years of education (p < 0.05) for each. In addition, lower income was also associated with worse reported health status, more medical conditions and less health insurance coverage. CAM therapy use varied by income quartile (lowest 43%, 37%, 44%, highest 48%; p < 0.05). The average annual out-of-pocket expenditures by CAM users increased with income quartile ($265, $440, $321, $505; p < 0.05). The authors concluded that higher income is associated with increased use of CAM therapies overall. After adjusting for other demographic variables and medical conditions, these differences become more dramatic.[19]

In summary, while income appears to be a barrier to CAM use, still, among the lowest income groups (less than $20 000 per year), an estimated 43% of respondents used CAM therapies and spent an average of $250 annually.

Relationship between choice of insurance plans and access to CAM benefits

Wolsko et al, utilizing the same national database, analyzed the data around the following issue: if presented with a choice of two insurance plans that were otherwise equivalent, would respondents choose the insurance plan offering CAM benefits or not?[20] Among eligible respondents, 69% reported that they would be more likely to sign up with that insurance plan, 25% were indifferent and 6.5% said that they would be less likely to sign up with that insurance plan. Wolsko et al concluded that insurance benefits for CAM services were desired by the majority of respondents who had used any type of CAM service during the past year. Extrapolation of these results to the US population suggests that there are, conservatively, 75 million US adults for whom the presence or absence of CAM insurance benefits may affect the selection of their insurer.[20]

CAM use among adults with anxiety or depression

Kessler et al, who used the same national data set as Eisenberg et al in their 1998 follow-up survey, explored the use of CAM therapies to treat anxiety and depression in a nationally representative sample of US adults.[21] Of the 2055 respondents in the 1997–98 telephone survey, 10.5% of respondents reported suffering from 'anxiety attacks' during the previous 12 months and 8.8% reported suffering from 'severe depression'; 57% of those with anxiety and 54% of those with depression reported using CAM therapies to treat these conditions during the previous year. These rates of CAM utilization were higher than those for all other conditions assessed other than treatment of back or neck problems. A wide variety of CAM therapies were used to treat anxiety and depression but most CAM therapy use was unsupervised, with only 20% of those with anxiety and 19% of those with depression seeing a CAM professional. The perceived helpfulness of CAM therapy in treating anxiety and depression was similar to the perceived helpfulness of conventional medical intervention. The authors concluded that CAM is used much

GENERAL TOPICS

more commonly than conventional therapies by people with self-defined anxiety attacks and severe depression. In light of recent reports of herb–drug interactions (including those attributed to interactions involving St John's wort, a botanical commonly used to treat depression), the authors encouraged opening up lines of communication between mental health professionals and their patients.[21]

The above-mentioned surveys are all based on nationally representative random samples of adult Americans. In addition, there have been a number of convenience samples investigating CAM therapy use among individuals with a particular condition or disease. Examples include surveys involving CAM therapy use among individuals with cancer,[22-31] rheumatologic disorders,[32-34] self-reported disability,[35] HIV,[36] inflammatory bowel disease[37] and rhinosinusitis,[38] as well as surgical patients[39] and patients in an emergency department.[40] These examples are not meant to be exhaustive but rather representative of convenience surveys performed on particular US patient populations over the past decade. Without exception, these surveys confirm the high prevalence of CAM therapy use among individuals with chronic and/or life-threatening illness.

Survey of courses involving CAM therapies at US medical schools

Wetzel et al described the prevalence, scope and diversity of medical school education in CAM therapy topics based on a mailed survey and follow-up letter to curriculum deans and faculty at each of the 125 US medical schools.[41]

Replies from the survey were received from 117 (94%) of the 125 US medical schools. Of those schools that replied, 75 (64%) reported the offering of elective courses in CAM topics and/or the inclusion of these topics in required courses. The majority of these courses were stand-alone electives. Educational formats included lectures, practitioner lecture and/or demonstration and patient presentations. Common topics included in these courses were chiropractic, herbal therapies, mind–body techniques, acupuncture and homeopathy. Wetzel et al concluded that there is tremendous heterogeneity and diversity in content, format and requirements among existing courses in CAM therapy topics at US medical schools.

Epidemiology of malpractice insurance claims for conventional and CAM practitioners

Studdert et al used data from malpractice insurers to analyze claims against chiropractors, massage therapists and acupuncturists for the period 1990–96.[42] They found that claims against these CAM practitioners occurred less frequently and typically involved injury that was less severe than claims against physicians (MDs, DOs) during the same period. They also reviewed relevant legal principles and case law to understand how malpractice law is likely to develop in this area.[42] Two textbooks by Michael Cohen[43,44] highlight a variety of CAM-related legal concerns from the vantage point of US legal statutes. Clearly, issues pertaining to malpractice liability relating to CAM will become increasingly important in the US and internationally during the coming decades.

Conclusion

The field of CAM has evolved with extraordinary rapidity in the United States during the decade 1990–2000. As summarized in this chapter, the epidemiology of CAM in the United States is now sufficiently robust to confidently predict that complementary and integrative medical therapies are and will be inextricable components of the US health-care delivery system well into the next century.

Epidemiologic research typically leads to a prioritization of research opportunities and a critical review of existing evidence. This is the position we now find ourselves in. The next phase in the evolution of CAM will likely involve large-scale, authoritative evaluation of individual CAM therapies as well as an assessment of models of integrative medical care for the prevention, treatment and management of disease. In addition, we can anticipate the application of additional resources to investigate plausible explanatory models for a range of CAM therapies.

Some elements of CAM may be found to be relatively safe, effective and capable of reducing overall health-care expenditures while others will not. Those approaches with attractive risk–benefit ratios will be incorporated into mainstream medical care and others will be avoided and/or proscribed. In addition, it is likely that individual therapies found to be useless and/or dangerous will be replaced by a new generation of 'complementary and alternative' medical interventions. As such, medical diversity will continue for generations to come. Given this prediction, it is useful to be reminded of an approach articulated by David Grimes: 'Doing everything for everyone is neither tenable nor desirable. What is done should, ideally, be inspired by compassion and guided by science and not merely reflect what the market will bear'.[45]

Note

Figures 6.2.3 and 6.2.5 reproduced with permission from the *JAMA*.

REFERENCES

1 Murray R H, Rubel A J. Physicians and healers – unwitting partners in health care. N Engl J Med 1992;326:61–64

2 Gevitz N. Three perspectives on unorthodox medicine. In: Gevitz N (ed) Other healers: unorthodox medicine in America. Baltimore: Johns Hopkins University Press, 1988, pp 1–28

3 Eisenberg D M, Davis R B, Ettner S L, Appel S, Wilkey S, Van Rompay M, Kessler R C. Trends in alternative medicine use in the United States, 1990–1997: results of a follow-up national survey. JAMA 1998;280:1569–1575

4 Eisenberg D M, Kessler R C, Foster C, Norlock F E, Calkins D R, Delbanco T L. Unconventional medicine in the United States: prevalence, costs, and patterns of use. N Engl J Med 1993;328:246–252

5 Ernst E, Resch K L, Mills S et al. Complementary medicine – a definition. Br J Gen Pract 1995;45:506

6 Angell M, Kassirer J P. Alternative medicine – the risks of untested and unregulated remedies (editorial). New Engl J Med 1998;339: 839–841

7 Fontanarosa P B (ed). Alternative medicine: an objective assessment. USA: American Medical Association, 2000

8 Fontanarosa P B, Lundberg G D. Alternative medicine meets science (editorial). JAMA 1998;280:1618–1619

9 Davidoff F. Weighing the alternatives: lessons from the paradoxes of alternative medicine. Ann Intern Med 1998;129:1068–1070

10 http://www.whccamp.hhs.gov

11 Fugh-Berman A. Herb–drug interactions. Lancet 2000;355:134–138

12 Ernst E. Second thoughts about safety of St. John's wort. Lancet 1999;354:2014–2016

13 Piscitelli S C, Burstein A H, Chaitt D, Alfaro R M, Falloon J. Indinavir concentrations and St. John's wort Lancet 2000;355:547–548

14 Nortier J L, Muniz Martinez M C, Schmeiser H H et al. Urothelial carcinoma associated with the use of a Chinese herb (*Aristolochia fangchi*). New Engl J Med 2000; 342:1686–1692

15 Paramore L C. Use of alternative therapies: estimates from the 1994 Robert Wood Johnson Foundation National Access to Care Survey. J Pain Symptom Manage 1997;13:83–89

16 Astin J A. Why patients use alternative medicine: results of a national study. JAMA 1998;279:1548–1553

17 Druss B G, Rosenheck R A. Association between use of unconventional therapies and conventional medical services. JAMA 1999; 282:651–656

18 Foster D F, Phillips R S, Hamel M B, Eisenberg D M. Alternative medicine use in older Americans. J Am Geriatr Soc 2000; 48:1560–1565

19 Foster D, Phillips R S, Davies R B, Eisenberg D. Income and alternative medicine use. J Gen Intern Med 2000; 15(suppl 1):67

20 Wolsko P M, Phillips R S, Davis R B, Eisenberg D. Choice of insurance plans offering alternative medicine benefits. J Gen Intern Med 2000;15(suppl 1):155

21 Kessler R C, Soukup J, Davis R B et al. The use of complementary and alternative therapies to treat anxiety and depression in the United States. Am J Psychiatr [in press]

22 Adler S R, Fosket J R. Disclosing complementary and alternative medicine use in the medical encounter: a qualitative study in women with breast cancer. J Fam Pract 1999;48:453–458

23 Burstein H J, Gelber S, Guadagnoli E et al. Use of alternative medicine by women with early-stage breast cancer. New Engl J Med 1999; 340:1733–1739

24 Cassileth B R, Lusk E J, Strouse T B et al. Contemporary unorthodox treatments in cancer medicine: a study of patients, treatments, and practitioners. Ann Intern Med 1984;101:105–112

25 Goldstein J, Chao C, Valentine E et al. Use of unproved cancer treatment by patients in a radiation oncology department: a survey. J Psychosoc Oncol 1991;9:59–66

26 Lee M M, Lin S S, Wrensch M R et al. Alternative therapies used by women with breast cancer in four ethnic populations. J Nat Cancer Inst 2000;92:42–47

27 Lerner I J, Kennedy B J. The prevalence of questionable methods of cancer treatment in the United States. CA Cancer J Clinic 1992; 42:181–191

28 Mooney K. Unproven cancer treatment usage in cancer patients who have received conventional therapy. Oncol Nurs Forum 1987;2(suppl):112

29 Newell S M. An investigation into the utility of the modified health belief model in predicting treatment compliance for advanced adult cancer patients in hospital outpatient clinics. Dissertation Abstracts Int 1985; 45:3201B

30 Richardson M A, Sanders T, Palmer J L, Greisinger A, Singletary S E. Complementary/alternative medicine use in a comprehensive cancer center and the implications for oncology. J Clin Oncol 2000; 18:2505–2514

31 VandeCreek L, Rogers E, Lester J. Use of alternative therapies among breast cancer outpatients compared with the general population. Alt Ther Health Med 1999;5:71–76

32 Rao J K, Mihaliak K, Kroenke K, Bradley J, Tierney W M, Weinberger M. Use of complementary therapies for arthritis among patients of rheumatologists. Ann Intern Med 1999;131:409–416

33 Nicassio P M, Schuman C, Kim J, Cordova A, Weisman M H. Psychosocial factors associated with complementary treatment use in fibromyalgia. J Rheumatol 1997;24:2008–2013

34 Cronan T A, Kaplan R M, Posner L, Blumberg E, Kozin F. Prevalence of use of unconventional remedies for arthritis in a metropolitan community. Arthritis Rheum 1989;32:1604–1607

35 Krauss H H, Godfrey C, Kirk J, Eisenberg D M. Alternative health care: its use by individuals with physical disabilities. Arch Phys Med Rehab 1998;79:1440–1447

36 Fairfield K M, Eisenberg D M, Davis R B, Libman H, Phillips R S. Patterns of use, expenditures, and perceived efficacy of complementary and alternative therapies in HIV-infected patients. Arch Intern Med 1998; 158:2257–2264

37 Rawsthorne P, Shanahan F, Cronin N C, Anton P A, Lofberg R, Bohman L, Bernstein C N. An international survey of the use and attitudes regarding alternative medicine by patients with inflammatory bowel disease. Am J Gastroenterol 1999;94:1298–1303

38 Krouse J H, Krouse H J. Patient use of traditional and complementary therapies in treating rhinosinusitis before consulting an otolaryngologist. Laryngoscope 1999; 109:1223–1227

39 Norred C L, Zamudio S, Palmer S K. Use of complementary and alternative medicines by surgical patients. AANA J 2000;68:13–18

40 Gulla J, Singer A J. Use of alternative therapies among emergency department patients. Ann Emerg Med 2000;35:226–228

41 Wetzel M S, Eisenberg D M, Kaptchuk T J. Courses involving complementary and alternative medicine at US medical schools. JAMA 1998;280:784–787

42 Studdert D M, Eisenberg D M, Miller F H, Curto D A, Kaptchuk T J, Brennan T A. Medical malpractice implications of alternative medicine. JAMA 1998; 280:1610–1615

43 Cohen M H. Complementary and alternative medicine: legal boundaries and regulatory perspectives. Baltimore: Johns Hopkins University Press, 1998

44 Cohen M H. Beyond complementary medicine: legal and ethical perspectives on health care and human evolution. Ann Arbor: University of Michigan Press, 2000

45 Grimes D A. Technology follies. The uncritical acceptance of medical innovation. JAMA 1993; 269:3030–3033

46 Woodwell D A. National Ambulatory Medical Care Survey: 1996 Summary. Advance data from vital and health statistics; no. 295. Hyattsville, MD: National Center for Health Statistics, 1997.

47 Schappert S M. National Ambulatory Medical Care Survey: 1990 Summary. Advance data from vital and health statistics; no. 213. Hyattsville, MD: National Center for Health Statistics, 1991

48 Health Care Financing Administration, Office of the Actuary, National Health Statistics Group. National health care expenditure projections tables. Available at: http://www.hcfa.gov/stats/NHE-Proj/tables/.

Complementary and Alternative Medicine: A European Perspective

Max H Pittler

The understanding of what precisely constitutes complementary and alternative medicine (CAM) differs considerably in Europe from that of other countries, such as the US. Different historical developments and traditions have meant that therapies such as herbal medicine, hydrotherapy and massage are firmly established in mainstream medicine in many European countries, while they are often classified as CAM outside Europe. In addition, some treatments such as the 'cure' (German *Kur*), which includes aspects of hydrotherapy and is considered a mainstream medical approach, are specific to some European countries. Despite these national differences and their implications for research, there is evidence, as in other parts of the world, for a substantial increase in the use and demand for CAM. To define requirements for the scientific investigation of CAM, education and regulation, information on the level of use among the general population and specific patient populations is of considerable importance. Although inconsistencies abound in many surveys it is possible to derive estimates and outline the development of CAM in Europe over time.

Usage

General adult population

Systematic reviews of survey data have suggested a frequent and increasing use of CAM among the general population.[1,2] A systematic review of surveys assessing random or representative population samples[1] identified one study which investigated the use of CAM in England.[3,4] In 1993 it was estimated that 8.5% of the adult population had visited at least one CAM provider of acupuncture, chiropractic, homeopathy, hypnotherapy, herbal medicine or osteopathy during the past 12 months. This figure was 10.6% in 1998 using similar methodology,[5] suggesting a slower rate of growth than that reported by Eisenberg and colleagues in the US over a similar time period.[6] This study suggested that inclusion of data for reflexology, aromatherapy and remedies purchased over the counter in the analysis increased the estimated one-year prevalence to 28.3%. In this sample, the frequency of use was greatest for osteopathy (4.3%) and chiropractic (3.6%). Other popular therapies included aromatherapy

(3.5%), reflexology (2.4%), acupuncture (1.6%) and herbal medicine (0.9%).[5]

Another survey of the UK general public, conducted in 1999, largely corroborated the above findings and estimated that 20% had used some form of CAM provided by practitioners or as remedies bought over the counter in the previous 12 months.[7] In Scotland, a random population survey suggested that the use of CAM had markedly increased in 1999 compared with 1993.[8] The use of acupuncture, for instance, increased from 6% in 1993 to 10% in 1999, while increases of 4% to 6% and 7% to 10% are suggested for herbal medicine and homeopathy respectively. Data from 192 individuals from Scotland who indicated that they would use CAM in the future suggested that osteopathy (45%), acupuncture (44%), aromatherapy (40%), chiropractic (33%), homeopathy (32%) and herbal medicine (25%) would be considered, confirming the popular demand for such therapies.[9]

Two surveys that assessed representative population samples from continental Europe were identified by a systematic review.[1] A study from Germany reported an overall prevalence rate of 65% in 1996, which compared to a corresponding figure of 52% in 1970.[10] While these figures are among the highest reported anywhere, the report lacks crucial details, preventing a critical appraisal of the data. Table 6.3.1 shows common conditions frequently treated with herbal medicinal products in Germany in 1997. Data from Austria suggested that acupressure was the most popular form of CAM in 1988.[11] The lifetime prevalence in this sample was relatively low and is reported for homeopathy (12.1%), reflexology (11.3%), acupuncture (9.6%) and chiropractic (9.5%). One reason for the relatively low figures reported may be the Austrian law, which prevents non-medically qualified CAM therapists practicing.

Few attempts have been made to estimate the consultation rate among European general populations. The most rigorous

Table 6.3.1
Conditions and frequencies of treatment with herbal medicinal products in Germany
(Institute for Demoscopy, Allensbach, Germany)

Condition	1997 (%)	1970 (%)
Common cold	66	41
Flu	38	31
Digestive or intestinal complaints	25	24
Headache	25	13
Insomnia	25	13
Stomach ulcer	24	21
Nervousness	21	12
Circulatory disorders	17	15
Bronchitis	15	12
Skin diseases	12	8
Fatigue and exhaustion	12	8

GENERAL TOPICS

study has been conducted in the UK. Its results suggested that about 4.2 million adults made 18 million visits to practitioners of one of six therapies (acupuncture, chiropractic, homeopathy, hypnotherapy, herbal medicine or osteopathy) in 1998. The National Health Service (NHS) provided about 10% of these contacts while the majority of non-NHS visits represented direct out-of-pocket expenditure.[5]

Patient populations

A number of systematic reviews of surveys have assessed the prevalence of CAM use among specific adult and pediatric patient populations.

AIDS or HIV-infected patients

Four surveys[12-15] assessing the overall prevalence of CAM use by individuals with AIDS or HIV infection were identified by a systematic review.[16] Studies from the UK[12,13] indicated that massage and dietary treatments were most popular, while those originating from Holland[14] and Switzerland[15] reported that homeopathy and vitamin supplementation were frequently used in this patient group. The reported overall prevalence in these studies ranged between 27% and 56% of the total study population.

Cancer patients

A systematic review of CAM use among patients with cancer identified a single investigation published in the 1970s, nine during the 1980s and 16 after 1990, indicating considerable interest in the subject.[17] Two of the reviewed surveys were conducted in the UK and assessed patients with various types of cancer.[18,19] These reported that 16–32% of respondents had used some form of CAM. Relaxation techniques, dietary interventions, visualization and homeopathy were among the most popular treatments. Fourteen other studies reported data from German-speaking countries and Scandinavia.[17] The use of CAM in these studies was highly variable and ranged between 9% and 62% of respondents. In studies conducted after 1990, the most commonly used complementary therapies were mind–body approaches, dietary interventions and herbal medicine.

Dermatologic patients

Five surveys of the use of complementary therapies by dermatologic patients were identified by another systematic review.[20] In the UK, a study published in 1998 suggested a lifetime prevalence of 69% among patients with psoriasis and reported dietary interventions, herbal medicine and acupuncture as the most popular treatments.[21] Surveys from Austria and Germany assessed patients with melanoma[22] and atopic dermatitis[23] respectively and suggested that homeopathy, acupuncture and diets were among the most frequently used treatments. Prevalence data, provided only for melanoma patients, indicated a point prevalence of 14%.[22] Studies from Norway and Sweden assessed pediatric patients with atopic dermatitis[24] and adult patients attending a dermatology outpatient clinic respectively.[25]

The latter suggested a lifetime prevalence of 35% with supplements, diets and herbal medicine being most popular.

Rheumatologic patients

The use of CAM in this patient group was assessed in seven surveys from Europe.[26] Four studies were conducted in the UK[27-30] with the remainder originating from the Republic of Ireland,[31] the former Yugoslavia[32] and Holland.[33] While studies from the UK and Ireland suggested dietary interventions, supplements and herbal medicine as the most frequently used therapies, on the European continent these were acupuncture, chiropractic and homeopathy. These studies reported that 30–81% of the patient populations had used some form of CAM.

Pediatric patients

A systematic review on the prevalence of CAM use among children retrieved three studies from Europe.[34] A questionnaire-based survey of 521 parents attending pediatric clinics in the UK suggested a frequency of CAM use of 15% of a community sample and 25% in a hospital sample, with an overall average of 21%.[35] Homeopathy, aromatherapy and osteopathy were among the most popular treatments. A study from Norway assessed patients aged 1–15 years with atopic dermatitis and psoriasis and reported a prevalence of 44% and 41% respectively, with herbal medicine and homeopathy as the most popular types of treatment.[24] This is corroborated by a small survey of children with acute lymphoblastic leukemia from Finland.[36]

The above data on the prevalence of CAM in European countries vary considerably. In random or representative samples of the general population, the one-year prevalence ranged between 11% and 28% in the UK, while prevalence rates as high as 65% have been reported on the European continent. The variation of these figures and those obtained for specific patient populations on a national level, as well as between countries, is not easily explained. In view of national differences, the complex problem of defining CAM and thus the array of therapies covered is one factor which has contributed to the variance in prevalence rates.[1] In addition, it is often unclear from the reports whether point prevalence, one-year or lifetime prevalence were assessed. Therefore, on the basis of the data available at present, it is concluded that the level of CAM use among the general population and specific patient populations is generally high and increasing. The true prevalence rates, however, remain uncertain in many countries.

Regulation

United Kingdom

In the UK, non-medically qualified practitioners are able to freely practice subject to minor limitations, which refer, for instance, to the treatment of venereal diseases, pregnancy, dentistry and veterinary medicine. This unregulated situation

GENERAL TOPICS

has existed since the 16th century. The passing of the Osteopaths' Act in 1993 followed by the Chiropractors' Act practically ended this situation and these Acts have been important initiatives in control over professional standards by restriction of title (i.e. not restriction of practice).[37] Osteopathy and chiropractic are the only two complementary professions that have achieved statutory regulation. Similar to the General Medical Council of the medical profession, the General Osteopathic Council and the General Chiropractic Council will be responsible for all aspects of professional regulation including ethics, disciplinary structures and insurance regulations. The Councils have the authority to remove practitioners from the register and prevent them from using the title 'chiropractor' or 'osteopath'.

Acupuncture is not regulated by statute so far, although initiatives are under way. The British Acupuncture Council, one of three regulatory bodies of professional acupuncturists, accepts only members who have completed training that has been independently accredited by the British Acupuncture Accreditation Board (BAAB). The BAAB was set up by acupuncture organizations and colleges to ensure that self-imposed criteria for educational standards are met. For medical doctors the regulating body is the British Medical Acupuncture Society, which offers a Diploma of Medical Acupuncture. For physiotherapists in the UK, the regulating body is the Acupuncture Association of Chartered Physiotherapists.

The main voluntary regulatory body for Western medical herbalists is the National Institute for Medical Herbalists, which accepts graduates of approved courses. Other bodies are the European Herbal Practitioner Association and the Register of Chinese Herbal Practitioners. Herbal medicinal products are available through pharmacies, health food shops and supermarkets and generally fall into three categories: licensed herbal medicinal products, herbal medicinal products that are exempt from licensing and food supplements.[38] Herbal medicinal products that are sold with therapeutic claims are regulated by the Medicines Control Agency (MCA) and are required to hold a product license. Those that are exempt from licensing also fall within the responsibility of the MCA. Food supplements are controlled by the Ministry of Agriculture, Fisheries and Foods.

There are two regulatory bodies in homeopathy. The Faculty of Homeopathy, which was incorporated by Act of Parliament in 1950 to train and examine medical doctors, and the Society of Homeopaths. The latter is the regulatory body mainly for non-medically qualified practitioners.

Continental Europe

In contrast to the situation in the UK, in some member states of the European Union such as Austria it is illegal for non-medically qualified therapists to practice any form of medicine.[39]

Other systems exist, for instance in Belgium, where steps have been taken to regulate CAM,[40] and in Germany, where officially registered non-medically qualified practitioners (*Heilpraktiker*) are able to practice alongside physicians.[41] The German *Heilpraktiker* has a similar therapeutic repertoire as a CAM practitioner in the UK. There is, however, more emphasis on diagnostic techniques and while CAM practitioners in the UK tend to specialize in one complementary therapy, *Heilpraktiker* normally use a wider range of different therapies. In addition, the situation in Germany differs from many other European countries in that some therapies which are considered complementary elsewhere (e.g. massage) are fully integrated into mainstream medicine. Many CAM therapies are practiced by medically qualified doctors, many of whom have received specialist training and hold diplomas qualifying them to use the title of naturopathic physician (*Arzt für Naturheilkunde*) in addition to their orthodox specialization.

Considering these national differences on regulatory issues, the harmonization process across the European Union is difficult indeed. Although the Treaty of Rome guarantees the free movement of professionals within its legislative borders, these issues prohibit its execution in practice. There have been repeated initiatives towards harmonization of non-medically qualified health practitioners,[42] which have subsequently been rejected[43] and currently it seems that a solution on the European level is distant. New and creative approaches towards solving these complex problems are warranted and awaited with some interest.

REFERENCES

1 Ernst E. Prevalence of use of complementary/alternative medicine: a systematic review. Bull WHO 2000;78:252–257

2 Harris P, Rees R. The prevalence of complementary and alternative medicine use among the general population: a systematic review of the literature. Compl Ther Med 2000;8:88–96

3 Thomas K J, Fall M, Williams B. Methodological study to investigate the feasibility of conducting a population-based survey of the use of complementary health care. Final report to the Research Council for Complementary Medicine. Unpublished, 1993

4 Vickers A. Use of complementary therapies. Br Med J 1994;309:1161

5 Thomas K, Nicholl J, Coleman P. Use and expenditure on complementary medicine in England – a population-based survey. Compl Ther Med 2000 (in press)

6 Eisenberg D M, Davies R B, Ettner S L, Appel S, Wilkey S, Rompay M V. Trends in alternative medicine use in the United States 1990–1997: results of a follow-up national survey. JAMA 1998;280:1569–1575

7 Ernst E, White A R. The BBC survey of complementary medicine use in the UK. Compl Ther Med 2000;8:32–36

8 Grampian Local Health Council. The use of complementary therapies in the Grampian population. Report of a population survey Unpublished, 2000

9 Emslie M, Campbell M, Walker K. Complementary therapies in a local care setting. Part 1: is there real public demand? Compl Ther Med 1996;4:39–42

10 Häußermann D. Wachsendes Vertrauen in Naturheilmittel. Dtsch Ärztebl 1997; 94:1857–1858

11 Haidinger G, Gredler B. Extent of familiarity with, extent of use, and success of alternative therapies in Austria. Öffentliche Gesundheitswesen 1988;50:9–12

12 Barton S E, Jadresic D M, Hawkins D A, Gazzard B G. Alternative treatments for HIV infection. Br Med J 1989;298:1519–1520

13 Barton S E, Davies S, Schroeder K, Artur G, Gazzard B G. Complementary therapies used by people with HIV infection. AIDS 1994;8:561

14 Wolffers I, De Morée S. Alternative treatments as a contribution to care of persons with HIV/Aids. Ned Tijdschr Geneeskd 1994; 138:307–310

15 Langewitz W, Rüttimann S, Laifer G, Maurer P, Kiss A. The integration of alternative treatment modalities in HIV infection – the patient's perspective. J Psychosom Res 1994;38:687–693

16 Ernst E. Complementary AIDS therapies: the good, the bad and the ugly. Int J STD AIDS 1997;8:281–285

17 Ernst E, Cassileth B R. The prevalence of complementary/alternative medicine in cancer. Cancer 1998;83:777–782

18 Burke C, Sikora K. Complementary and conventional cancer care: the integration of two cultures. Clin Oncol (Roy Coll Radiol) 1993;5:220–227

19 Downer S M, Cody M M, McCluskey P et al. Pursuit and practice of complementary therapies by cancer patients receiving conventional treatments. Br Med J 1994; 309:86–89

20 Ernst E. The usage of complementary therapies by dermatological patients: a systematic review. Br J Dermatol 2000;142:857–861

21 Clark C M, McKay R A, Fortune D G et al. Use of alternative treatments by patients with psoriasis. Br J Gen Pract 1998;48:1873–1874

22 Söllner W, Zingg-Schir M, Rumpold G et al. Attitude towards alternative therapy, compliance with standard treatment and need for emotional support in patients with melanoma. Arch Dermatol 1997;133:216–220

23 Augustin M, Zschoke I, Buhrke U. Attitudes and prior experience with respect to alternative medicine among dermatological patients: the Freiburg Questionnaire on attitudes to naturopathy (FAN). Forsch Komplementärmed 1999;6(suppl):26–29

24 Jensen P. Use of alternative medicine by patients with atopic dermatitis and psoriasis. Acta Derm Venereol 1990;70:421–424

25 Berg M, Arnetz B. Characteristics of users and nonusers of alternative medicine in dermatologic patients attending a University hospital clinic: a short report. J Alt Compl Med 1998;4:277–279

26 Ernst E. Usage of complementary therapies in rheumatology: a systematic review. Clin Rheumatol 1998;17:301–305

27 Pullar T, Capell H A, Miller A, Brooks A. Alternative medicine: costs and subjective benefit in rheumatoid arthritis. Br Med J 1982;285:1629–1631

28 Higham C, Ashcroft C, Jayson M I V. Non-prescribed treatments in rheumatic diseases. Practitioner 1983;227:1201–1205

29 Struthers G R, Scott D L, Scott D G I. The use of alternative treatments by patients with rheumatoid arthritis. Rheumatol Int 1983; 3:151–152

30 Dimmock S, Troughton P R, Bird H A. Factors predisposing to the resort of complementary therapies in patients with fibromyalgia. Clin Rheumatol 1996;15:478–482

31 Cassidy M, Jacobs A, Bresnihan B. The use of unproven remedies for rheumatoid arthritis in Ireland. Irish Med J 1983;76:464–465

32 Krajnc I. Alternative medicine in the treatment of rheumatic diseases. Lijec Vjesn 1993; 115:35–39

33 Visser G J, Peters L, Raser J J. Rheumatologists and their patients who seek alternative care, an agreement to disagree. Br J Rheumatol 1992;31:485–490

34 Ernst E. Prevalence of complementary/alternative medicine for children: a systematic review. Eur J Pediatr 1999;158:7–11

35 Simpson N, Pearce A, Finlay F, Lenton S. The use of complementary medicine by children. Ambulatory Child Care 1998;3:351–356

36 Möttönen M, Uhari M. Use of micronutrients and alternative drugs by children with acute lymphoblastic leukemia. Med Pediatr Oncol 1997;28:205–208

37 Maxwell R J. The Osteopaths' Bill. Br Med J 1993;306:1556–1557

38 Anderson L A. Herbal medicinal products: regulation in the UK and European Union. In: Ernst E (ed) Herbal medicine – a concise overview for professionals. Oxford: Butterworth Heinemann, 2000

39 Ernst E. Heilpraktiker – ein deutsches Phänomen. Fortschr Medizin 1997;115:38–41

40 Watson R. Belgium is to regulate complementary medicine. Br Med J 1999;318:1372

41 Ernst E. Außenseiter, Schulmedizin, und nationalsozialistische Machtpolitik. Dtsch Ärzteblatt 1995;92:104–107

42 Hege H. Das Lannoye-Papier. Alternativmedizin im Europäischen Parlament. Dtsch Ärzteblatt 1995;92:1543–1544

43 Watson R. European complementary medicine proposal watered down. Br Med J 1997; 314:1641

Why Patients Use Complementary and Alternative Medicine

Clare Stevinson

Investigations of the use of complementary and alternative medicine (CAM) generally address three points:

- the *extent* to which it is used (prevalence)
- the *people* who use it (patient characteristics)
- the *reasons* for using it (motives).

Some forms of CAM have a long history but given the considerable and continual advancements in orthodox medicine, might have been expected to have gradually fallen into obscurity. However, the indications are that the reverse is true.

The popularity of CAM

Survey data suggest that CAM is used by a sizable proportion of both adult and pediatric populations in a number of countries.[1,2] The most authoritative estimates of prevalence exist for the United States (42% during 1997),[3] Australia (49% in 1993)[4] and the United Kingdom (20% in 1998).[5] Figures reported for several European nations in the early 1990s are between 20% and 50%.[6] The data from the United States demonstrate an increase in use during the last decade[3] and it is reasonable to assume that this is reflected elsewhere. Surveys have also provided information on the characteristics of people using CAM. Compared with non-users, they are more likely to be female,[3-5,7] better educated,[3,4,8] have higher incomes[3,4,8] and suffer from chronic (mainly musculoskeletal) conditions.[3,7,8]

Given the growing popularity of CAM and the fact that the majority of this use represents 'out-of-pocket' expenditure,[3] the issue of why people use it is both relevant and intriguing. Although the question itself is a simple one, the answer is undoubtedly more complex. In fact, there are probably as many different reasons as there are users. One important finding that has been reported consistently is that the majority of CAM use does not occur instead of orthodox medical care, but in addition to it.[9,10] Patients report using orthodox medicine for some complaints and CAM for others or in particular cases, they may choose to use CAM alongside conventional treatment. Although the literature on the subject is quite limited and the reasons for the popularity of CAM are not fully understood, a number of explanations have been proposed.

GENERAL TOPICS

395

Explanations for CAM use

Furnham[11] summarized the main hypotheses relating to why people use CAM (Box 6.4.1). Some he described as 'push' factors. These include dissatisfaction with or outright rejection of orthodox medicine through prior negative experiences or a general anti-establishment attitude. For these reasons, patients are 'pushed' away from conventional treatment in search of alternatives. Other factors 'pull' or attract patients towards CAM. These include compatibility between the philosophy of certain therapies and patients' own beliefs and a greater sense of control over one's own treatment.

Three of these hypotheses were tested by Astin in a preliminary attempt to develop explanatory models that account for the increasing use of complementary medicine.[12] He predicted that dissatisfaction with conventional care, need for personal control over treatment and philosophical congruence with own beliefs would distinguish CAM users from non-users. 1035 US residents were surveyed about their use of CAM, health status, values and attitudes to conventional medicine and the results were subjected to multiple logistic regression analyses. These indicated that only philosophical congruence was predictive of CAM use. Rather than being 'pushed' towards alternatives to conventional medicine due to disillusionment, participants were 'pulled' towards CAM because it is seen as more compatible with their values, worldview, spiritual/religious philosophy or beliefs about health and illness. Borrowing from Ray[13] the notion of 'value subcultures', the author found that those respondents who could be identified as 'cultural creatives' were

Box 6.4.1
Possible factors contributing to CAM use

Push factors

- Dissatisfaction with orthodox medicine
  - ineffective
  - adverse effects
  - poor communication
    with doctor
  - insufficient time with
    doctor
  - waiting lists
- Rejection of orthodox
  medicine
  - anti-science or anti-
    establishment attitude
- Desperation
- Cost of private orthodox
  medical care

Pull factors

- Philosophical congruence
  - spiritual dimension
  - emphasis on holism
  - active role of patient
  - explanation intuitively
    acceptable
  - natural treatments
- Personal control over
  treatment
- Good relationship with
  therapist
  - on equal terms
  - time for discussion
  - allows for emotional
    factors
- Accessible
- Increased well-being

more likely to be users of CAM. These individuals tend to be at the cutting edge of cultural change and innovation in society. They are identifiable by their interests in environmentalism, feminism, globalism, esoteric forms of spirituality, self-actualization, altruism and self-expression and a love of the foreign and exotic. According to Ray, this subgroup of the American population has increased hugely since the late 1960s and represents almost one quarter of the adult population.

The persuasive appeal of CAM

The features of CAM that foster the philosophical congruence perceived by patients were discussed by Kaptchuk & Eisenberg.[14] They suggest that certain fundamental premises of most forms of CAM contribute to its persuasive appeal. One of these is the perceived association of CAM with _nature_. It is inextricably linked with certain terminology: natural rather than artificial; pure versus synthetic; and organic as opposed to processed. This relationship is not restricted to plant-based medicines; rather, the metaphor of nature pervades other forms of CAM. Another fundamental component of CAM is _vitalism_. The enhancement or balancing of 'life forces', 'qi' or 'psychic energy' is central to many forms of CAM. For patients, there is intuitive appeal in this non-invasive notion of healing from within. The _science_ of CAM is a further important aspect in its attraction. Many therapies have long intellectual traditions and sophisticated philosophies, with training involving many years of study of complex systems and concepts. This contributes to the credibility and authority of the scientific label. The science of CAM is less dependent on the principles of objectivity and clinical experimentation than positivist science. The approach tends to be person centered, relying on observation, self-knowledge and human awareness. The language is one of unity and holism in contrast to the distant, reductionist terminology of normative science. Human experience, rather than being marginalized, is made the central element of CAM science. A fourth element in the appeal of CAM is _spirituality_. This bridges the gap between the domain of medical science, with its search for truth and strict causality, and the domain of religion, with its moral freedom and self-chosen values. CAM offers a satisfying unification of the physical and spiritual.

Underlying motives

Other proposed explanations for use of CAM refer to underlying reasons rather than deliberate patient motives. One of these is that patients using CAM are essentially neurotic so are drawn towards the touching/talking approach of many therapies. While levels of neurosis are reported to be high in patients visiting CAM therapists[15] and higher than those visiting a general practitioner (GP),[16] this may be nothing more than a reflection of the nature of the conditions being treated. CAM practitioners mainly see patients with chronic or incurable disorders in whom the incidence of neurosis is likely to be high. However, a study of 480 US breast cancer patients found an association between poorer mental health and depression and use of CAM following surgery,[17] suggesting that those with greater psychosocial stress may be more likely to turn to CAM.

Another suggestion is that patients with a better understanding of the workings of the human body are attracted to CAM therapists because diagnosis and treatment involve more discussion and explanation than offered by orthodox medical practitioners. Again, although one study did show that patients visiting CAM therapists had greater knowledge of human biology than those visiting a GP,[18] there is no clear causal relationship. It is possible that CAM therapists attempt to educate their patients on biological or physiological processes, making enhanced knowledge a consequence rather than a cause of their choice. Furthermore, better understanding of the human body may simply be a reflection of the higher levels of education that have been consistently reported for CAM users.

The limitations of survey data

There are various limitations to the use of surveys in attempting to understand what motivates patients to use CAM, particularly some of those mentioned above.[16,18] First, a comparison of patients visiting a CAM therapist with those visiting a GP is not necessarily the same as a comparison of people who do and do not use CAM. The patients visiting the GP on the day of the survey may be equally likely to consult a CAM therapist another day for a different complaint, and vice versa. Without knowing the purpose of the visit, an examination of patient variables is meaningless. Only a comparison of patients consulting different practitioners for the same condition would provide relevant information.

Second, this approach only tackles explanations for use of CAM practitioners rather than CAM use in general. These may well be two separate questions. People who purchase a homeopathic or herbal product off the shelf may have very different motives from those who visit a homeopath or herbalist. Similarly, the act of learning a relaxation technique or self-massage from a book is not necessarily the same as visiting a therapist to learn these techniques. Many people who self-treat with CAM may not even contemplate visiting a CAM therapist. It seems reasonable to suggest that these represent different forms of CAM usage and different motives may underlie them. This draws attention to the wider problem of referring to CAM in such general terms. The term encompasses a vast number of very different therapies and approaches and it is possible that motives for using them are highly therapy-specific. Reasons for participating in yoga, for example, may not be readily generalizable to mega-vitamin supplementation. Understanding of why people use CAM would probably be enhanced by separate investigations of different modalities.

A third weakness of many surveys is their indirect approach to identifying patient motives. Although attempting to address the question of *why* patients use CAM, they actually contribute more to the issue of *who* uses it. Rather than directly asking patients about their reasons for using CAM, there is a tendency to examine patient characteristics, beliefs and attitudes and from them make assumptions about motives.[19,20] Just because a survey finds that patients visiting a CAM therapist display skepticism about conventional treatments according to questionnaire items[16] does not necessarily mean that they chose to consult the CAM therapist due to disenchantment with orthodox medicine. As well as the assumption that measuring attitudes necessarily reveals motives, there are problems regarding causality. Do patients visit a CAM therapist because of particular attitudes or beliefs or do they hold those attitudes or beliefs as a result of visiting the therapist? More valid answers could be derived from directly questioning patients about their motives for using CAM.

Direct investigations of patient motives

One specific example of an attempt to address the question directly was a qualitative study in the US of 22 patients self-medicating with the herb St John's wort for depression.[21] The coherent themes emerging from the interviews were:

- desire to take control of own health
- perception that their condition was not serious and did not require medical treatment
- belief that St John's wort was safe while prescribed anti-depressants were dangerous
- perception of St John's wort as an effective and easily accessible option, compared with lack of confidence in and barriers to orthodox medical care for depression.

Another study that directly addressed patient motives was conducted with patients suffering from inflammatory bowel disease in Canada.[22] Questionnaire data from 134 patients revealed that side effects and ineffectiveness of orthodox treatments were the main reasons for seeking CAM. Follow-up in-depth interviews confirmed the importance of side effects in decisions to try CAM, along with an attempt to improve their quality of life and have a greater control over their own treatment. A questionnaire study of 442 Norwegian patients with atopic dermatitis and psoriasis[23] also found that ineffectiveness and side effects of their conventional treatment were among the main reasons for trying CAM. However, the strongest motivation was a keenness to try all available options. This particular reason was also cited the most in a survey of 211 general practice patients from Austria, Germany and England who were asked why they thought people used CAM.[24] Using CAM as a 'last hope' was also one of the most common answers in this study.

GENERAL TOPICS

Patients who turned to CAM as a last resort could be clearly differentiated from those who embraced CAM for its compatibility with their own beliefs in a UK-based study.[25] Interview and questionnaire data from 38 patients attending a CAM center revealed two discrete patient types. Those who sought CAM as a last resort because no conventional treatments had proved effective for their complaint had similar scores to the general population on locus of control. Furthermore, they maintained faith in the principles of orthodox medicine and displayed little initial commitment to the values or philosophies of CAM. The other type of patient chose CAM because it matched his or her own beliefs about health and illness. These individuals showed a greater internal locus of control and skepticism about orthodox methods, as well as commitment to CAM.

The role of the therapeutic relationship

This study[25] also found that 68% of patients reported a better relationship with the CAM practitioner than with their own GP and this finding was not related to their commitment to CAM. The specific reasons given for this were that practitioners were more friendly and personal, treated the relationship more like a partnership and provided more time for the consultation. Satisfaction with the therapeutic encounter was also greater with CAM practitioners than GPs in a survey of arthritis sufferers in the UK,[26] although interestingly 'friendliness' was rated higher in GPs. Again, satisfaction with the time spent on the patient was higher with CAM practitioners, as it also was in a Spanish study of CAM use by patients with somatoform disorder.[27] The duration of CAM consultations is invariably longer than with orthodox medicine. A comparison of physicians using homeopathy with those practicing conventional medicine reported that the former spent more than twice as long on patient consultations.[28] As well as leading to greater satisfaction with patients, this may be one of the key factors in the success of CAM. A clinical trial of homeopathy for premenstrual syndrome reported a response rate of 47% in a pre-treatment placebo wash-out phase,[29] which the authors suggested may have been due largely to the depth and intimacy of the homeopathic interview.

Shopping for health

Despite the limitations of the existing literature on the motives for CAM use, a few consistent findings have emerged. It is clear that in general, CAM does not replace orthodox medical care. Rather, it serves as a substitute in some particular situations and as an adjunct in others, while being disregarded when not considered appropriate for the condition in question. This has led to CAM use being described as 'shopping for health'.[11] Rather than being specifically 'pushed' or 'pulled' towards CAM, patients simply perceive it as one of a range of treatment options available to them and exercise their freedom of choice and discriminating power accordingly. The desire to try all available options may be for some an attempt to leave no stone unturned as they become increasingly desperate for an effective treatment. However, for others it may simply reflect opportunism and experimentation. The finding that CAM use is associated with higher levels of income may support the concept of CAM as a commodity for those that can afford it. Intriguingly, a strong positive correlation was reported between sale data of BMW cars (a possible measure of affluence) and use of herbal remedies in the US.[30]

Barriers to CAM

'Shopping for health' is not a particularly new concept. A UK study of CAM users in 1989 concluded that interviewees had an eclectic approach to health care which could be described as 'consumerist'.[31] In modern, consumer-oriented societies this seems entirely reasonable and perhaps it is more pertinent to ask why people don't use CAM. One study of 90 fibromyalgia patients in the UK actually addressed this question.[32] Those that did not make any use of CAM cited two reasons: lack of information and expense. A qualitative study involving 36 Canadian breast cancer patients[33] also investigated why some individuals chose not to use CAM. The main reasons were lack of information, skepticism about efficacy and fear of therapies being harmful. Some patients who wanted to use CAM did not actually do so because they encountered certain barriers. These mainly related to the cost of therapies, lack of access and lack of time to devote to the therapy. A subsequent questionnaire study by the same research group of 411 breast cancer survivors confirmed these findings.[34] Cost and lack of information were the most common barriers stated, with fear of harm, lack of time and lack of access also cited. Only a small percentage reported fear of their physician's disapproval as a barrier.

Directions for future research

According to the most authoritative paper on the subject,[12] CAM use in the general population is influenced more by philosophical attraction than negative attitudes to orthodox medicine or desire for personal control of health. However, individual studies in specific populations suggest that these other factors are important for patients. There may prove to be interesting differences in motivation for using CAM between particular patient groups depending on the nature and severity of their condition and the existence of effective conventional treatments. Differences between individual therapies and between patients of different nationalities are also worth investigating. Greater insights could be generated by exploring the reasons for not using CAM and differentiating between those *never* using CAM and those *no longer* using CAM. Despite the interest in examining dissatisfaction with orthodox medicine, there has been little investigation of disillusionment with CAM. A further issue for future research is the change in motives over time. As orthodox medicine continues to advance and questions about efficacy and safety of CAM begin to be properly answered by rigorous research, it is possible that the factors motivating patients to use CAM today will be entirely different from those in the future.

REFERENCES

1 Harris P, Rees R. The prevalence of complementary and alternative medicine use among the general population: a systematic review of the literature. Compl Ther Med 2000;8:88–96

2 Ernst E. Prevalence of complementary/ alternative medicine for children; a systematic review. Eur J Pediatr 1999;158:7–11

3 Eisenberg D M, Davis R B, Ettner S L, Appel S, Wilkey S, Rompay M V, Kessler R C. Trends in alternative medicine use in the United States, 1990–1997. Results of a follow-up national survey. JAMA 1998;280:1569–1575

4 MacLennan A H, Wilson D H, Taylor A W. Prevalence and cost of alternative medicine in Australia. Lancet 1996;347:569–573

5 Ernst E, White A. The BBC survey of complementary medicine use in the UK. Compl Ther Med 2000;8:32–36

6 Fisher P, Ward A. Complementary medicine in Europe. Br Med J 1994;309:107–111

7 Bullock M L, Pheley A M, Kiresuk T J, Lenz S K, Culliton P. Characteristics and complaints of patients seeking therapy at a hospital-based alternative medicine clinic. J Alt Compl Med 1997;3:31–37

8 Blais R, Maiga A, Aboubacar A. How different are users and non-users of alternative medicine? Can J Pub Health 1997;88:159–162

9 Kranz R, Rosenmund A. Über die Motivation zur Verwendung komplementärmedizinischer Heilmethoden. Schweiz Med Wochenschr 1998;128:616–622

10 Druss B G, Rosenheck R A. Association between use of unconventional therapies and conventional medical services. JAMA 1999;282:651–656

11 Furnham A. Why do people choose and use complementary therapies? In: Ernst E (ed) Complementary medicine: an objective appraisal. Oxford: Butterworth Heinemann, 1996

12 Astin J. Why patients use alternative medicine. Results of a national survey. JAMA 1998;279:1548–1553

13 Ray P H. The emerging culture. American Demographics 1997; February (available at www.demographics.com)

14 Kaptchuk T J, Eisenberg D M. The persuasive appeal of alternative medicine. Ann Intern Med 1998;129:1061–1065

15 Davidson J, Rampes H, Eisen M, Fisher P, Smith R, Malik M. Psychiatric disorders in primary care patients receiving complementary medicine. Compr Psychiatr 1998;39:16–20

16 Furnham A, Smith C. Choosing alternative medicine: a comparison of the beliefs of patients visiting a general practitioner and a homoeopath. Soc Sci Med 1988;26:685–689

17 Burstein H J, Gelber S, Guadagnoli E, Weeks J C. Use of alternative medicine by women with early-stage breast cancer. New Engl J Med 1999;340:1733–1739

18 Furnham A, Forey J. The attitudes, behaviours and beliefs of patients of conventional versus complementary (alternative) medicine. J Clin Psychol 1994;50:458–469

19 Hentschel C, Kohnen R, Hauser G, Lindner M, Hahn E G, Ernst E. Complementary medicine today: patient decision for physician or magician? A comparative study of patients deciding in favour of alternative therapies. Eur J Phys Med Rehab 1996;6:144–150

20 Mitzdorf U, Beck K, Horton-Hausknecht J et al. Why do patients seek treatments in hospitals of complementary medicine? J Alt Compl Med 1999;5:463–473

21 Wagner P J, Jester D, LeClair B, Taylor T, Woodward L, Lambert J. Taking the edge off: why patients choose St. John's wort. J Fam Pract 1999;48:615–619

22 Hilsden R J, Scott C M, Verhoef M J. Complementary medicine use by patients with inflammatory bowel disease. Am J Gastroenterol 1998;93:697–701

23 Jensen P. Alternative therapy for atopic dermatitis and psoriasis: patient-reported motivation, information source and effect. Acta Derm Venereol 1990;70:425–428

24 Ernst E, Willoughby M, Weihmayr T. Nine possible reasons for choosing complementary medicine. Perfusion 1995;8:356–359

25 Finnigan M D. The Centre for the Study of Complementary Medicine: an attempt to understand its popularity through psychological, demographic and operational criteria. Compl Med Res 1991;5:83–88

26 Resch K L, Hill S, Ernst E. Use of complementary therapies by individuals with 'arthritis'. Clin Rheumatol 1997;16:391–395

27 Garcia-Campayo J, Sanz-Carrillo C. The use of alternative medicines by somatoform disorder patients in Spain. Br J Gen Pract 2000; 50:487–488

28 Jacobs J, Chapman E H, Crothers D. Patient characteristics and practice patterns of physicians using homeopathy. Arch Fam Med 1998;7:537–540

29 Chapman E H, Angelica J, Spitalny G, Strauss M. Results of a study of the homeopathic treatment of PMS. J Am Inst Homeopath 1994;87:14–21

30 Ernst E. Alternative views of alternative medicine. Ann Intern Med 1999;131:230

31 Sharma U M. Alternative choices of healing in North Staffordshire. Compl Med Res 1989; 3:1–4

32 Dimmock S, Troughton P R, Bird H A. Factors predisposing to the resort of complementary therapies in patients with fibromyalgia. Clin Rheumatol 1996;15:478–482

33 Boon H, Brown J B, Gavin A, Kennard M A, Stewart M. Breast cancer survivors' perceptions of complementary/alternative medicine (CAM): making the decision to use or not to use. Qual Health Res 1999; 9:639–653

34 Boon H, Stewart M, Kennard M A et al. Use of complementary/alternative medicine by breast cancer survivors in Ontario: prevalence and perceptions. J Clin Oncol 2000;18:2515–2521

Legal and Ethical Issues in Complementary and Alternative Medicine

Michael H. Cohen

Introduction

As complementary and alternative medical (CAM) therapies increasingly penetrate conventional health care, physicians and other health-care providers find themselves providing (or being asked to provide) care at the borderland of medicine, ethics, public policy and law. Whereas historically, many physicians and patients shunned a dialogue concerning use and potential applicability of CAM therapies in mainstream care, such dialogue is now flourishing, both in the US and internationally.

Discussions about CAM are enriching the physician–patient encounter, educating various players in the health-care arena about the role of nutrition, herbal medicine, mind–body interactions and other phenomena in mainstream care and contributing to a greater foundation of world medical knowledge. Such dialogue is also leading physicians to reconsider their moral, ethical and legal obligation to be aware of the best available evidence emerging from CAM, to present such evidence to the patient in meaningful terms and to confront therapeutic issues and choices from a more comprehensive, unified perspective on health and the possibility for human healing.

This chapter explores and outlines the regulatory boundaries of such an obligation.

Background of the regulatory structure

In the US, the law governing integration of CAM into conventional medical care is underdeveloped. The law provides no official definition of 'complementary and alternative medicine'. Rather, a body of legislative codes and judicial decision making at the federal, state and even municipal levels is emerging which, taken as a whole, creates the basic regulatory framework for physician integration of CAM.[1]

Some of the legal doctrines traditionally applied in health-care law remain applicable, with some modification, to the practice and integration of CAM; for example, as discussed below, basic principles of malpractice and requirements of informed consent. Other legal rules, such as the potential liability associated with physician referrals to CAM providers who lack independent state licensure (e.g. massage therapists in states such as California), require reconceptualization.[2]

One reason the law in this field is nascent is that regulatory structures governing CAM emerged out of the sectarian rivalries, destructive competition and attempts at medical monopolization during the late 19th and early 20th centuries.[3] Legal authority typically follows consensus medical opinion in setting the parameters of health-care law; thus, legal authority to date has mirrored the historical perspective of majority interests in biomedicine in treating patient use of CAM as deviant, suspect or marginal.[4]

It was only in the late 20th century, for example, that decisions by US courts gave tangible recognition to allegations that the American Medical Association and other groups had engaged in a conspiracy to preserve a professional monopoly;[5] recognized a strong consumer autonomy interest in the selection and purchase of dietary supplements;[6] allowed physicians a defense to malpractice when patients knowingly, voluntarily and intelligently made a decision to utilize a CAM therapy over conventional care;[7] and otherwise affirmed the rights of CAM providers to practice and patients' rights to make autonomous therapeutic choices outside biomedicine.

Similarly, the late 20th century also saw the establishment of a National Center for Complementary and Alternative Medicine at the National Institutes of Health and, concomitantly, a flurry of federal and state statutes aimed at increasing consumer access to CAM.[8] Today, new and emerging government institutions, professional organizations, scientific publications, decision makers in legislatures and agencies (and public attitudes) are creating a complex and shifting medical and legal environment governing the integration of CAM into conventional care.

In this rapidly changing environment, three of the key regulatory areas that highlight scientific considerations of evidence-based practice are licensing, professional discipline and malpractice and informed consent.

Regulation through professional licensure

The requirements for professional practice vary by complementary and alternative modality and practitioner internationally. In the USA, professional licensure is governed by state law pursuant to the Tenth Amendment to the US Constitution, which leaves states free to regulate matters of health, safety and welfare affecting their citizens. Each state has enacted a medical licensing statute which prohibits the unlicensed practice of medicine. Typically, such statutes define such practice as including one or more of the following:

- diagnosing, preventing, treating and curing disease
- holding oneself out to the public as able to perform the above
- intending to receive a gift, fee or compensation for the above
- attaching such titles as MD to one's name

- maintaining an office for reception, examination and treatment
- performing surgery
- using, administering or prescribing drugs or medicinal preparations.[9]

In most states, therefore, CAM providers who lack licensure could be viewed as 'diagnosing' and 'treating' patients and thus as practicing medicine unlawfully. Courts have interpreted medical practice acts broadly where state legislatures have failed to create separate licensure for providers such as midwives, naturopaths, homeopaths, hypnotherapists, faith healers, providers of colonic irrigation, nutritionists, iridologists and even those offering ear piercing, tattooing and massage.[10]

An example is <u>Stetina v State</u>, which involved a non-medical provider of health care lacking independent licensure.[11] The defendant, Stetina, was a nutritionist who practiced iridology. An undercover investigator visited Stetina and she prescribed colonic irrigation and various nutritional remedies. On appeal from an injunction barring her from practice, Stetina argued that her conduct, which aimed at helping individuals follow proper nutritional advice, was outside the purview of the Medical Practice Act and that in any event, most physicians did not address nutrition and thus her practice was complementary. The Indiana Court of Appeals disagreed and held that Stetina was practicing medicine without a license.

Thus, unlicensed providers have had little success arguing that the prohibition in medical licensing statutes against unlicensed medical practice exempts a non-medical, holistic healing practice. Their typical remedy is to lobby state legislatures for licensure or, more infrequently, to lobby for an exemption from the medical licensing statute.

Because licensure is controlled by state legislatures, physician views of the scientific evidence favoring or disfavoring use of a particular CAM modality have been relevant but not dispositive. Legislatures will take consensus medical views of safety and efficacy into account but social, political and larger policy considerations typically dictate the outcome. To put the matter simply: 'Legislative recognition trumps medical recognition'.[12]

Although legislatures can decide which providers they wish to license and how broadly to define the legislatively authorized scope of practice for such providers, physicians in the USA will be liable for malpractice if they refer patients to a 'known incompetent'.[13] The fact that the CAM provider to whom the physician has referred a patient is licensed by the state will not necessarily protect the physician from liability. Among other things, the physician still has an obligation to exercise reasonable care in selecting the provider, to determine that the referral is clinically justifiable and to ascertain that the provider is offering therapies within legally authorized practice boundaries and is only utilizing therapies accepted as safe within the provider's own profession.[14]

Regulation through professional discipline

Professional discipline similarly is governed by state law in the USA and typically is written into the licensing statutes. Physicians are prohibited from engaging in 'unprofessional conduct'. Generally, unprofessional conduct (or 'professional misconduct') includes such acts as obtaining the license fraudulently, practicing the profession fraudulently, beyond its authorized scope, with gross incompetence or with gross negligence, practicing while impaired by alcohol or drugs or while convicted of a crime, permitting or aiding an unlicensed person to perform activities requiring a license or failing to comply with relevant rules and regulations.[15] In many states, unprofessional conduct also includes 'any departure from, or the failure to conform to, the standards of acceptable and prevailing medical practice ... irrespective of whether or not a patient is injured thereby'.[16] The breadth of such statutory language has left physicians who use complementary and alternative treatments, even together with conventional care, open to state medical board disciplinary action.

In re Guess,[17] for example, involved a licensed physician practicing family medicine who administered homeopathic remedies to his patients when conventional treatment failed. The Board of Medical Examiners of North Carolina charged Guess with 'unprofessional conduct', alleging that his use of homeopathic medicines departed from community standards. There was no evidence that Guess's homeopathic treatments had harmed patients and in fact, patients testified that homeopathy had helped them after biomedicine had failed to provide relief. The North Carolina Supreme Court, after a series of appeals, nonetheless affirmed the revocation of Guess's licensure.

As Guess suggests, although the licensee may appeal, a court will not reverse the medical board decision to revoke licensure, unless there is no rational basis for the exercise of discretion complained of or the action is arbitrary and capricious. Thus, relatively few medical board decisions result in published judicial opinions overturning the decision.[18]

Proponents of greater freedom for health-care consumers have responded by lobbying state legislatures to enact statutes protecting physicians from professional discipline merely for offering patients CAM. By and large, such legislative efforts have succeeded. For example, New York's legislation addresses 'concerns regarding the treatment of non-conventional physicians in the professional medical conduct process by recognizing the role of legitimate non-conventional medical treatments in the practice of medicine' and 'secures the rights and freedoms of patients to choose their own medical treatments'.[19] The bill permits the 'physician's use of whatever medical care, conventional or nonconventional, which effectively treats human disease, pain, injury, deformity, or physical condition'.[20]

Similarly, North Carolina's legislation amends the disciplinary provisions of its medical licensing act to provide that:

The Board shall not revoke the license of or deny a license to a person solely because of that person's practice of a therapy that is experimental, nontraditional, or that departs from acceptable and prevailing medical practices unless, by competent evidence, the Board can establish that the treatment has a safety risk greater than the prevailing treatment or that the treatment is generally not effective.[21]

Likewise, Oklahoma's bill states: 'The Board shall not revoke the license of a person otherwise qualified to practice allopathic medicine within the meaning of this act solely because the person's practice of a therapy is experimental or nontraditional'.[22] These statutes legislatively expand patient access to CAM by safeguarding physicians against professional disciplinary proceedings based solely on medical board antipathy to complementary and alternative therapies.

While medical licensing statutes make no mention of different levels or hierarchies of evidence, the notion of evidence-based practice is implicit in the policing role that state medical boards continue to play pursuant to the disciplinary provisions of the licensing statutes. If, for example, a physician ignores necessary conventional care and instead offers the patient an ineffective CAM therapy, hoping for a cure based solely on anecdotal evidence, a medical board would likely conclude that the physician engaged in professional misconduct. Because of the failure to follow community standards of care and even minimal professionally agreed norms regarding levels of proof justifying the selection of a therapy, the board's determination well might be upheld in court, state 'medical freedom' legislation notwithstanding.

If, on the other hand, the physician continued to monitor the patient conventionally and utilized due care in selecting and delivering a therapy that had reasonable clinical evidence of safety and/or promise of efficacy, a conclusion of professional misconduct would be less likely. Thorough documentation, reasonable reliance on best scientific evidence justifying a therapy and continued conventional monitoring will help protect the physician against undue medical board action. In short, at least as far as professional discipline is concerned, physicians' legal and ethical obligations are more likely to coincide with a narrower range of scientifically acceptable options and less likely to follow broader legislative or populist notions.

Regulation through malpractice and the informed consent obligation

Malpractice typically is defined as unskillful practice that fails to conform to a standard of care in the profession and results in patient injury. The definition is problematic for physicians integrating complementary and alternative treatments. Courts may look to a lack of general medical acceptance of specific modalities or to a lack of Food and Drug Administration approval as indicative of failure to follow the standard of care. Further, courts may tend to locate the cause of patient injury in the CAM treatment, since the treatment differs from the medical norm and may have an unknown or inadequately explained mechanism of action.

A number of medical malpractice defenses can be adapted to physician inclusion of CAM in treatment protocols. Most promising are the respectable minority defense and assumption of risk. The first protects physicians if their conduct conforms to that adopted by a respectable minority within the profession; the second enables patients to knowingly, intelligently and voluntarily assume the risk of treatments outside the medical model and provides that if they do, physicians will have a viable defense to malpractice.[23] If the CAM practice in question is evidence based and thus thoroughly justified by the literature, a good case can be made that the physician is following a respectable minority within medicine in offering the therapy.

An important case supporting the assumption of risk defense is Schneider v Revici.[24] Here the patient learned that a lump had been found in her breast, refused a biopsy and consulted a physician for nutritional and other alternative methods of cancer treatment. Although the physician advised surgery, he acceded to the patient's request for treatment upon her signing a consent form by which she assumed the risk that the non-conventional cancer therapy would not cure her condition. The Second Circuit held that express assumption of risk by virtue of the unambiguous consent form could be a complete defense to the patient's malpractice claim. The court stated:

We see no reason why a patient should not be allowed to make an informed decision to go outside currently approved medical methods in search of an unconventional treatment. While a patient should be encouraged to exercise care for his own safety, we believe that an informed decision to avoid surgery and conventional chemotherapy is within the patient's right to determine what shall be done with his own body.[25]

As CAM increasingly enters mainstream health care, such therapies will begin to be considered to fall within provision of informed patient decisions, thus reducing the risk that physicians will incur malpractice liability merely for providing such therapies. Physicians still will have to use due care, however, in the selection and execution of such therapies.[26]

GENERAL TOPICS

A second basis for the imposition of malpractice liability is inadequate informed consent. The informed consent obligation requires the physician to disclose to the patient, among other things, the risks and benefits of a recommended therapy and all reasonable and feasible options.

In assessing whether a specific failure to disclose has violated the informed consent obligation, many US courts look to whether the reasonable patient would find the information material to a decision to undergo or forego treatment. In other words, if the reasonable patient would have decided to forego a conventional therapy (for example, chemo-therapy) in favor of a CAM therapy (for example, an herbal or nutritional protocol), the physician's failure to disclose the possibility of such an alternative could violate the informed consent obligation and hence constitute malpractice.[27] Other US courts judge materiality by the reasonable physician standard: non-disclosure violates informed consent only if the reasonable physician would have disclosed the information in question.

The reasonable physician standard should be guided by scientific rules regarding best evidence, whereas such rules of evidence are less significant if courts use the reasonable patient standard.[28] In other words, because best evidence rules are relevant to the physician and less important to the patient, such rules will control the physician's decision to disclose only where the physician's reasonable judgement and not the patient's, governs the legal obligation of informed consent.

Evolution of law

Many physicians are beginning to recognize that health and disease correlate with not only biochemical and physiological influences but also nutritional, environmental, social, mind–body and spiritual factors. The question is whether legal and regulatory structures will evolve to support this broader, more inclusive system of health care by recognizing the many legitimate facets of the person's search for wholeness. Internationally, there is a crucial need to provide leadership in legal and regulatory developments to serve hospitals, academic medical centers, educational institutions and federal, state and local governments who are creating law and setting policy.

Developments in law parallel paradigmatic shifts in health care; regulatory goals adjust to meet the changing social consciousness. While rules of best evidence are established by science, their application in clinical settings is molded by legal and ethical considerations, refined by physician–patient dialogue and broadened by transcultural perspectives on the nature of healing. The more evidence-based practices open to the challenges raised by policy decisions involving CAM therapies, the more that shared perspectives may contribute to new views of learning, being, consciousness and health.

REFERENCES

1 Cohen M H. The emerging field of law and complementary and alternative medicine Orange County Lawyer 2000;30:42

2 Cohen M H. Beyond complementary medicine: legal and ethical perspectives on health care and human evolution. Ann Arbor: University of Michigan Press, 2000, pp 55–58

3 Cohen M H. Complementary and alternative medicine: legal boundaries and regulatory perspectives. Baltimore: Johns Hopkins University Press, 1998, pp 15–23

4 Cohen 1998, p 23 (citing cases)

5 Wilk v American Medical Association, 719 F.2d 207 (7th Cir. 1983), cert. denied, 467 U.S 1210 (1984), on remand. 671 F. Supp. 1465 (N.D. Ill. 1987), aff'd, 895 F.2d 352 (7th Cir.1990)

6 Pearson v Shalala, 164 F.3d 650 (D.C. Cir. 1999), reh'g en banc denied, 172 F.3d 72 (D.C. Cir. 1999)

7 Schneider v Revici, 817 F.2d 987 (2d Cir. 1987)

8 See, e.g., Dietary Supplement Health and Education Act of 1994, Pub. L. No. 103-417, 108 Stat. 4325, 21 U.S.C. §§ 301 et seq. (1994); proposed Access to Medical Treatment Act, H.R. 746, § 3(a) (Feb. 19, 1997); S. 578, 105th Cong., 1st Sess. (Apr. 18, 1997)

9 Cohen 1998, p 26–29

10 See id. at 29–31 (citing cases)

11 513 N.E.2d 1234 (Ind. Ct. App. 1987)

12 Eisenberg D M, Cohen M H, Hrbek A, Grayzel J. Credentialing complementary and alternative medical providers. Ann Intern Med (submitted)

13 Cohen 2000, p 50

14 Id., 57; Cohen M H. Malpractice considerations affecting the clinical integration of complementary and alternative medicine. Current Practice of Medicine 1999;87:2

15 See, e.g., New York Educ. L. § 6509

16 In re Guess, 393 S.E.2d 833 (N.C. 1990) (quoting N.C. Gen. Stat. § 90–14(a)(6)), cert. denied, Guess v. North Carolina Bd. of Medical Examiners, 498 U.S. 1047 (1991), later proceeding, Guess v. Board of Medical Examiners, 967 F.2d 998 (4th Cir. 1992)

17 See Guess, 393 S.E.2d at 833

18 Cohen 1998, p 88

19 NY State Assembly Mem. in Support of Legislation (Bill No. 5411-C (Assembly), 3636-C (Senate) (1994)

20 New York Educ. L. § 6527(4)(e)

21 N.C. Gen. Stat. § 90-14(a)(6)

22 Okla. Stat. Ann. tit. 59, § 509.1(d)

23 Cohen 1998, pp 56–65

24 817 F.2d 987 (2d Cir. 1987)

25 Id. at 992

26 Cohen 2000, p 30

27 Cohen 2000, p 43

28 Ernst E, Cohen M H. Informed consent in complementary and alternative medicine. Arch Intern Med 2001 (in press)

Safety Issues in Complementary and Alternative Medicine

Edzard Ernst

Throughout this book we have placed much emphasis on safety issues. In particular, we have alerted the reader to the risks associated with specific therapies and we have attempted to evaluate the risk–benefit profile of complementary and alternative medical (CAM) treatments in comparison with that of conventional options. Direct toxicity, interactions, contraindications, etc. have therefore been given a prominent place.

More general aspects of safety issues related to CAM have, however, been somewhat neglected. The following discussion is aimed at filling this gap.

Problems with unregulated food supplements

In the US, Canada and the UK herbal medicinal products (HMPs) are, by and large, marketed as food supplements. As such no rigorous regulation comparable to the pharmaceutical sector applies. In particular, the necessity for a manufacturer to demonstrate safety and quality of the marketed product is far less.

Table 6.6.1 shows some of the contaminants that have been found in HMPs which have obvious safety implications.

Table 6.6.1
Contaminants that have been found in herbal medicines

Type of contaminant	Examples
Microorganisms	*Staphylococcus aureus*, *Escherichia coli* (certain strains), *Salmonella*, *Shigella*, *Pseudomonas aeruginosa*
Microbial toxins	Bacterial endotoxins, aflatoxins
Pesticides, herbicides	Chlorinated pesticides (e.g. DDT, DDE, HCH-isomers, HCB, aldrin, dieldrin, heptachlor), organic phosphates, carbamate insecticides and herbicides, dithiocarbamate fungicides, triazin herbicides
Fumigation agents	Ethylene oxide, methyl bromide, phosphine
Radioactivity	Cs-134, Cs-137, Ru-103, I-131, Sr-90
Heavy metals	Lead, cadmium, mercury, arsenic

Adulteration of HMPs with non-declared herbs or conventional drugs is a further problem with unregulated HMPs of dubious quality. It pertains in particular to Asian HMPs. For instance, when 2609 Chinese herbal medicines were collected and analyzed in Taiwan, 24% of them were shown to be adulterated with synthetic drugs like acetaminophen, hydrochlorothiazide, indomethacin, phenobarbital, theophylline and corticosteroids.[1]

Underdosing is another problem with HMPs. Whenever herbal food supplements from the US market are analyzed by independent experts, the findings reveal that in a substantial proportion of them, the active ingredient content differs marginally from label claims (e.g. [2]).

Problems with unregulated providers of CAM

In most countries, CAM providers are predominantly non-medically qualified practitioners. Most of these are probably adequately trained to do what they do. However, in the absence of adequate regulations, some providers will not adhere to adequate standards of clinical practice. This can have obvious safety implications.

With depressing regularity we hear of cases where CAM providers have delayed or hindered access to potentially life-saving conventional treatment (e.g. [3,4]). The best-researched example in this respect is probably the advice of some CAM providers against any type of immunization.[5]

Similar problems relate to CAM providers ignoring contraindications to treatment. If, for instance, a bleeding abnormality is a contraindication against chiropractic manipulation, how will the average chiropractor exclude such an abnormality before treating a new patient?

Changing or omitting prescribed treatments might be another problem. There is preliminary evidence that a significant proportion of CAM providers have the unfortunate habit of doing this,[6] which could be associated with important risks.

Some CAM providers could also be unable to adequately diagnose medical problems while patients are in their care. One could imagine a patient being treated for headache which reveals increasingly clearer signs of a sinister underlying cause. If these signs are missed, valuable time for adequate, perhaps life-saving treatment could be lost.

Another problem could be the use of diagnostic techniques which are either in themselves not risk free or invalid. An example for the first scenario is the overt overuse of some chiropractors of X-ray diagnosis.[7] An example of the second scenario is the use of iridology which would lead to false-negative or false-positive diagnosis.[8]

Basically these concerns relate to the (lack of) competence of CAM providers. The only acceptable way to eliminate such concerns is to adequately train and regulate all health-care professionals who employ CAM.

GENERAL TOPICS

Problems with users of CAM

The attitude of the consumer towards CAM may constitute a risk which is independent of CAM providers. For instance, when users of HMPs were interviewed about their behavior *vis à vis* an adverse effect of a herbal versus a synthetic 'over-the-counter' drug, the results suggested that about one quarter would consult their doctor for a serious adverse effect of conventional medication while less than 1% would do the same in relation to a herbal remedy.[9]

A further risk unrelated to CAM providers but nevertheless associated with CAM might lie in the plethora of lay books on CAM now available in every high street bookstore. Preliminary evidence[10] suggests that this lay literature has the potential to put the health of the reader at risk if the advice from these books is adhered to by seriously ill individuals. Similarly, we have shown that a significant proportion of the UK daily press reports about CAM in a much more favorable tone than about mainstream medicine.[11] This could lead to distrust in the latter, unjustified trust in the former or both and thus put the health of the reader at risk.

Conclusion

CAM is associated with complex safety concerns which are often difficult to resolve. Awareness and vigilance are, however, invariably a valuable first step towards minimizing the risks to our patients.

REFERENCES

1 Huang W F, Wen K C, Hsiao M L. Adulteration by synthetic therapeutic substances of traditional Chinese medicines in Taiwan. J Clin Pharmacol 1997;37:334–350

2 Gurely B J, Gardner S T, Hubbord M A. Content versus label claims in ephedra-containing dietary supplements. An J Health Syst Pharm 2000;57:1–7

3 Coppes M J, Anderson R A, Egeler R M, Wolff J E A. Alternative therapies for the treatment of childhood cancer. New Engl J Med 1998;339:846

4 Oneschuk D, Bruera E. The potential dangers of complementary therapy use in a patient with cancer. J Palliat Care 1999;15:49–52

5 Ernst E. Attitude against immunisation within some branches of complementary medicine. Eur J Pediatr 1997;156:513–515

6 Moody G A, Eaden J A, Bhakta P, Sher K, Mayberry J F. The role of complementary medicine in European and Asian patients with inflammatory bowel disease. Public Health 1998;112:269–271

7 Ernst E. Chiropractors' use of X-rays. Br J Radiol 1998;71:249–251

8 Ernst E. Iridology – not useful and potentially harmful. Arch Ophthalmol 2000;118:120–121

9 Barnes J, Mills S, Abbot N C, Willoughby M, Ernst E. Different standards for reporting ADRs to herbal remedies. Br J Clin Pharmacol 1998;45:496–500

10 Ernst E, Armstrong N C. Lay books on complementary/alternative medicine: a risk factor for good health? Int J Risk Safety Med 1998;11:209–215

11 Ernst E, Weihmayr T. UK and German media differ over complementary medicine. Br Med J 2000;321:707

Economic Issues in Complementary and Alternative Medicine

Adrian White

Introduction

Complementary and alternative medicine (CAM) users and practitioners often claim that the integration of CAM would inevitably lead to cheaper health care because it reduces the need for expensive consultations, high technology investigations and costly treatment with drugs or surgery. Most CAM treatment only involves talking or touching and some simple products which are often available naturally. However, CAM usually demands a considerable amount of professional time, which is a major cost of any health-care provision. The fundamental questions are whether CAM can substitute for conventional care at less expense or whether it can provide additional improvements to health and health-related quality of life, improvements which justify the extra expense.

The public currently seems to believe that the benefits of CAM are worth paying for in addition to conventional medicine. In the US, Eisenberg and colleagues, using the results of a telephone survey of 2055 adults, estimated conservatively that the total annual 'out-of-pocket' expenditure on all CAM therapies was in the region of $27 billion.[1] This sum is in addition to costs reimbursed by insurers. It is similar to the sum spent out of pocket on all US physician services. In Australia, MacLennan and colleagues estimated that annual expenditure of $AU621 million on CAM far exceeded the total amount patients contributed to the cost of pharmaceutical drugs each year.[2] In the UK, the annual expenditure on CAM for the whole UK population was estimated to be in the region of £1.6 billion per annum, even though conventional medicine is available free to all.[3] This represents about 4% of the public expenditure on health. In each of these countries, this money is spent by members of the public in addition to their personal contribution to health insurance schemes.

Health insurance providers in some countries (e.g. UK, US) are also increasingly willing to include some CAM in their provision, although it is rare to offer unlimited reimbursement for CAM treatment. This trend may be in the expectation of savings in future health-care costs or, more likely, because of competition for subscribers. In Germany, by contrast, various forms of CAM are becoming less frequently offered by insurance companies, as the recession makes rationing of resources necessary.

415

Costs of CAM

Consultation costs

In this book, it has not been possible to provide current charges for treatment with individual therapies since these vary extensively, both within and between countries. Charges comprise practitioner fees, which depend on the length of training together with indemnity and professional fees, plus the overhead costs of treatment room facilities. Charges are not regulated in any CAM therapy, although some professional organizations make recommendations or issue guidelines and insurance bodies may have upper limits for reimbursement. In general, charges are governed by market principles, in some cases distorted by the common but false assumption that the most expensive therapies are the most effective. Individual therapists (for example, some spiritual healers) may offer their services for free.

Treatment from a CAM practitioner usually takes longer than normal primary care physician appointments and may be repeated over a course of treatments. A survey of UK practitioners of acupuncture, chiropractic, homeopathy and osteopathy[4] found considerable differences between the normal patterns of consultation of different practitioners (Table 6.7.1). These factors may have financial implications for patients in terms of travel costs and time lost from work.

Product costs

In addition to consultation costs, patients need to be aware that they may have to pay for medicinal products. Homeopathic remedies, which are made by repeatedly diluting mother tinctures, have very low product costs. However, patients may be charged in addition to the consultation. Herbal remedies, on the other hand, often have shelf prices that are surprisingly similar to the conventional drugs with which they compete. For example, in the UK the over-the-counter price of St John's wort, from a reputable manufacturer, is similar to that of a modern antidepressant drug and much higher than the price of standard

Table 6.7.1 **Average characteristics of consultations, based on a survey of 98 CAM practitioners in UK[4]**

	Acupuncture	Chiropractic	Homeopathy	Osteopathy
Duration of first appointment (min)	75	30	90	40
Duration of subsequent appointments (min)	60	15	45	30
Number of consultations in first year	7.0	8.3	4.75	4.75

tricyclic drugs. Prices may fall when development costs have been recovered, although impending demands for standardization and evidence of effectiveness and safety would add to costs for the foreseeable future. Contract prices for health service providers may be lower than over-the-counter prices. Nutritional supplements also have a reputation for high prices. Acupuncture needles are cheap and in the UK even disposable needles cost less per item than an ibuprofen tablet purchased over the counter. Needles are usually, though not invariably, included in the charge for treatment.

Other costs

Other potential costs of CAM mainly relate to adverse effects. These are likely to be rare, but may be dramatic. For example, stroke from spinal manipulation or a pneumothorax from acupuncture lead to loss of income, expenses of hospitalization and (intangible) costs of pain and suffering. Other adverse effects are likely to be unrecognized at present because of a lack of awareness of CAM and may only be revealed over time. A recent example of this is the discovery of interactions between St John's wort and various conventional drugs, including warfarin.[5]

CAM diagnostic methods may give patients false-positive diagnoses that generate anxiety, which may possibly incur its own treatment costs. They may also produce false-negative diagnoses that may delay conventional treatment, potentially increasing suffering and costs of treatment. A further cost, that is difficult to assess, is the time that a patient may need to spend with a conventionally trained physician, nurse or pharmacist after a CAM therapy has proved unsuccessful, in order to 'unlearn' some of the theoretical constructs and misperceptions that have been delivered along with the therapy.

Benefits of CAM

Direct benefits

There are standard methods of assessing the value of treatments in financial terms. One method is to ask what patients would be willing to pay for a given percentage chance of improvement in the condition. When considering the benefits of CAM, it is necessary to include all aspects of perceived benefits, such as adequate consultation time and personal satisfaction with the treatment process, in addition to the straightforward outcome of symptom relief. Other possible benefits that have been claimed for CAM but are difficult to measure include health benefits from lifestyle changes and from the management of stress. These are likely to have a long time course and require prolonged studies. For example, the reduction in death rate associated with vegetarian diet was investigated in a cohort followed over a period of 17 years.[6]

Substitution of costs of conventional health care

CAM is only likely to be integrated within existing health care if it can be shown to substitute for the health costs that would otherwise be incurred. Costs that may potentially be reduced by CAM include (expensive) physician consultations in both primary and secondary care and other treatment costs such as drugs and surgery. It is also possible that CAM may be used where investigations might otherwise be performed, for example where these are being arranged largely for reassurance. Furthermore, several CAM therapies may alleviate stress which may be the underlying cause of functional conditions which otherwise demand medical care.

Another area where CAM may lead to considerable savings is the prevention of adverse effects of drugs. It has been estimated that on average one in 1200 persons taking NSAIDs for at least 2 months will die from gastroduodenal complications who would not have died had they not taken NSAIDs.[7] In comparison, 32 000 treatments with acupuncture (for a variety of indications) were only associated with one life-threatening event – a reflex anoxic seizure (own data).

Financial consequences of CAM: the evidence

The financial consequences of using CAM have been systematically reviewed.[8] The studies have tested two models: global provision of CAM for health care and individual CAM therapies for specific indications.

Global provision of CAM

Several authors have shown that the treatment costs incurred by naturopathic physicians are lower than those of conventional physicians (e.g. [9]). This evidence is easily collected but is of little value. The populations compared are dissimilar, since naturopathic physicians are likely to attract a particular group of patients and patients may even choose different physicians for different illnesses. Serious conditions that require expensive conventional investigation and treatment will severely distort the comparison. Global comparisons of different existing services also take no account of the success of treatment by the two different methods.

The question whether open access to CAM increases or reduces health-care costs has been addressed by an RCT.[10] A representative sample of 7500 policy holders in the database of a Swiss health insurance provider was selected at random and offered free cover for CAM, as well as retaining normal orthodox medical cover. The remaining 670 000 subscribers acted as the control group. Over the 3 years of the study, there were no significant differences between the total medical costs of the two groups. This might imply that CAM saved costs but in fact less than 1% of the experimental group used CAM exclusively for any episode of illness and so the authors conclude that CAM was not a substitute for orthodox care. This may simply reflect uncritical usage of CAM as a luxury. There was no attempt to establish referral protocols or to educate 'gate-keepers' to ensure the most effective use of CAM. The conclusions that can be drawn from this study are limited, because the uptake of CAM changed by a similar amount in both groups. The most useful lessons from this study have been about the methodology for such research.

Individual CAM therapies for specific indications

Spinal manipulative therapy for back pain

Spinal manipulation for back pain is one area where the cost implications could be large and have therefore been researched. Retrospective analyses of workers' compensation claims appeared to show that patients treated by manipulation incurred lower health costs than patients treated with conventional management.[11]

However, like was not compared with like, as the two groups were different in important ways, including their risk factors for back pain and their insurance cover for chiropractic. Moreover, these results are not generalizable. A more rigorous study prospectively examined the costs of treatment of back pain by various therapies at the patient's choice.[12] If hospital costs are excluded from the analysis (as chiropractors do not have admitting rights), the average costs per episode were about $280 for care by chiropractic, orthopedist and osteopath and $120 for care by general practitioner. Clinical outcomes of treatment were not reported and so cannot be compared.

One prospective controlled trial[13] compared the outcomes and costs in 1633 back pain patients who self-referred to orthopedic physicians, chiropractors, primary care physicians or HMO (health maintenance organisation) provider. Patients were followed up by telephone for 24 weeks. There were no differences between the groups for the time taken to recover normal function and to return to work but there were marked differences in their costs. Most expensive were orthopedists ($746) and chiropractors ($697), the former because of high consultation costs, use of diagnostic procedures and use of physical therapy, the latter because of use of radiographs and the large number of office visits (average about 12). The average cost of care by primary care physician was $491 and by HMO provider $435. Patient satisfaction was highest with chiropractic care. Although the participating practitioners were selected at random, this study lacks some rigor because the patients were not allocated at random. However, it gains from reflecting what actually happens in normal life.

An RCT investigated five different treatment methods in 250 chronic back pain patients who worked for an automobile manufacturer and had already undergone laminectomy.[14] They received one intensive course of:

- physical agents including hot packs, ultrasound and TENS
- joint manipulation by the Maitland method

- low-technology home exercises
- exercises using apparatus, or
- standard care.

They were followed up for at least 1 year. Only the exercise regimes produced improvements in Oswestry scores. They were also associated with significantly longer pain relief than the other treatments. Simple, low-technology home exercises were most cost-effective.

Two other pragmatic RCTs have examined the economic aspects of chiropractic care as an integral part of the study. In the first,[15] 321 patients with back pain were randomly allocated to receive chiropractic, the McKenzie method of physical therapy or minimal intervention (provision of an educational booklet). There was slightly greater dysfunction after 12 months in the group who had minimal intervention but there were no other clinically meaningful differences for bothersomeness or missed work between the groups at any stage over the following 2 years. Average total costs of care over 2 years were $429 for chiropractic, $437 for physical therapy and $153 for the booklet group. In the second RCT, 323 patients with acute back or neck pain in primary care were randomized to receive either chiropractic or physiotherapy.[16] There were no significant differences in pain score, Oswestry score, return to work or recurrence of pain over the following year. The costs of the two treatments were the same, as were the costs for all health-care utilization and indirect costs of days off work.

One RCT of 741 patients with back pain recruited in the UK found that private chiropractic management was more expensive than hospital outpatient care (£165 v £111) but more effective as measured by the Oswestry score over 3 years.[17,18] This was a pragmatic study of two methods of management, rather than a test of manipulation. Economic modeling on the basis of this study suggested that, for the approximately quarter of back pain patients in whom it is not contraindicated, manipulative therapy would be more expensive than standard hospital outpatient care but the reduction in days lost from work would more than cover the extra expense and society would gain overall.[17]

Acupuncture for chronic pain

There is no rigorous evidence on the economic consequences of providing acupuncture. One retrospective study[19] measured the costs of acupuncture for 65 carefully selected patients with pain and then compared these with the equivalent costs of hospital outpatient referral, using the actual treatment costs of similar cases. The clinical results of treatment were satisfactory (nearly four fifths of patients gained 70% pain relief, as measured by visual analog scale). Estimated savings were in the region of £260 per patient. Two RCTs compared the potential savings in medical costs from the benefits of using acupuncture compared with no additional treatment. One suggested acupuncture may reduce the costs of caring for stroke victims[20] and the other that it may reduce the need for replacement surgery for arthritis of the knee.[21] The cost element of these studies was not prospective and therefore not reliable. A further study suggested that acupuncture together with lifestyle changes and shiatsu for patients with angina might save costs compared to bypass surgery or angioplasty.[22] However, the two groups were not truly comparable.

Other therapies

The available evidence does not allow clear statements of the economic consequences of any other CAM therapy. *Gingko biloba* treatment for intermittent claudication is comparable to pentoxifylline in terms of effectiveness,[23] but the over-the-counter price is no less than the conventional drug. Total costs may be lower, however, since *Gingko biloba* is associated with fewer adverse effects. One herbal medicine that may offer savings is saw palmetto which improves symptoms in benign prostatic hyperplasia and is comparable to finasteride.[24] An economic model (unpublished) suggests that the cumulative cost of this herb will remain less than the cost of either transurethral resection (discounted at 6% per annum) or treatment with finasteride. However, it should be stressed that the long-term effectiveness of saw palmetto has yet to be established.

Conclusion

Although there may be some optimism that CAM might save costs of managing disease, there is not enough evidence to make specific recommendations for its use based on cost. This partly reflects the difficulty of performing sound and relevant cost evaluation studies, not least because of the many relevant but intangible benefits. Much of the data currently available relates to chiropractic in the treatment of back pain. It is noteworthy that early, non-rigorous studies suggested that chiropractic could lead to cost savings but these have been refuted by the majority of subsequent, more rigorous evidence. It is likely that careful selection of appropriate patients will be necessary to achieve the best chance of cost savings with CAM.

REFERENCES

1 Eisenberg D M, Davis R, Ettner S L, Appel S, Wilkey S, Rompay M V. Trends in alternative medicine use in the United States, 1990–1997. JAMA 1998;280:1569–1575

2 McLennan A H, Wilson D H, Taylor A W. Prevalence and cost of alternative medicine in Australia. Lancet 1996;347:569–573

3 Ernst E, White A R. The BBC survey of complementary use in the United Kingdom. Compl Ther Med 2000;8:32–36

4 White A R, Resch K-L, Ernst E. A survey of complementary practitioners' fees, practice, and attitudes to working within the National Health Service. Compl Ther Med 1997; 5:210–214

5 Rey J M, Walter G. Hypericum perforatum (St John's Wort) in depression: pest or blessing? Med J Aust 1998;169:583–586

6 Key T J A, Thorogood M, Appleby P N, Burr M L. Dietary habits and mortality in

11 000 vegetarians and health conscious people: results of a 17 year follow up. Br Med J 1996;313:775–779

7 Tramèr M R, Moore R A, Reynolds D J, McQuay H J. Quantitative estimation of rare adverse events which follow a biological progression: a new model applied to chronic NSAID use. Pain 2000;85:169–182

8 White A R, Ernst E. Economic analysis of complementary medicine: a systematic review. Compl Ther Med 2000;8:111–118

9 Chaufferin G. Improving the evaluation of homeopathy: economic considerations and impact on health. Br Homeopath J 2000; 89(suppl):S27–S30

10 Sommer J H, Burgi M, Theiss R. A randomized experiment of the effects of including alternative medicine in the mandatory benefit package of health insurance funds in Switzerland. Compl Ther Med 1999;7:54–61

11 Stano M. A comparison of health care costs for chiropractic and medical patients. J Manip Physiol Ther 1993;16:291–299

12 Shekelle P G, Markovich M, Louie R. Comparing the costs between provider types and episodes of back pain. Spine 1995; 20:221–227

13 Carey T S, Garrett J, Jackman A, McLaughlin C, Fryer J, Smucker D R. The outcomes and costs of care for acute low back pain among patients seen by primary care practitioners, chiropractors, and orthopedic surgeons. The North Carolina Back Pain Project. New Engl J Med 1995;333:913–917

14 Timm K E. A randomized-control study of active and passive treatments for chronic low back pain. J Orthop Sports Phys Ther 1994; 20:276–286

15 Cherkin D C, Deyo R A, Battie M, Street J, Barlow W. A comparison of physical therapy, chiropractic manipulation, and provision of an educational booklet for the treatment of

patients with low back pain. New Engl J Med 1998;339:1021–1029

16 Skargren E I, Carlsson P G, Oberg B E. One-year follow-up comparison of the cost and effectiveness of chiropractic and physiotherapy as primary management for back pain. Spine 1998;23:1875–1884

17 Meade T W, Dyer S, Browne W, Townsend J, Frank A O. Low back pain of mechanical origin: randomised comparison of chiropractic and hospital outpatient treatment. Br Med J 1990;300:1431–1437

18 Meade T W, Dyer S, Browne W, Frank A O. Randomised comparison of chiropractic and hospital outpatients management for low back pain: results from extended follow up. Br Med J 1995;311:349–351

19 Lindall S. Is acupuncture for pain relief in general practice cost-effective? Acupunct Med 1999;17:97–100

20 Johansson B B. Has sensory stimulation a role in stroke rehabilitation? Scand J Rehabil Med 1993;29(suppl):87–96

21 Christensen B V, Iuhl I U, Vilbek H, Bulow H H, Dreijer N C, Rasmussen H F. Acupuncture treatment of severe knee osteoarthrosis: a long-term study. Acta Anaesthesiol Scand 1992;36:519–525

22 Ballegaard S, Johannessen A, Karpatschof B, Nyboe J. Addition of acupuncture and self-care education in the treatment of patients with severe angina pectoris may be cost beneficial: an open, prospective study. J Alt Compl Med 1999;5:405–413

23 Pittler M H, Ernst E. The efficacy of Gingko biloba extract for intermittent claudication. A meta-analysis of randomized clinical trials. Am J Med 2000;108:276–281

24 Wilt T J, Ishani A, Stark G, MacDonald R, Lau J, Mulrow C. Saw palmetto extracts for treatment of benign prostatic hyperplasia: a systematic review. JAMA 1998;280:1604–1609

Postscript

Our main aim has been to provide state-of-the-art information and evidence on CAM as a practical reference resource, in a way that is accessible to busy physicians and other health-care professionals. Despite persistent suggestions that the RCT is not an appropriate or feasible method for testing CAM, we have found large numbers of RCTs that cover almost every form of therapy, demonstrating that CAM can be tested in a rigorous manner. As in all branches of medicine, inevitably some evidence is negative but the overriding conclusions are that some forms of CAM are frequently supported by evidence and therefore do have a role in modern health-care.

The writing of this book has been a major, fascinating and novel task for us as authors and contributors. We have ourselves learnt a great deal from the experience. We intend to continue the project, to update and expand the evidence base. We recognize that there will inevitably be errors and omissions and that not all readers will agree with every recommendation we make. We invite your constructive criticism and feedback with a view to improving future editions of this book.

GENERAL TOPICS

423

Appendix

Search Strategy for Clinical Evidence

1   exp Alternative medicine/
2   exp essential oil/ or exp lavender oil/
3   aromatherap$.tw.
4   exp "oils, volatile"/
5   exp Essential oil/
6   (essential adj oil$).tw.
7   (volatile adj oil$).tw.
8   exp Massage/
9   massage.tw.
10   (therapeutic adj touch).tw.
11   reflexolog$.tw.
12   (spiritual adj healing).tw.
13   (healing adj (touch or technique$)).tw.
14   exp Relaxation/
15   (relaxation adj technique$).tw.
16   exp meditation/ or exp transcendental meditation/
17   meditation.tw.
18   exp Yoga/
19   yoga.tw.
20   exp Hydrotherapy/
21   hydrotherapy.tw.
22   exp Spa treatment/
23   (spa adj medicine$).tw.
24   exp Autogenic training/
25   (autogenic adj training).tw.
26   exp Herbal medicine/
27   (herbal adj medicine$).tw.
28   exp Chinese herb/
29   (chinese adj herb$).tw.
30   (herbal adj drugs).tw.
31   (herbal adj remed$).tw.
32   (herbal adj preparation$).tw.
33   exp Medicinal plant/
34   (medicinal adj plant$).tw.
35   (plant adj medicine$).tw.
36   exp Traditional medicine/
37   (tradition$ adj medicine$).tw.
38   exp Ayurvedic drug/
39   (ayurvedic adj medicine$).tw.
40   ayurvedic.tw.
41   exp ginseng/ or exp ginseng polysaccharide/ or exp ginseng saponin/
42   ginseng.tw.
43   (panax adj quinquefolius).tw.
44   eleutherococcus.tw.
45   exp chamomile/ or exp chamomile oil/
46   chamomile.tw.
47   (chamomilla adj recutita).tw.
48   exp echinacea/ or exp echinacea extract/ or exp echinacea purpurea extract/
49   echinacea.tw.
50   exp Tanacetum parthenium/
51   feverfew.tw.
52   (tanacetum adj parthenium).tw.
53   exp garlic/ or exp garlic extract/ or exp garlic oil/
54   garlic.tw.
55   (allium adj sativum).tw.
56   exp Ginkgo biloba extract/
57   gingko.tw.
58   exp kava/ or exp kava extract/
59   kava.tw.
60   (piper adj methysticum).tw.
61   (saw adj palmetto).tw.
62   (serenoa adj repens).tw.
63   exp Saint johns wort/
64   (st adj john's adj wort).tw.
65   (saint adj john's adj wort).tw.
66   exp hypericum extract/ or exp hypericum perforatum extract/
67   hypericum.tw.
68   exp Hypericin/
69   hypericin.tw.
70   exp Valerian/
71   valerian.tw.
72   (valeriana adj officinalis).tw.
73   exp aloe/ or exp aloe arborescens extract/ or exp aloe barbadensis

extract/ or exp aloe emodin/ or exp aloe vera extract/ or Aloe emodin anthrone/
74 aloe.tw.
75 exp peppermint/ or exp peppermint oil/
76 peppermint.tw.
77 (mentha adj x adj piperita).tw.
78 exp Aesculus hippocastanum/
79 horsechestnut.tw.
80 (horse adj chestnut).tw.
81 horse-chestnut.tw.
82 (aesculus adj hippocast$).tw.
83 anthroposophy.tw.
84 (anthropos$ adj medicine$).tw.
85 ((toxic or poisonous) adj plant$).tw.
86 exp acupuncture/ or exp acupuncture analgesia/
87 acupunct$.tw.
88 (acupuncture adj anesthesia).tw.
89 (acupuncture adj points).tw.
90 (acupuncture adj therapy).tw.
91 exp Acupressure/
92 acupressure.tw.
93 exp Manipulative medicine/
94 chiropract$.tw.
95 osteopath$.tw.
96 exp Homeopathy/
97 hom?eopath$.tw.
98 naturopathy.tw.
99 pharmacognosy.tw.
100 exp Chinese medicine/
101 (chinese adj (traditional adj medicine)).tw.
102 (chinese adj traditional adj medicine).tw.
103 (chinese adj medicine).tw.
104 ((flower or remedy or remedies) and bach).tw.
105 (remed$ and flower).tw.
106 (flower adj essence$).tw.
107 (homeopathic adj formularies).tw.
108 (homeopathic adj pharmacopoeias).tw.
109 exp diet therapy/
110 (diet adj therap$).tw.
111 exp Vegetarian diet/
112 vegetarian$.tw.
113 vegan$.tw.

114 exp macrobiotic diet/
115 (macrobiotic adj diet$).tw.
116 (megavitamin or megamineral).tw.
117 (holistic adj health).tw.
118 exp Hypnosis/
119 hypnosis .tw.
120 exp ginseng/ or exp ginseng polysaccharide/ or exp ginseng saponin/
121 ginseng.tw.
122 (panax adj quinquefolius).tw.
123 eleutherococcus.tw.
124 exp chamomile/ or exp chamomile oil/
125 chamomile.tw.
126 (chamomilla adj recutita).tw.
127 exp echinacea/
128 echinacea.tw.
129 exp tanacetum parthenium/
130 feverfew.tw.
131 exp garlic/ or exp garlic extract/ or exp garlic oil/
132 garlic.tw.
133 (allium adj sativum).tw.
134 exp ginkgo biloba extract/
135 gingko.tw.
136 exp kava/
137 kava.tw.
138 ginkgo.tw.
139 (piper adj methy$).tw.
140 exp sabal/
141 (saw adj palmetto).tw.
142 (serenoa adj repens).mp. [mp=title, abstract, heading word, trade name, manufacturer name]
143 exp saint johns wort/
144 (st adj johns adj wort).tw.
145 (st adj john's adj wort).tw.
146 (john's adj wort).tw.
147 (john's adj wort).tw.
148 hypericum.tw.
149 exp hypericin/
150 hypericin.tw.
151 exp valerian/
152 valerian.tw.
153 valeria$.tw.
154 exp aloe/ or exp aloe emodin/ or exp aloe emodin anthrone/
155 aloe.tw.

156 exp peppermint/ or exp peppermint oil/
157 peppermint.tw.
158 piperita.tw.
159 exp aesculus hippocastanum/
160 horse?chestnut.tw.
161 horsechestnut.tw.
162 chestnut.tw.
163 exp ginseng/ or exp ginseng polysaccharide/ or exp ginseng saponin/
164 ginseng.tw.
165 exp electroacupuncture/
166 electroacupuncture.tw.
167 iridology.tw.
168 exp kinesiology/
169 kinesiology.tw.
170 kirlian.tw.
171 (pulse adj diagnosis).tw.
172 radionics.tw.
173 exp thermoregulation/
174 (thermo adj regulation).mp. [mp=title, abstract, heading word, trade name, manufacturer name]
175 (tongue adj diagnosis).tw.
176 (alexander adj technique$).tw.
177 biofeedback.tw.
178 (craniosacral adj therapy).tw.
179 kampo.tw.
180 (european adj herbs).tw.
181 (tibetan adj herbs).tw.
182 (indian adj herb$).tw.
183 (european adj herb$).tw.
184 (tibetan adj herb$).tw.
185 hypnotherapy.tw.
186 (nutritional adj therapy).tw.
187 (tai adj chi).tw.

188 (autologous adj blood adj ther$).tw.
189 (colon adj therapy).tw.
190 (colour adj therapy).tw.
191 feldenkrais.tw.
192 exp music therapy/
193 (music adj therap$).tw.
194 (ozone adj therapy).tw.
195 rolfing.tw.
196 shiatsu.tw.
197 exp spa treatment/
198 (spa adj treatment).tw.
199 or/ 1-198
200 trial$.tw.
201 exp clinical trial/ or exp phase 1 clinical trial/ or exp phase 2 clinical trial/ or exp phase 3 clinical trial/ or exp phase 4 clinical trial/
202 (randomised adj controlled adj trial$).tw.
203 (randomized adj controlled adj trial$).tw.
204 exp peer review/ or exp professional standards review organization/ or exp review/ or exp utilization review/
205 review.tw.
206 exp meta analysis/
207 (meta adj analysis).tw.
208 meta-analysis.tw.
209 or/200-208
210 exp [name of condition/]
211 [name of condition].tw.
212 210 or 211
213 199 and 212
214 limit 213 to human
215 214 and 209

Index

Page numbers in **bold** indicate major references. Page numbers in *italic* indicate tables.